The Complete Book *of* Breastfeeding

The Complete Book of Breastfeeding

FOURTH EDITION

Sally Wendkos Olds, Laura Marks, MD,
& Marvin Eiger, MD

WORKMAN PUBLISHING · NEW YORK

Library of Congress Cataloging-in-Publication Data is available.

ISBN: 978-0-7611-5113-5

Workman books are available at special discounts when purchased in bulk for premiums and sales promotions as well as for fund-raising or educational use. Special editions or book excerpts also can be created to specification. For details, contact the Special Sales Director at the address below or send an e-mail to specialsales@workman.com.

Workman Publishing Company, Inc.
225 Varick Street
New York, NY 10014-4381
www.workman.com

Printed in the United States of America

First printing July 2010

10 9 8 7 6 5 4 3 2 1

CREDITS

Cover photograph: Deborah Ory

Interior illustrations: Wendy Wray; reference provided by Medela p. 52 and by Dee Kassing p. 135.

Original photography: Deborah Ory p. 96, 105, 106, 107, 108, 109, 158, 317, 354, 355.

Interior photos: age fotostock: Tetra Images p. 75; Phototeque Oredia p. 101; Deloche p. 345; Juice Images p. 379; Ben Welsh p. 381. Alamy Images: Bubbles Photo Library p. 14; thislife pictures p. 36; Photofusion Picture Library p. 270; Picture Partners p. 299; llOver photography p. 337; Phototake Inc. p. 338; Peter Banos p. 371. Getty Images: ustus Butera p. 4; Jupiterimages p. 32, 98; Kin Images p. 150. Robin Holland: p. 156. erfile: Jerzyworks p. 193. Medela: p. 241, 329. Mother and Baby Picture Library: Spain p. 213. Photo Researchers, Inc.: Phanie p. 93.

nks to Glamourmom LLC for providing nursing tank tops and to Medela for rsing stools and nursing bras.

As always, to our children,
who have taught us so much
and from whom we keep learning:

Nancy and Dorri Olds
Jennifer Olds Moebus
Jacob, Becca, and AJ Marks
Michael and Pamela Eiger

Thanks from the Authors

Again, the fourth edition of this book owes so much to our friends, colleagues, and family members who shared their knowledge, their experience, and their time to make this edition of *The Complete Book of Breastfeeding* even more helpful than the three that built the foundation for this one.

We're especially grateful for the medical advice we've received from doctors whose commitment to breastfeeding has made them authorities in the field. Two have given us help not only on this edition, but also on the ones that came before. They have kept us current on the science of lactation. Dr. Lawrence M. Gartner, former and founding chair of the American Academy of Pediatrics' section on breastfeeding, was there at the beginning—even before the first edition was published—when he brought Sally in to speak to his pediatric residents and interns about breastfeeding. Dr. Cheston M. Berlin Jr. has been our go-to expert, edition after edition, for many questions about the impact of medications and other substances on breast milk.

We owe a special debt to Karen M. Zeretzke, MEd, IBCLC, RLC, and Melissa Clark Vickers, MEd, IBCLC. They brought their knowledge of breastfeeding, based upon their years of experience as lactation consultants, La Leche League leaders, and nursing moms, to read through the manuscript, ask questions, make comments, and offer suggestions. The book is better for their considerable input.

We want to extend thanks to Laura's colleagues in the Willows Pediatric Group: Isis Bartels, MD; Peter Czuczka, MD; Jeffrey Owens, MD; Jonathan Sollinger, MD; and Janet Woodward, MD; Susan Amster, PA-C; Heather Buccigross, PA-C; and Sue Demelis, PA-C; lactation consultant Cathy Peters, IBCLC, RLC; and to all the wonderful nurses in the practice. A special thank-you to lactation consultant Cathy Peters, IBCLC, RLC, who provided invaluable feedback on the manuscript and was available at a moment's notice for consultation. And, of course, to all our patients, who have helped us while we were helping them.

We're also grateful to the following people, some of whom reviewed various parts of the manuscript for this edition and made it better through their help, and all of whom contributed expertise and information. We thank Matthew Anderson, MD, MSc; Myrna L. Armstrong, EdD, RN, FAAN; Jimmie Lynne Avery; Cathy

Bastian, MA, RD, IBCLC; James Belisle, MD; Nils Bergman, MD; Brandi Campbell; Rona Cohen, RN, MN, IBCLC; Betty Crase, IBCLC; Mark D. Cregan, PhD; Annie Crombie; Cullen Curtiss; Bronwen Epstein; Sue Freedman; Donna T. Geddes, PhD; Sandra Gordon; Karleen D. Gribble, PhD; Dr. Ellen Homewood; Elizabeth Hormann, IBCLC; Sari Kalin; Dee Kassing, IBCLC; Kathleen Kendall-Tackett, PhD, IBCLC; Miriam H. Labbok, MD, IBCLC, RLC; Judy S. LaKind, PhD; Ruth Lawrence, MD (current chair of the American Academy of Pediatrics section on breastfeeding); Debbie Linchesky and Susan Martin of the American Academy of Pediatrics; Cheryl A. Lovelady, PhD; James McKenna, MD; Rachel Mennell; Kevin Milligan; Nancy Mohrbacher, IBCLC; Brian Palmer, DDS; Nina Planck; Mitra Pikwer; Kathleen M. Rasmussen, ScD, RD; Brian D. Rinker, MD; Tanya Roberts, BSEd, IBCLC; Jen Russo; Diane Sam; Hugh Sampson, MD; Katherine Shealy, MPH, IBCLC, RLC; Christina Smillie, MD; Alison Smith; Amy Spangler, MN, RN, IBCLC; Diane L. Spatz, PhD, RNC; Sandra Steingraber, PhD; James Trussell, PhD; Charlotte Vallaeys; Frederick vom Saal, PhD; Claire-Dominique Walker, PhD; Laura Weinberg; Wenjun Zhou; and Diana Zuckerman, PhD.

We owe a huge debt of gratitude to Peter Workman, president of Workman Publishing Company, who with his wife, Carolan, saw the need for this book so many years ago and has supported it through every edition. We also appreciate the many extensive efforts of the Workman staff. Our editors Suzanne Rafer and Erin Klabunde devoted endless hours to shepherding the book along. The Workman team included project editor Mary Wilkinson, production editors Beth Levy and Judit Bodnar, designer Yin Ling Wong, photo editor Anne Kerman, photo coordinator Danielle Hark, and typesetter Barbara Peragine. Wendy Wray captured the beauty and the how-tos of breastfeeding in her illustrations.

We're grateful to our agent, Linda Konner, not only for being our champion but for being the matchmaker who brought Laura and Sally together, and thus helped to create a working and personal relationship that has enriched both our lives.

Our thanks would not be complete if we didn't recognize the consistent and loving support of our spouses, David Mark Olds and David Marks, and Carol Eiger, who were supportive of our project, generous with helpful suggestions, and flexible in accommodating their schedules to ours.

We also want to acknowledge the many individuals and organizations who provided invaluable help for the first three editions. While we appreciate everyone's input, we take full responsibility for the book you hold in your hands, and we hope it helps you and your family to enjoy this special time in your life.

Contents

INTRODUCTION xvii

CHAPTER ONE

Will You or Won't You? 1

30-Day Guarantee. 2
Why Breastfeed? Why Not?. 2
Benefits for the Baby. 3
Disadvantages of Formula-Feeding 5
American Academy of Pediatrics Statement on Breastfeeding. 7
Some of the Ways Breastfed Babies Differ from Formula-Fed Babies. 10
From Sally Olds: A Mother's Enjoyment 16
Importance of Breastfeeding for the Mother. 16
The WIC Program 19
When Breastfeeding May Not Be an Option 21
Reasons Women Give for Not Wanting to Breastfeed 22
A History Lesson: How Our Society Has Influenced Women 24
Today's Society and Breastfeeding 25
What Will You Do? 28

CHAPTER TWO

Questions You May Have About Breastfeeding 29

CHAPTER THREE

The Miracle of Lactation 44

The Development of Your Breasts. 45
The Anatomy of Your Breasts. 49
How Your Baby Gets Your Milk: The Let-Down Reflex 53
Signs of an Active Let-Down Reflex 56
Menstruation, Ovulation, and Pregnancy. 57
Human Milk: The Ultimate Health Food. 58

CHAPTER FOUR

Before Your Baby Comes 63
Choosing Your Health Care Providers 64
Types of Health Care Provider 64
Questions to Ask Health Practitioners 70
Choosing Where You'll Give Birth 74
The Ten Steps to Successful Breastfeeding in a Baby-Friendly Hospital 76
Packing Your Bag 78
Choosing When You'll Give Birth 79
Prenatal Classes 79
Preparing Your Breasts 80
Who Will Mother You? 83
To Grandmas: How You Can Help 85

CHAPTER FIVE

Your Baby Is Here 89
The Ideal Beginning 90
Recommendations for Successful Breastfeeding from the American Academy of Pediatrics 91
Breastfeeding in a Hospital or Birthing Center 92
The First Nursing 93
A Gift That You Don't Want 95
Cesarean Birth 96
Mother-Baby Contact 97
Hospital Help 98
Hospital Hindrance 99
Speak Up in the Hospital 100
Newborn Health Measures 101

CHAPTER SIX

Breastfeeding Begins 103
Bringing Your Baby to the Breast: Positive Positioning 104
What Makes a Good Position for Breastfeeding? 107
How Your Baby Gets Your Milk 111
How to Tell When a Baby is Actively Suckling 113
Waking a Sleepy Baby 116
How Frequently Should You Nurse Your New Baby? 117
How Long Should Early Nursing Periods Last? 119

Burping Your Baby.. 120
Bowel Movements 122
Your Baby's First Posthospital Doctor's Visit 122
Your Baby's Weight After Birth 123
Is My Baby Getting Enough Milk?................................. 124
Judging Intake by Output 125
Jaundice in Infants... 127
When to Seek Immediate Help.................................. 130
Exclusive Pumping... 133
Bottle-Feeding the Breastfed Baby................................. 133
How to Bottle-Feed the Breastfed Baby............................. 134

CHAPTER SEVEN

You Are a Nursing Family

You Are a Nursing Family..................................... 138
Breastfeeding at Home.. 140
Tips on Relaxing Before and/or During Feedings.......................... 145
The Popular Pacifier 147
If You Have "Too Much" Milk................................... 148
Breast Milk Bonus 148
Babywearing... 149
When Your Baby Cries 150
The Colicky Baby 151
Ways to Comfort a Crying Baby................................. 152
Sleeping Arrangements.. 157
Sleep and Lack of It: Night Feedings 161
Encouraging a Baby to Give Up Nighttime Nursing 162
Ways to Guard Your Rest 164
Diapers, Revisited... 165
What Is Your Baby Like? 166
How to Discourage Biting..................................... 168
Cutting Down on Spitting Up 170
What Will You Call It? 171
Life as Part of a Nursing Family.................................. 171

CHAPTER EIGHT

Diet, Exercise, and Your Health

Diet, Exercise, and Your Health................................. 172
Diet: What You Eat, What You Drink 173
Guidelines for Healthy Eating 174

The Healthy Eating Pyramid 175
Avoiding Harmful Environmental Substances 182
Losing Weight: How Much, How Soon? 186
What the Labels Usually Mean 187
Exercise: How Much, How Soon? 189
An Exercise Guide for the Nursing Mother 192
How Do You Feel—and Why Do You Feel This Way? 195
Ways to Boost Your Postpartum Morale 198
Differences Between Postpartum Blues and Postpartum Depression 201

CHAPTER NINE

Confident, Comfortable Nursing at Home and Away 203

Care of Your Breasts 204
Finding the Right Nursing Bra 206
How You Look 209
Going Out with Your Baby 212
Nursing in Public 212
Flying with Your Nursing Baby 214

CHAPTER TEN

Drugs and the Nursing Mother 217

Resources and Information about Drugs and Breastfeeding 219
Drugs During Childbirth 220
Medicines 221
Medicines That Can Usually Be Taken Safely by Nursing Mothers 224
Medicines That Should Not Be Taken by Nursing Mothers 225
Medicines That Require a Temporary Cessation of Breastfeeding 226
Medicines of Concern 226
Birth Control 229
Herbs and Other Natural Remedies 229
Recreational and Hard Drugs 230
Minimizing the Effect of Nicotine on Your Nursing Baby 231

CHAPTER ELEVEN

Pumping, Expressing,
and Storing Breast Milk 235

What Kind of Pump Do You Need? 236

Choosing a Pump 237

Principles That Apply to All Methods of Collecting Milk 243

A Note of Caution about Bisphenol A (BPA). 245

How to Handle Expressed and Pumped Breast Milk 247

Storing Collected Breast Milk 248

Offering Expressed Milk to Your Baby 251

CHAPTER TWELVE

The Working Nursing Mother

The Working Nursing Mother 253

Finding Support 254

Planning Ahead: While You're Pregnant and Still on the Job 255

Employer-Supported Lactation Programs 258

Planning Ahead: While You're on Your Maternity Leave 260

Tips for Feeding a Baby from a Cup 263

Your Baby's Feedings While You're at Work 265

Back at Work 269

Wardrobe Tips for the Working Breastfeeding Mother 272

CHAPTER THIRTEEN

Breastfeeding: A Sexual Passage

Breastfeeding: A Sexual Passage 275

Sexy? Or Not So Sexy? 276

Resuming Sexual Activity 277

Pelvic Floor (Kegel) Exercises 279

You and Your Relationship 281

The Five Phases of Female Sexuality 282

Female Sexuality 282

The Sensuous Nature of Breastfeeding 284

Birth Control 286

Contraception for the Nursing Mother 288

Your Partner Is Still Your Lover 292

CHAPTER FOURTEEN

Especially for Dad or Partner 297
Breastfeeding's Benefits for You, the Father 298
Becoming a Father 299
The Father's Importance in the Family 300
Boot Camp for New Dads 302
Your Baby's Mother Is Still Your Lover 304
Rolling Up Your Sleeves 305
How a "Breastfeeding" Father Can Nurture a Baby 306
You Can Be a Complete Father 307
Getting Support for Yourself 309

CHAPTER FIFTEEN

Preventing and Treating Nursing-Related Problems 310
Disagreement with Your Doctor 311
Engorgement (Hard, Swollen Breasts) 312
Ways to Relieve Engorgement 313
Sore Nipples 314
Thrush 319
Clogged Duct (Plugged Duct, "Caked" Breasts) 321
Breast Infection (Mastitis) 322
Galactocele (Milk-Retention Cyst) 324
Sudden Increase in Baby's Demand 324
The Baby Who Gains Too Slowly 325
Helping the Older Baby Who Isn't Gaining 326
Nursing Supplementers 328
The Baby Who Gains Too Fast 330
Temporary Rejection of the Breast ("Nursing Strike") 331
When an Older Baby Refuses the Breast 333

CHAPTER SIXTEEN

Special Situations 335
Breastfeeding Your Preterm (Premature) Infant 336
Separation of Mother and Baby 346
If Your Baby Gets Sick 346
If You Get Sick 347
If You Have Had Breast Surgery 351
Piercing and Tattooing 353

Twins and More 354

Nursing Through a Pregnancy and Tandem Nursing Afterward 356

Milk Banks 357

Breastfeeding Another Woman's Baby 358

Relactation and Nursing an Adopted Baby 359

Succeeding at Induced Lactation or Relactation 360

Babies with Special Needs 362

CHAPTER SEVENTEEN

Beyond Breastfeeding 365

Vitamins 366

Recommended Vitamin and Mineral Supplementation

for Breastfed Babies 367

Weaning Your Child 368

Extended Breastfeeding 371

"When Are You Going to Stop Nursing?" 372

How Should You Wean? 373

Suggestions for Weaning the Older Child 375

How Weaning Affects You 377

Other Food and Drink 379

Offering Solid Foods 382

Staying Close with Your Child 384

APPENDIX I: BREASTFEEDING AND THE LAW 385

APPENDIX II: RESOURCE APPENDIX: HELPFUL ORGANIZATIONS AND

SOURCES OF INFORMATION 389

APPENDIX III: WEBSITE APPENDIX 401

APPENDIX IV: A COMPARISON OF COW'S MILK AND HUMAN MILK 405

INDEX 408

Here We Go Again

If you were living at some other time or in some other place, you might not need this book. You might even wonder about its purpose, since you would be getting much of the information in these pages from your mother, your aunts, your older sisters, and your neighbors. They would share with you their breastfeeding experiences and those of their mothers before them. As you saw them suckling their infants, you would pick up the "tricks of the trade" without even realizing it. It would never occur to you that you would not nurse your baby, because every baby that you had ever seen would have been fed at his mother's breast—except in the extremely rare case when a mother was too ill to nurse.

The paragraph above appeared as the introduction to the original edition of this book, published in 1972. It's one of the very few paragraphs that were carried over to the second edition, published in 1987, and the third edition, which came out in 1999.

So much has changed in the years since *The Complete Book of Breastfeeding* was first conceived. The year 1971 (when the first edition of this book was being researched and written) marked the lowest rate of breastfeeding in the history of this country. Only one in four women even began to breastfeed their babies. Now, thirty-nine years later, we're happy to report that that percentage has reversed, so that three out of four women begin to nurse. But some of these mothers stop nursing sooner than they would like to because they encounter problems along the way. It's good to know that in almost all cases, problems can be resolved with the right information and support.

You're more likely now to get that information and support than you were in earlier years. Today's doctors learn more in medical school about breastfeeding and are more convinced of its value than earlier generations were. More hospitals are putting in place more policies that promote breastfeeding rather than interfere with it. Lactation consultants serve on the staffs of many hospitals and pediatric practices, and many practice independently. And the Internet is abuzz with websites and blogs that offer advice, sell nursing-related products, and offer chances for moms to share their experiences and learn from one another. Still, it's sometimes hard to navigate all these streams of advice.

Breastfeeding is easy; there's nothing complicated about it. And there's no single best way to do it. Still, it's a skill that both you and your baby need to learn. Nursing a baby may fulfill an instinctual drive, but you need to learn all the how-to's—basics like how to hold your baby, how to help your baby latch on, how to tell when your baby is getting enough milk. And you need help while you're learning. Succeeding at breastfeeding depends on knowing when you need help, what kind you need, and how to find it. Some mothers intuitively know what to do and breeze into breastfeeding with no questions and no problems. But most new moms have questions about all aspects of infant care, including breastfeeding, the way you'd have questions about anything you're doing for the first time.

A Note About Language

Since babies come in two sexes, we write about them accordingly, alternating gender pronouns throughout the book.

We made another linguistic decision by alternating references to "your husband," "your partner," and "your baby's father." Today's families come in many different forms. It's likely that many readers of this book are married, but that quite a few are not. You may be living with an adult who is neither your husband nor your baby's father. Your partner may be male or female. You may be part of a big extended family. Or you may be raising your child alone. No matter what your personal situation may be, you can get help from these pages.

Even today you're unlikely to have grown up in a culture in which it's taken for granted that when you had babies this is how you would feed them. We, the authors of this edition—a pediatrician and a medical writer who nursed our own children—have aimed to stand in for the women in that kind of culture, to present as much help as we can in a single, easy-to-reference place. We want you to continue to tell us what so many of your mothers have said: "Your book was my bible."

To make the book more relevant to today's families, we have introduced new topics, expanded on others, incorporated the most recent research and most effective practices, and revised throughout to make all the information in these pages as up-to-the-minute as possible. Although, as we said, there's no one "best way" to breastfeed, there are certain practices that seem to make the course of nursing go more smoothly for most mothers and babies. These are the practices that we describe and recommend in these pages. However, every baby is unique, every mother is unique, and every family situation is unique. You may find that you and your baby do better by doing things differently from what we recommend. If it works for you—do it, with our blessing.

The three essential tools for a happy breastfeeding experience are knowledge, confidence, and determination. You need to know what to do, feel confident that you're doing the right thing for your baby and yourself, and be determined to persist in the face of any temporary obstacles. We want to help you develop all three of these tools.

This journey may be among the most exhilarating of your life. Enjoy the ride!

SALLY WENDKOS OLDS
Port Washington, New York

LAURA M. MARKS, M.D.
Westport, Connecticut

CHAPTER ONE

Will You or Won't You?

"I truly believe breastfeeding was made to be wonderful not only for the baby, but also for the mother. Within five minutes of being born, Jacob latched on and started nursing. I was just so amazed that my body has the ability to provide all the nutrients for my little bundle of joy."

KATIE Lansdale, Pennsylvania

Today, in the twenty-first century, you have a choice in the way you feed your baby. You can decide whether you want to feed your baby the natural way, with the milk produced by your own body—the way mothers have done from time immemorial—or whether you will provide your baby's nourishment in a bottle of infant formula. Many factors will enter into your decision: the customs of your community; the attitudes of your doctor, your husband or life partner, your friends and family; your lifestyle, including your work commitments; your personality; your feelings about mothering; your knowledge about breastfeeding; and how much emotional and practical support you receive.

Keep in mind that if you decide to formula-feed right away, it's much harder, and sometimes impossible, to change your mind later on. Initiating breastfeeding after only a week has gone by requires a great deal of determina-tion, persistence, and patience. It has been done by mothers who found that their babies needed breast milk to sur-vive and by women who discovered that bottle-feeding has its own problems. But it is *not* as simple as breastfeeding from the beginning. (For information about relactation, see Chapter 16.)

30-Day Guarantee

We hope that once you read this chapter and see the impor-tance that breastfeeding holds for you, your baby, and the world you live in—and all the advantages you'll miss out on if you formula-feed—you'll decide to nurse. Look on it as a thirty-day money-back guarantee. You will most likely find breastfeeding gratify-ing for both you and your baby and go on to nurse well beyond those initial thirty days.

But suppose you begin to nurse your baby and you have to or decide to stop. You haven't lost anything and you haven't invested in anything. The stores will always have those bottles, nipples, sterilizers, and formulas. You haven't made a lifelong commitment. You can easily change your mind.

Meanwhile, you have given your baby the wonderful substance of colostrum, which is like an injection of antibodies at the most vulnerable time of your baby's life, right after birth. And while exclusive breastfeed-ing (that is, giving nothing but breast milk) for at least the first six months confers the most benefits on both you and your child, some breastfeeding is better than no breastfeeding for both of you.

Why Breastfeed? Why Not?

For many years in the United States, the nursing mother was the nonconformist, a member of a minority group, a hippie. By 1971, for-mula-feeding had become the norm in this country, with only 25 percent of women nursing. Since then, the long-term trend away from breastfeeding has been reversed. This book was first published in 1972, and we like to think that the advice and encourage-ment it offered helped to accelerate the trend toward the rediscovery of breastfeeding.

You probably have heard many of the reasons why breastfeeding is important for babies. You may not be as aware of its importance for you. One of the prime benefits for the mother is the all-around good feeling you're likely to derive from the experience. In talking about their breastfeeding experiences, women often emphasize how good it feels (or felt)—emotionally, physically, and intellectually. When a woman has breastfed one baby, she almost always nurses the next.

Women who have bottle-fed one baby and nursed another tend to feel closer to their nursing infants in the early months of life. One mother told us, "I never knew what I was missing by not nursing my first baby. I loved him and I enjoyed him, yes, but I never got so many of the *extras* that I get from this one—that little hand that touches my skin as she's nursing, the way she'll pull away from the breast, smile at me, and go right back again, the happiness that I feel at being able to give her what she wants."

The nursing pair—mother and baby —forge an especially close and interdependent relationship. Your baby depends upon you for sustenance and comfort, and you look forward to feeding times to gain a pleasurable sense of closeness with your infant. If a feeding time is too long delayed, it's hard on both of you—on your baby because of hunger and on you because of uncomfortably full breasts. Each of you needs the other, yearns for the other, is intimate with the other in a very special way. Because of this unique symbiotic relationship, many women (including both authors of this book) consider the period of nursing among the most fulfilling times of their lives.

Also, nursing can be an intensely pleasurable, sensuous activity. Finally, knowing all the health benefits that breastfeeding confers on both mother and baby affirms a woman's conviction that she is making the best possible decision for herself and her baby.

Benefits for the Baby

The basic fact about breastfeeding is not just that it's better than anything else—it's normal. It's the way babies are meant to be fed, and any other way of feeding them involves a deviation from this norm. Sometimes women have to, or decide to, deviate—but at least you should know what you're deviating from, and why breastfeeding is the gold standard of infant feeding. Let's see why.

The Importance of Breastfeeding for Infant Nutrition

Human breast milk is the ultimate health food for human infants. Nursing your baby is the first proactive measure you can take for your child's health. For at least the first six months, breast milk is the only food most babies need. Even

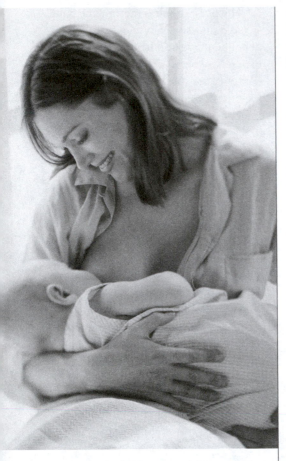

Both mom and baby treasure these special moments.

after your baby begins to eat other foods in the latter half of the first year, breast milk continues to supply protective immunity, as well as such vital nutrients as essential fatty acids, lactose (the predominant sugar in milk), and the correct balance of proteins. (See Chapter 3 for more about this ideal food.) All these elements are important for proper growth of brain cells.

Worldwide, there's a new awareness of the problems caused by overweight. Bottle-fed babies tend to develop more fat than breastfed babies, and the longer a woman breastfeeds (up to nine months), the lower the odds of her baby's being overweight. However, even babies breastfed for only a month or two are less likely to become obese by the time they go to elementary school. This protection against becoming overweight may persist into the teenage years and adulthood. And the higher rates of obesity among African American teenagers and those in lower socioeconomic circumstances have been attributed to lower breastfeeding rates by black and low-income mothers. Breastfed children of overweight or diabetic mothers are less likely to become obese themselves. Fortunately, more mothers in these groups are breastfeeding these days. And the Special Supplemental Nutrition Program for Women, Infants, and Children (WIC) recently changed its practices to encourage breastfeeding (see box on page 19).

How does breastfeeding discourage gaining too much weight? For one thing, bottle-feeding mothers who see milk left in the bottle tend to encourage their babies to drain the last drop, while breastfeeding mothers usually assume that their babies know when they have had enough. When the baby stops suckling, the mother takes him off the breast. But there are several other theories. One explanation lies in the difference between the high-protein milk produced at the beginning of a feeding (fore milk) and the high-fat milk produced at the end (hind milk). The richness of the hind milk (which some call "baby's dessert") may

Disadvantages of Formula-Feeding

❖ You need to have enough formula on hand at all times. If you run out, your baby is in trouble. And so are you!

❖ You need to sterilize bottles and nipples before first use and wash them thoroughly before every later use.

❖ You need to be sure that your baby's bottles do not contain BPA (bisphenol A), which is used to make polycarbonate, a clear and rigid plastic. For more information and ways to determine this, see page 245.

❖ If you leave home with your baby, you need to take formula, bottles, and nipples, and be able to clean everything thoroughly.

❖ Ready-to-feed formulas (both cow's milk and specialty formulas like soy and hypoallergenic) are expensive, with the cost likely to run about $1,500 a year.

❖ You need to be sure to use formula before its date of expiration.

❖ You have to throw out any open or prepared formula left out of the refrigerator longer than one hour.

❖ Prepared bottles of formula can be kept refrigerated for only 24 to 48 hours, depending on the type of formula.

❖ Formula does not provide the baby with important antibodies against infection and illness.

❖ Formula is the same at every feeding, unlike breast milk, which changes as your baby's needs change (more on this on page 8).

❖ Formula is not digested as readily as breast milk, so formula-fed babies are more likely to have gas, diarrhea, and constipation.

❖ Formula-fed babies get sick more often, requiring more doctor visits and more time you have to take off from work.

make the baby feel full and send a signal that mealtime is over.

Other explanations for breastfed children's lower rates of obesity point to the higher concentrations of insulin in the blood of formula-fed babies, possibly because they are overfed, or possibly because the production of leptin, a hormone related to appetite and overweight, may be influenced by breastfeeding.

Even before birth, your baby becomes familiar with different tastes and smells in the amniotic fluid. And then after birth, the variety of tastes and smells that pass through your milk accustoms your child to the foods of your particular culture. Breastfed children tend to like vegetables more than formula-fed infants do when they're first introduced to them, probably because breastfed babies become more familiar with the varied flavors that pass through the milk of their vegetable-eating mothers. Thus, by encouraging a diverse and healthy diet, breastfeeding can offer health protection later, when babies will be more receptive to new foods.

While your breast milk varies from day to day, depending on whether you have eaten pad Thai, pasta primavera, or chicken with broccoli, commercial formula tastes and smells the same, day after unvarying day. Consequently, the formula-fed baby misses out on the rich and varied sensory experiences transmitted through a mother's milk.

Importance of Breastfeeding for Health in Childhood and Adulthood

In developing countries, the survival rate of the breastfed baby may be six times greater than that of her formula-fed cousin. And even among the children of middle- or upper-class parents in highly developed countries, breastfed babies are healthier and have better chances for survival.

In technologically developed countries like the United States, where sanitary conditions are generally good, the gap in health between the breastfed and the formula-fed baby is narrowed considerably. In addition, modern medical techniques can now vanquish many of the illnesses that used to be fatal to infants. Still, it's better to prevent disease than to cure it. And there's a great

deal of evidence that breast milk does indeed have preventive and protective powers, even in the most advanced countries. According to a 2010 report, if 90 percent of U.S. mothers breastfed exclusively for six months, more than 900 infants' lives would be saved in one year.

Breastfed babies make fewer visits to doctors' offices and hospitals than formula-fed babies do, especially for diarrhea and other gastrointestinal disorders, rashes, and respiratory infections. Recent research in Argentina concluded that breastfeeding helps babies cope better with infections. Breastfed infants are also less likely to suffer from diaper rash, a common problem in infancy, apparently because their higher level of fecal acidity helps protect them against the yeast infections that can lead to diaper rash.

Breastfed babies also seem to be protected in varying degrees from a number of other illnesses (see the box opposite). When they do get sick, their illnesses are likely to be less severe and their recovery faster. The presence of the nutrient DHA in breast milk also seems to enhance children's vision. Although this fatty acid is added to some formulas, the consensus so far is that there's no benefit to the supplements—in fact, they may pose a risk of illness for the baby (see page 9).

Breastfeeding's advantages are most striking during the first six months of life, very evident during the first two years, and still apparent later in life. Thus mother's milk is a gift that lasts a lifetime. Breastfeeding seems to protect against breathing disorders that

American Academy of Pediatrics Statement on Breastfeeding

In the strongest, best-documented statement it has ever issued about the value of breastfeeding, the American Academy of Pediatrics states:

> Research in developed and developing countries of the world, including middle-class populations in developed countries, provides strong evidence that human milk feeding decreases the incidence and/or severity of a wide range of infectious diseases, including bacterial meningitis, bacteremia [bacteria in the blood], diarrhea, respiratory tract infection . . . otitis media [middle ear infection], urinary tract infection, and late-onset sepsis [bacterial poisoning] in preterm infants. In addition, postneonatal infant mortality rates in the United States are reduced by 21 pecent in breastfed infants. . . .
>
> Some studies suggest decreased rates of sudden infant death syndrome [SIDS]* in the first year of life and reduction in incidence of insulin-dependent (type 1) and noninsulin-dependent (type 2) diabetes mellitus, lymphoma, leukemia, and Hodgkin's disease, overweight and obesity, hypercholesterolemia, and asthma in older children and adults who were breastfed, compared with individuals who were not breastfed.

"Breastfeeding and the Use of Human Milk."
—American Academy of Pediatrics Section on Breastfeeding (2005)

*SIDS is the sudden and unexpected death of an infant under one year of age, with the onset of the lethal episode apparently occurring during sleep, that remains unexplained after a thorough investigation.

can occur when children are asleep, and it also enhances lung function. Children who have been breastfed for at least four months have stronger lung function later in childhood, too: They can exhale more air after taking a deep breath and can blow it out faster. There is also evidence that breastfeeding may increase a child's bone mineral density (which protects against fractures), and that it protects against such respiratory diseases as bronchitis, pneumonia, and asthma during middle childhood.

Breastfeeding may even help to prevent various illnesses in adulthood. Having been breastfed as a baby lowers a woman's risk for breast cancer, both before and after menopause. Breastfed babies are less likely to be obese or suffer heart disease later in life: They are 55 percent more likely to have high levels of HDL (high-density lipoprotein), the "good" cholesterol that protects against heart disease.

The greatest health differences between breastfed and formula-fed babies show up when babies are fed exclusively by either method. The differences narrow in proportion to the amount of formula or other foods given in addition to breast milk.

Ease of Digestibility of Breast Milk

Most infant formulas use cow's milk as their base. The chart in Appendix IV compares human milk with cow's milk. Babies can digest human milk more easily than the milk of any other animal, probably because human milk contains an enzyme to aid in its own digestion. Breast milk forms softer curds in the infant's stomach than cow's milk does and is more quickly assimilated. About half the protein in cow's milk is wasted, passing through the baby's body and making extra work for the baby's excretory system. Iron and zinc are also absorbed better by breastfed babies.

Breastfed babies are less apt to get diarrhea, and they don't become constipated, since breast milk cannot solidify in the intestinal tract to form hard stools. While your breastfed baby may soil all his diapers in the early days or go several days without a bowel movement later on, neither situation necessarily indicates intestinal upset (see Chapter 6).

Human Milk for Human Babies

In country after country, language after language, the most common way that young children call their mothers is with the two syllables *ma-ma*. This universal word probably gave rise to the Latin word for breast, *mamma*. And, in 1758, the importance of a mother's ability to nurture her babies from her breasts was scientifically acknowledged for perhaps the first time, when the Swedish botanist Carolus Linnaeus coined the name *mammalia* for the class of animals designed to breastfeed their young. No doubt he chose this particular female trait because he considered it so significant. As indeed it is.

Each mother's milk is custom-designed for her own baby. Women develop specific antibodies against bacteria and viruses that are found in their own lungs and intestines. These antibodies also appear in their milk. Thus, they manufacture the mix of antibodies that is best for their own babies. The perfect match between a baby and her mother's milk is most dramatic in the case of premature infants: The milk of a woman who has delivered early is higher in protein and in fat than the milk of a mother of a full-term baby and is, therefore, better suited to the special growth needs of her preterm baby.

Also, breast milk changes in composition from feeding to feeding, from day to day, and from month to month. The fat content in breast milk changes during the course of a feeding: As noted earlier, the milk a baby gets at the beginning of a feeding (fore milk) is higher in protein, whereas the milk later in the feeding (hind milk) is higher in fat. The fat content in breast milk also varies at different times of day, partly in response to what the mother has eaten. As lactation progresses, the amount and kind of proteins in breast milk change to meet different stages of a baby's growth, with very high protein levels at the beginning when the baby needs to grow rapidly, and lower levels later on when normal growth slows down. Formula, however, remains the same at every feeding.

Human milk contains at least 100 ingredients that are not in cow's milk, and while artificial formulas try to imitate mother's milk, they can never duplicate it exactly. No manufacturer has ever officially claimed that a formula product is just as good as or better than breast milk, and none is likely to make such an audacious claim. In fact, the Food Standards Agency in Great Britain plans to bar infant formula makers from making claims that their products approximate breast milk. As one team of researchers wrote, "Formula milk is just a food, whereas breast milk is a complex living nutritional fluid that contains antibodies, enzymes, and hormones, all of which have health benefits."

We're constantly discovering new ingredients in mother's milk. One is mucin, an acid-based protein that prevents intestinal illness in nursing animals. Another important element in breast milk is DHA, an omega-3 fatty acid that aids brain and eye development in newborns. As we said earlier, DHA is now added to some formulas. A recent study, however, found that breastfed babies have better stereoscopic (three-dimensional) vision than formula-fed babies, even when the

bottle babies received formula with DHA. Reports presented to the U.S. Breastfeeding Committee in 2008 also charged that new additives of laboratory-produced oils containing DHA and ARA (an omega-6 fatty acid) in some formulas have caused diarrhea and other problems in infants who received them. At this writing, the jury is still out on these claims.

With breast milk, the whole is greater than the sum of its parts. We don't know all the constituents in breast milk and how they work together. Through trial and error, formula manufacturers have learned that many ingredients are essential for babies' nutrition. Who knows what other ingredients will be identified in mother's milk for formula makers to try to imitate?

How Breastfeeding Protects Against Disease

In some countries around the world, especially in parts of Africa, China, South America, and the Middle East, mothers put breast milk in their children's eyes or on a boy's recently-circumcised penis to prevent or treat infections. A Swedish study provides scientific evidence supporting these folk treatments: It reports that a compound in breast milk destroys skin warts. And there is much more evidence supporting breastfeeding's disease-protection benefits.

For example, mother's milk transmits immunoglobulin A (IgA) proteins,

Some of the Ways Breastfed Babies Differ from Formula-Fed Babies

The milk of each species is designed to further the optimal development of the young of that species. What, then, are some of the differences between babies fed human milk and babies fed formulas based on the milk of other animals?

✧ Breastfed babies grow differently. Formula-fed babies not only grow longer and fatter, but they also develop bigger and heavier bones during the first year of life, probably due to the larger amounts of calcium in cow's milk. Formula-fed babies may grow faster than nature intended them to: Bigger is not necessarily better. The growth charts issued by the World Health Organization (WHO) in the 1970s were based on a limited sample of children in the United States, most of whom had been formula-fed. According to these standards, many breastfed children were thought not to be growing properly. Then, after intensive study, WHO published new growth charts in 2006 based on the breastfed child as the norm for growth and development.

✧ The bacteria in their intestinal tracts are strikingly different. Bifidobacteria and lactobacilli are two types of bacteria more common in the systems of breastfed babies. Bifidobacteria strengthen the immune system, helping to prevent diarrhea, and lactobacilli heal wounds and protect against viruses. These beneficial bacteria, which are present in only small numbers in the stools of formula-fed babies, prevent the growth of certain harmful bacteria.

✧ Lysozyme, another substance found only in the stools of breastfed infants, also protects against harmful microorganisms.

✧ Human milk contains more cholesterol than does formula, and animal studies suggest that exposure to cholesterol early in life may help to program the individual to metabolize cholesterol more efficiently in adulthood, offering some protection against heart disease. Breastfed infants have higher cholesterol levels at first than do formula-fed babies, but the higher levels are not unhealthy. The difference disappears after weaning.

which are antibodies against pathogens (disease-causing organisms) to which the mother has been exposed. These IgA proteins are unique: They line the baby's respiratory and intestinal surfaces, forming a protective coating that prevents many bacterial and viral agents from invading the baby's body and causing disease. Since various versions of this unique protein fight specific organisms, your breastfed baby is protected during the vulnerable first few months, until his own immune system matures.

The mechanism behind this protection lies in a change in the body of a nursing mother. Before you became pregnant, cells producing antibodies against intestinal infections went through your circulatory system into your intestine. When you began to lactate, some of these antibody-producing cells moved into your mammary glands. So when your baby nurses, these antibodies go straight to his intestine, protecting him while he builds up his own immunity.

Breast milk also contains other protective substances. Eighty percent of the cells in breast milk are macrophages, cells that in other parts of the body are known to kill bacteria, fungi, and viruses and to help stop the growth of cancer cells. The mystery is that the macrophages in human milk are inactive. (Again, we see why it's impossible to make a formula that duplicates human milk exactly. There's too much that science does not know about why human milk does such a good job helping babies grow.)

In addition, the complex sugars in all human milk are thought to protect a baby against pathogens to which the mother has *not* been exposed, but to which the baby may have been, including some that cause diarrhea and ear infections. They do this by preventing the first step in infection, the binding of a pathogen to the infant's cells. This may account for the fact that even babies who are genetically susceptible to middle-ear infections are less likely to get these infections if they have been breastfed.

Other elements in breast milk also confer protection. Some benefits of breastfeeding, though, are procedural: The milk in your breast cannot be contaminated by the harmful bacteria that can multiply in animal milk left out of the refrigerator for too long. It's always served in a clean container. It can't be overdiluted to save money. It can neither be counterfeited nor prepared incorrectly (both of which have occurred from time to time in baby formulas). And human milk has no expiration date.

The breastfed baby is a beautiful illustration of teleology, the ultimate purpose of design in nature. For example, a newborn baby placed facedown on his mother's body typically can find his own way to her breast and the nipple and begin to nurse. Also, newborn babies see best at a distance of between twelve and fifteen inches, precisely the usual distance of a baby's eyes from the face of a nursing mother. And neuroscientists point to the importance of repeated experience, as in gazing intently at a loving face, in aiding babies' brain development. Suckling at the breast even helps a baby develop hand-to-eye coordination, especially when the mother switches from one breast to the other. As Aristotle said so many centuries ago, "There is reason behind everything in nature."

Even though we don't know the precise reasons for, or the significance of, all the differences between the baby nourished at the breast and the baby fed by formula, it seems logical to assume that the best first food for your baby is the kind you provide yourself. As Dr. Paul György, MD, the pioneering researcher who discovered vitamin B$_6$, said more than 80 years ago, "Human milk is for the human infant; cow's milk is for the calf." As two nurses proposed more recently, breast milk substitutes should carry a label stating: WARNING: THIS PRODUCT IS INFERIOR TO HUMAN MILK.

Importance of Breastfeeding to Protect Against Allergic Reactions

Although many babies do well on formulas, some have an allergic reaction like indigestion or diarrhea. As a breastfeeding mother, you won't have to experiment with different milk and nonmilk formulas, since no baby is allergic to breast milk. However, some breastfed babies do develop allergic reactions like vomiting, diarrhea, skin rash, or hives to something in the mother's diet that's transmitted through her milk. But it's usually possible for the mother to identify and stop eating that particular food for the duration of nursing (see Chapter 8).

Also, breastfeeding reduces the likelihood of such allergic reactions as eczema and other skin ailments, as well as celiac disease (an intolerance to gluten, a protein found in many grains). It also protects against asthma, unless the mother has asthma herself. Nursing, then, is particularly important if you have a family history of allergy. Cow's milk allergy is fairly

common, and babies are protected from this as long as they're feeding only on breast milk and their mothers significantly reduce or eliminate cow's milk products from their own diets.

The earlier a baby with a predisposition to allergy receives cow's milk, the greater the risk of developing an allergy. The best protection for babies with a family history of allergy is exclusive breastfeeding for at least four months. After this time, breastfeeding should continue, with vigilance regarding the introduction of other foods.

Importance of Breastfeeding for Brain Development

Although many factors affect how well people do in school and in other areas of life, several studies have suggested that adults who were breastfed achieve higher IQ scores than formula-fed children. Some researchers believe that this cognitive advantage may result from the presence in breast milk of certain fatty acids that promote lasting brain development.

Recent research has shown a fascinating interaction between heredity and environment: Breastfed children who have a certain gene that affects the body's absorption of fatty acids score higher on IQ tests than children who have the gene and received only formula. Children without this gene didn't show this advantage. This evidence strongly suggests the presence of some substance in human milk that affects mental development.

One recent study of bed wetters found that they were twice as likely to have been formula-fed as a comparison group who did not wet their beds. The dry-at-night children tended to have been nursed for longer than three months.

Importance of Breastfeeding for Tooth and Jaw Development

Suckling at the breast is good for your baby's tooth and jaw development. Babies at the breast use different muscles to get food than do those drinking from a bottle. The nursling (nursing baby) has to draw much or all of the areola (the darker area around the nipple) into her mouth and move her jaws up and down. The tongue also moves up and down, creating a vacuum and a pressure that helps to extract milk. To accomplish this task, your baby has been endowed with jaw muscles that, relative to her size, are three times stronger than yours. As these muscles are strenuously exercised in suckling, their constant activity encourages a well-formed jaw and palate and straight, healthy teeth.

One factor accounting for many dental malformations that eventually send children to the orthodontist or the speech therapist is an abnormal feeding pattern known as tongue thrust. This is common among bottle-fed babies, but almost nonexistent among the breastfed. As we explain in the box on page 111, the breastfed baby works her gums and lower jaw quite vigorously to get the milk, whereas bottle-fed babies don't have to exercise their jaws so energetically, since light sucking alone produces a rapid flow. In fact, the formula often flows so freely that the baby has to learn how to protect herself from a very fast flow so that she won't choke. She pushes her tongue forward against the bottle nipple's holes to stem the flow to a level that she can easily handle. Many dentists believe that such a forward tongue thrust can result in mouth breathing, lip biting, and gum disease.

Furthermore, since breastfed babies do more of the sucking that babies need, they're less likely to suck their thumbs. Bottle-fed babies have to stop sucking on the nipple as soon as the bottle is empty to avoid taking in air. Your baby at the breast can continue in this blissful pastime until you or she decide she's been at the well long enough.

Of course, many bottle-fed babies do not develop dental problems, and some breastfed babies do. Still, this is one more realm in which breastfeeding remains superior to bottle-feeding.

One fascinating study of historical skulls in several museum collections found that the skulls from periods of time before the widespread introduction of rubber nipples and baby bottles showed almost universally well-developed mouth formations, compared with more recent skulls, which showed more dental formation problems.

Constant Availability of Breast Milk

Another advantage your nursling enjoys is the virtually constant availability of milk. His dinner is always ready, and it's always at the right temperature. He doesn't have to struggle to get milk from an artificial nipple with scanty holes, nor does he have to gulp furiously to keep up with a gush from extra-large ones. No hurricane or flood, no car breakdown, no workers' strike, no emergency of any kind can keep food away from him. You don't have to worry about running short when you're out with your baby.

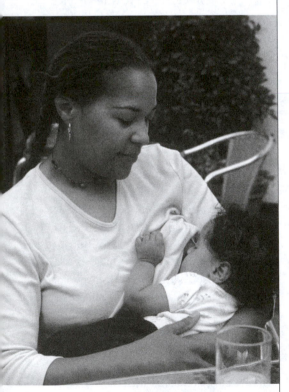

No matter where mom and baby are, baby's meal is ready.

As long as mother is near, so is your child's sustenance.

Here's one remarkable survival story: In December 2006, a mother and two children, aged seven months and four years, were trapped for nine days in a snowed-in car in subfreezing temperatures miles from any town. When rescued, both children were in good condition as a result of being breastfed, even though the mother had had very little to eat herself. If they had not had access to their mother's breast milk, the result would undoubtedly have been disastrous.

Emotional Gratification from Breastfeeding

When you nurture your baby at your breast, you cannot be tempted—even on your busiest days—to lay your baby down with a propped bottle. You have to draw her close to you for every single feeding. While bottle-feeding mothers can also show their love for their babies by holding and cuddling them at feeding times, in actual practice they tend to do less of this. And while they can hold their babies next to their bare skin when they offer the bottle, to simulate the body contact of nursing, they rarely do.

Research has proved the value of the sense of touch in many different settings. This basic element of breastfeeding is one of the most gratifying aspects of the experience, to both mother and baby. Dr. Nils Bergman, MD, a South African pediatrician, developed the concept known as kangaroo mother care (more about this in Chapter 16). Under this paradigm, a baby is held skin-to-skin with the mother 24 hours a day. Although this form of care was originally developed for premature babies, Dr. Bergman points out the many pluses of skin-to-skin care for full-term babies as well. These include improved breathing, heart rate, temperature control, nutrition, and protection from infection.

This close, early physical contact that's part of breastfeeding may be responsible for breastfed children's ability to deal better with stress. Various studies have shown that: Ten-year-old children who were breastfed as infants experienced less anxiety about their parents' marital problems than formula-fed children; newborns who were breastfed during routine heel-prick or needle-stick blood tests experienced less pain than those fed sugar water in bottles; and babies who receive immunization shots while actively nursing show fewer signs of discomfort than babies who are not breastfeeding.

Babies also gain a sense of well-being from secure handling, and nursing mothers often seem more confident. Whether the woman who's sure of her maternal abilities is more likely to breastfeed—or whether the experience of being a good provider infuses her with self-confidence—is hard to determine. Some nursing mothers seem more likely to know how to soothe their babies when they're upset, maybe because the very act of putting them to the breast is so comforting

that they don't have to search for other means of solace. The breast is more than a pipeline for getting food into your baby. It's warmth, it's reassurance, it's comfort.

Infants seem to recognize and become attached to their nursing mothers very early: When one-week-old babies are presented with breast pads that their own mothers have worn and with pads worn by other nursing women, they seem to prefer their mothers' smell. They turn their heads more often, and are more likely to make sucking motions, toward their own mothers' breast pads.

However, we do need to point out the conclusions of researchers who have, over the past seventy years, conducted studies that tried to correlate methods of infant feeding with later personality development. Their findings: As important as early feeding experiences may be to a child's later development, there are so many variables in parent-child relationships that it's impossible to claim definitively that any one factor, including breastfeeding, is, in and of itself, a prescription for healthy adjustment.

Still, psychiatrists and other students of human and animal nature do state categorically that babies gain a sense of security from the warmth and closeness of the mother's body. Also, it seems logical that the more intimate interaction between the breastfeeding mother and child, the warm skin-to-skin contact, and the more immediate satisfaction of the nursing baby's hunger would make for healthier psychological development.

From Sally Olds: A Mother's Enjoyment

When I was nursing my first baby, I was struck by how much information was available about the benefits breastfeeding conferred on babies, but I felt I had really discovered something when I realized how many advantages it held for mothers. My first published article, "Nursing Is Good for Mothers, Too," appeared in a small-circulation baby-care magazine.

Nancy, my first baby, is now a mother herself (who nursed her own daughters), but my memories of Nancy's infancy are still vivid. I remember so clearly hearing her lusty cry, picking her up and holding her next to my heart, inhaling her incredibly sweet new-baby fragrance, feeling the tingling in my breasts that told me my milk was letting down for her, and looking at her with a heart full of joy as she suckled eagerly.

I thought—and wrote—in that first article, "There's something very right about a system that makes one human being so happy about being responsible for another. I could never have the same good feeling of accomplishment by relying on the neighborhood store or the dairy for my baby's milk. Knowing that I was giving her something no one else could give her created a tie between us that became one of my deepest joys."

As I watched Nancy's little legs become chubby and dimpled, and as I laughed at the little-old-lady look that her double chin gave her, any doubts about the quality of "my formula" vanished. And so I went on to nurse my second and third daughters.

Importance of Breastfeeding for the Mother

Your primary reason for wanting to breastfeed is probably your awareness that it will be better for your baby. You may not have realized how much better it is for you, too.

Breastfeeding Is Good for Your Figure

Nursing your baby will help you to regain your figure more quickly after childbirth, since the process of lactation causes the uterus (which has increased during pregnancy to about twenty times its normal size) to shrink more quickly to its prepregnancy size. During the early days of nursing, you can feel your uterus contracting while your baby suckles. (The sensation feels like menstrual cramps.) As he nurses, he stimulates your pituitary gland to secrete the hormone oxytocin, which causes uterine contractions. These contractions hasten your uterus's return to its former size, while helping to expel excess tissue and blood. The uterus of the mother who doesn't breastfeed always remains somewhat larger than it was before she became pregnant.

Also, since breastfeeding uses up so many calories, you may be able to lose weight while eating more. A number of research studies have found that nursing mothers, who generally eat more than women who feed their babies formula, lose more weight over the first year after childbirth. This is particularly true if they nurse for at least six months, and especially if they nurse exclusively, not feeding their babies any formula at all. Not only do nursing women shed pounds—they lose more fat from their bodies, especially the hips and thighs, which affects how they look as well as how much they weigh. (For more about the impact of breastfeeding on the mother's weight, see Chapter 8.)

Furthermore, despite what many people believe, nursing does not break down the connective tissues in your breasts. Changes in the breasts that occur, such as a loss of firmness, are the results of pregnancy, weight gain, heredity, and maturity, not lactation. (See Chapter 2 for more on this.)

Breastfeeding Is Convenient

Even today, when formula comes ready-mixed in nursing bottles, breastfeeding is easier than formula-feeding. No efficiency expert has been able to outdo nature's way of feeding an infant. Your baby's daily batch of food prepares itself in its own permanent containers.

It's so easy just to wake up in the morning, pick up your baby, and put her to your breast. You don't have to scrub and sterilize bottles and nipples. You don't have to pad barefoot into a chilly kitchen to fetch a bottle. You never have to make up an extra bottle at the last minute or throw out formula that your baby doesn't want. Working on the time-honored principle of supply and demand, your breasts produce the amount of milk your baby wants. Your actively lactating breasts are never empty, so that no matter how often your baby is hungry, they will be able to supply milk.

You'll find it easier to go visiting or traveling with your baby, since you won't have to take along bottles, nipples, powders, or heavy cans of formula. Nor will you have to worry about refrigeration, dishwashing facilities, or changes in the water supply.

Breastfeeding Is Important for Your Health

Not surprisingly, the natural way of infant feeding is good for your health also. First, you reap benefits right after your baby's birth; then you gain an advantage from the continued suspension of your periods; and in later life, you appear to have some protection from both breast and ovarian cancer, type 2 diabetes, heart problems, rheumatoid arthritis, and osteoporosis. Some of these later health benefits may be due to long-term changes in a woman's immune system induced by breastfeeding.

✤ **Postpartum:** Breastfeeding your infant within the first hour of birth offers you three health benefits: (1) It helps to prevent postbirth hemorrhaging; (2) it facilitates the expulsion of the placenta; and (3) it speeds up the process of involution by which your uterus returns to its prepregnancy size. This process is the mechanism that protects new mothers from hemorrhage.

✤ **Welcome breaks:** Every mother of a newborn needs enough rest. (Try telling this to your baby!) The physiological changes of pregnancy, the hard work of labor and delivery, and the demanding care of a new baby all deplete your energy. When you breastfeed, you're forced to relax during feedings, since you can't prop a bottle or turn the baby over to someone else while you run around doing chores. Your baby's feeding times are your enforced rest times.

✤ **Respite from menstruation:** As an exclusively breastfeeding woman, you probably won't menstruate for at least six months after childbirth, and possibly longer if you're feeding your baby solely with breast milk. This is the only time in your reproductive life when you're not losing iron through your period or through nourishing a baby in

your womb. Although you do provide iron in your milk, the amounts taken from your body are much less than you would be losing through your menstrual periods. Thus, this is a chance to build up your stores of iron and to correct any anemic tendencies you may have.

✤ **Cancer:** The risk of ovarian cancer is directly related to a woman's lifetime number of ovulations. The fewer times in your life you ovulate, the lower your risk may be for ovarian cancer. Lactating women tend to resume ovulation later after childbirth.

Another major health benefit of breastfeeding is its role in lowering the risk of breast cancer for both premenopausal and postmenopausal women. Breast cancer is the second leading cancer killer among women (after lung cancer), and breastfeeding is one of the few actions that you can take to reduce your risk. One medical researcher concluded that if all mothers nursed for a total of two years (with one or more babies), the incidence of breast cancer in the United States would drop by 25 percent. The protective effect is strongest among women who nurse for longer durations. According to one analysis, breast cancer risk decreases by 2 percent for each five months of breastfeeding.

✤ **Osteoporosis:** Osteoporosis is a thinning of the bones that causes "widow's humps" and bone fractures, and this is one more condition for which breastfeeding may offer protection. Women who breastfeed tend to have increased bone mineral density later in life, and denser bones are a protective factor against fractures of the hip and other sites—a major health risk for older women. Women over 65 who have breastfed have half the risk for bone fractures as women who did not nurse their babies. The longer a woman's lifetime lactation, the lower her risk of fracture.

❖ **Postpartum depression:** Breastfeeding can protect women's mental health by lowering stress and anxiety levels, contributing factors to postpartum depression.

❖ **Rheumatoid arthritis:** New research shows that women who breastfeed for 13 months or more are less likely to develop rheumatoid arthritis (RA) later in life, probably because of the hormones involved in lactation. The longer a woman nurses, the lower her risk of developing RA.

❖ **Type 2 diabetes:** The longer a woman breastfeeds, the lower her risk of diabetes. For every year a woman nurses a baby (either one baby or the total time she spent nursing more than one), she is 15 percent less likely to develop type 2 diabetes in the next fifteen years. Lactation improves the body's ability to process insulin and metabolize blood sugar.

❖ **Heart disease:** A recent study of almost 100,000 women showed that breastfeeding protects against heart attacks. Women who had spent at least two years of their lives breastfeeding were 19 percent less likely to have heart attacks than those who had never nursed. Doctors think this may be due to better regulation of body fats and more weight loss.

❖ **Lowered blood pressure:** Recent research has shown that breastfeeding

The WIC Program

The federally subsidized governmental program known as WIC (Special Supplemental Nutrition Program for Women, Infants, and Children) gives financial aid to mothers who qualify. Only about half of low-income WIC mothers begin to nurse. In view of the cost-saving nature of breastfeeding, the fact that these women are less likely than more affluent women to breastfeed is troubling. There's cause for optimism, though: The current figure reflects an increase in breastfeeding among low-income women, largely because of the WIC program's increased emphasis on encouraging new mothers to breastfeed.

The increase in nursing among low-income women saves everyone money—as taxpayers. The government spends an estimated $578 million a year to pay for formula for babies in the WIC program, plus office visits and prescriptions for sick children, who are more likely to be formula-fed.

mothers experience a drop in blood pressure during a nursing session and just before a feeding during at least the first six months of nursing.

Breastfeeding Is Economical

Breastfeeding saves you money. (And it could save us *all* money—if 90 percent of U.S. moms breastfed exclusively for six months, the nation would save $13 billion a year.) If you already eat right, you don't have to change your diet. You just need to eat a little extra food to make up for the calories you expend in producing and giving milk. (See Chapter 8 for more about diet during pregnancy and lactation.) This will cost you less than you'd have to pay for bottles, nipples, sterilizing equipment, and formula. For the average family, formula takes twice the bite from the family budget as does extra food for mom.

Breastfed babies also tend to be healthier, which means fewer days the parents need to miss from work and fewer doctors' visits.

Breastfeeding Is More Aesthetic

If you have a sensitive nose, you'll appreciate the fact that your breastfed baby smells sweeter. Both bowel movements and excess milk spit up after feedings smell mild and inoffensive, unlike the strong, nose-wrinkling odors emitted by the formula-fed baby. And

they're less likely to stain clothing—baby's and yours.

Breastfeeding Helps to Control Fertility

Breastfeeding acts as a natural—although not totally reliable—means of spacing children. While your baby is under six months of age and receiving nothing but breast milk—no solid foods or formula at all—and is still being nursed during the night, you are less likely to become pregnant than is the non-nursing or partially nursing mother. This is because the fully lactating woman rarely ovulates. This is the basis of the Lactational Amenorrhea Method (LAM) of child spacing (details in Chapter 13).

Nursing a baby is not a guarantee against pregnancy, however. Although you are less likely to conceive while you're nursing, you still might become pregnant. If you want to plan the size and spacing of your family, you need to use some form of contraception. (See Chapter 13 for birth control methods suitable for nursing women.)

Breastfeeding Is Earth-Friendly

At a time when so much of our existence seems unsettlingly unnatural—with pollutants in the air we breathe, the clothes we wear, and the foods we eat—more and more of us are striving to recapture some of the natural joys of life on Earth. When you breastfeed your baby, you know you're giving her the natural food intended just for her. Its purity is not tainted by synthetic compounds, preservatives, or artificial ingredients. Cow's milk is very likely to come from cows that have been treated with artificial growth hormone and antibiotics to encourage greater production; the effects of this treatment on health, the environment—and the welfare of cows—are unknown. Despite occasional sensational headlines about chemicals in breast milk, research has shown that even in an industrial world, breastfeeding is still superior to formula (see Chapter 8 for a detailed discussion of this topic).

If you're concerned about your child's environment, you can appreciate

When Breastfeeding May Not Be an Option

Breastfeeding may be either inadvisable or impossible if you:

❖ Have had surgery or trauma to the breasts that has severed the ducts. (In some cases, the ducts have been known to reconnect, however, so you could give nursing a try if you closely monitor your baby's weight and hydration status.)

❖ Are so ill that you can't be with your baby and are too sick to pump your breasts.

❖ Are taking any of the small number of medications that could be harmful to your nursing baby (see Chapter 10).

❖ Live in a developed country and are infected with HIV (human immunodeficiency virus) that can be passed to the baby through breast milk. HIV is linked to AIDS (acquired immune deficiency syndrome). Although a new drug in widespread use in the developing world greatly reduces the risk of HIV transmission during breastfeeding, the American Academy of Pediatrics and most public health advocates in developed countries advise against breastfeeding by an HIV-positive mother when a safe alternative is available.

❖ Have insufficient tissue in the milk-producing glands in the breasts. This very rare condition affects fewer than 2 percent of women and usually can be detected in a prenatal breast examination (an important reason why your obstetrician should examine your breasts before you give birth). In this kind of situation, the baby can still be put to the breast, if she is receiving appropriate supplements to ensure proper nutrition for growth and development.

❖ Have a baby who has a condition or illness that makes it impossible to nurse. In such cases, your pumped or expressed breast milk may be given to the baby, if the baby is being closely monitored for proper growth and development.

Reasons Women Give for Not Wanting to Breastfeed

❖ They're embarrassed about the idea.

❖ They're modest and want neither to nurse publicly nor have to run into another room whenever people are around. (See suggestions in Chapter 9 for nursing discreetly.)

❖ They're uncomfortable thinking about body secretions of any kind.

❖ They are afraid of being tied down. (See Chapter 9 for suggestions on going out with and without your baby.)

❖ They have to go back to work and don't want to start something they think they can't finish. (See suggestions for working moms in Chapter 12.)

❖ They want the baby's father to share more equally in the baby's care. (For ways this can be done, see Chapter 14.)

❖ They're afraid of ruining their figures. (They won't, as seen in Chapters 2 and 3.)

❖ Their husbands or partners don't want them to.

❖ They think they're too nervous. (Nervous moms can breastfeed, too.)

---

the ecological superiority of breastfeeding. Feeding formula entails the use and disposal of innumerable bottles and cans (as many as 450 million for every 3 million babies) of formula, the cardboard cartons that package them, and the baby's bottles and nipples, either after one use or after a few months. Manufacturing the packaging uses paper, plastic, and metal—and creates toxins. One study estimated that producing about 2 pounds of formula in Mexico costs about 12 square yards of rain forest.

The fertilizer used to grow feed for dairy cows, along with their sewage, pollutes rivers and other waters, affecting all ecosystems dependent upon these water sources. Then there's the energy used to transport the milk and to heat it in the home, and the soap or detergents and water used to wash all that equipment. It all adds up.

Why Some Women Decide Against Breastfeeding

The reasons why women decide not to breastfeed are almost as varied as the arguments in its favor. There are a very few instances when a woman is physiologically unable to nurse her baby, as indicated in the box on page 21. Fortunately, such cases are

✥ They think they don't have the right kind of breasts. (Virtually everyone has the right kind.)

✥ They're afraid they won't know whether their baby is getting enough to eat. (To judge baby's intake, see Chapter 6.)

✥ They're afraid that they will have to restrict or radically change their diet. (Your milk will be good even if your diet isn't. See Chapter 8 for food talk.)

✥ They think that breastfeeding plunges women back into traditional roles, negating many societal advances made over the past several decades toward equality of the sexes. (Some of the strongest proponents of breastfeeding are feminists.)

✥ The whole business just seems too complicated. (It sometimes is, in the beginning, but nursing soon becomes easier than formula-feeding. See Chapter 6.)

✥ Occasionally, there is a reason that goes unspoken, but that often influences a woman's decision not to breastfeed. For a woman who has suffered sexual abuse at some time in her life, among its many painful vestiges can be feelings of shame and embarrassment concerning bodily sensations. Unless she understands where these feelings are coming from, she may be so uncomfortable with her body that she shrinks from breastfeeding. (Breastfeeding lets a woman reclaim the beauty of her body.)

extremely rare. Virtually every healthy woman can breastfeed her baby if she wants to.

Why do some women choose not to breastfeed? This question has no simple answer. Some of the most common reasons given are listed in the box above. All of these concerns are answered in this book.

None of these reasons exists in a vacuum. Most were born in history, either society's or the individual's. Many stem from a lack of knowledge, others from a lack of support, even today. The problem with breastfeeding is that there's not much money to be made from it, so its "marketing strategy" is less effective than those of

manufacturers of formula, baby foods, and other products, which spend millions on advertising and promotion. While it's up to each individual woman to examine her own personal reasons for her choice, we can take a look at some relevant societal trends.

Parents are greatly influenced by cultural norms, that is, by what a society considers usual, typical, and normal behavior. In the following pages we take a look at some societal norms that have decreased the practice of breastfeeding.

In the next chapter, we'll answer some of the questions that are most often on women's minds, and we'll deal with these issues throughout this book.

A History Lesson: How Our Society Has Influenced Women

For most of human history, breast-feeding was the only way to nourish an infant. Then, over the past century and a half, western society underwent cultural changes that caused women to consider breastfeeding just one of two options for feeding babies. Let's see what some of these changes were and how they affected mothers' choices.

Rigid Beliefs About Child Rearing

At the beginning of the last century, psychologists, psychiatrists, and physicians were convinced that babies developed best if they were raised according to certain hard-and-fast rules. Doctors ordered mothers not to feed—or even pick up—their babies more often than every four hours, no matter how piercing or pathetic the infants' wails. Bottle-feeding was far better adapted to these practices. Breastfeeding requires flexibility, not rigidity; understanding of a baby's needs, not the ability to tell time; and an intuitive response, not an adherence to a cultural fad. Also, because the child-care experts insisted that only they knew what was best for children, mothers believed them—and lost confidence in their own

capabilities. And lack of confidence itself can sabotage breastfeeding.

Thus for about fifty years—from the 1920s until the 1970s—the United States served as the laboratory for the largest and most dangerous uncontrolled "scientific experiment" in history, perpetrated on subjects who, because they were infants, could not give their informed consent. The feeding method that had sustained our species for millions of years was discredited and abandoned, with no evidence to justify this wholesale rejection.

Changing Status of Women

At the same time mothers were being intimidated in the nursery, during the Roaring Twenties, they were becoming more assertive outside the home. Demonstrating to gain the right to vote, bobbing their hair, and daring to carve out their own careers, women were eager to free themselves from their traditional roles in the house. The baby bottle became an instant symbol of emancipation.

Furthermore, as the quality of formulas improved during the 1930s, the act of giving a bottle achieved a certain status of its own. Women who wanted to be modern wanted to bottle-feed. Unfortunately, this urge to keep up, to be cutting-edge, has wooed many poor women in both developed and developing countries around the world away from the breast, often with disastrous results. When money is scarce, mothers dilute formula and babies starve; when refrigeration and sanitation are inadequate, formula becomes contaminated and babies fall ill. The World Health Organization (WHO, the public health arm of the United Nations), governments of many nations, and numerous private health organizations have mounted major campaigns around the world to encourage women to go back to safe, healthy breastfeeding.

Sexualization of Breasts

During the flapper era of the 1920s in the United States, women bound and flattened their breasts. Then, by the 1940s, pin-up photos were gracing barracks walls, exhibiting the new ideal of feminine beauty—a pretty young woman with large breasts. Molded into fashionably pointed (and highly unnatural) shapes by the brassieres of the day, breasts became purely decorative in nature, valued for their sexiness and forgotten for their function. This cultural attitude contrasts with that of many societies around the world, which do not view the mammary gland as erotic or sexual.

Embarrassed by the sexual nature of their breasts, many women shyly shrank away from touching them or using them in nonsexual ways. Many men jealously looked upon their wives' breasts as their own property and resented the idea of those breasts being seen by anyone else, even their infant children. One recent survey found that a mother's perception that the baby's father had negative feelings about breastfeeding often led her to choose formula-feeding.

More recently, as nudity has become more prevalent in the media, many women have become more comfortable with the notion of baring their breasts, at least to the extent required for nursing. As we'll see in Chapter 9, it's possible to nurse so discreetly that observers can't even tell what you're doing, which sets to rest a concern of many women and men.

Today's Society and Breastfeeding

In the twenty-first century, the age-old practice of breastfeeding still has societal obstacles to overcome, but for the most part it is reclaiming its original status as the best way to feed babies.

First, the Bad News

It's ironic that a society that equates motherhood with apple pie balks at linking motherhood with mother's milk, as seen in the following events:

❖ Even today, women breastfeeding in public are sometimes asked to cover up more completely or to leave the establishment. You should know that nursing in public is not illegal anywhere in the United States. (More about this in the Legal Appendix.)

❖ The word *breast* was held obscene in 1995, when America Online (AOL) banned the word from its online chat groups, thus making any discussion of breast health or breastfeeding impossible, unless subscribers used other (more colorful?) terms or synonyms. (AOL changed its stance on this, after much protest by users.)

❖ A 2004 survey by the American Dietetic Association found that fewer than half of almost 4,000 respondents said that women should have the right to breastfeed in public places.

❖ The August 2006 cover of a magazine marketed to new mothers showed a nursing baby and part of the mother's breast—and in a poll of more than 4,000 readers (mostly women), one fourth of the responses were negative, calling the photo "inappropriate."

❖ In 2006 and 2007, public "nurse-ins" were held around the country after breastfeeding mothers were harassed at Victoria's Secret, Starbucks, Toys "R" Us, and other stores. In 2008, a mother who tried to nurse her crying eight-month-old in a beauty salon, covering herself and her baby with the salon smock, was told to leave with her hair half-cut.

❖ In 2008, a cyber nurse-in was held on Facebook, after the site had removed photos of women nursing their babies. More than 134,000 women (including the authors of this book) joined the protest group "Hey Facebook, Breastfeeding Is Not Obscene!" And more than 11,000 took part in the virtual nurse-in, some displaying art of the Madonna nursing the infant Jesus.

❖ Greeting cards offering congratulations on a new baby, television shows, and movies all trumpet the baby bottle as the symbol for infant care, routinely assuming that babies will be fed with formula.

❖ Too many physicians, nurses, and hospital personnel are uninformed and unenthusiastic about the value of breastfeeding, equating it with formula and implying that there's little difference between the two feeding methods. And too many hospitals send new mothers home with samples of baby formula. A recent British survey of 500 new mothers of sick or premature babies found that only 33 percent were told about potential breastfeeding problems and how to overcome them, more than 10 percent were not shown how to position the baby for nursing, and 5 percent felt under pressure from hospital staff to stop breastfeeding and switch to formula.

No wonder so many women are confused or embarrassed by the idea of breastfeeding!

Now the Good News

Today's woman is more comfortable with her body than in times past, is concerned with fitness and health for herself and for her family, and is less embarrassed to be herself. Our ideals of beauty have changed from the heavily made-up, elaborately coiffed look of yesterday to the healthy, natural look of today. Thus, the contemporary woman is more likely to want to feed her baby in the healthiest and the most natural way.

In fact, the modern counterparts of those feminists who moved away from breastfeeding—the well-educated middle- and upper-class women who set trends—are now among its staunchest supporters. Many women see their choice to breastfeed as a liberating one, one that challenges ingrained practices in the workplace and society in general.

Furthermore, society has changed in many ways. As new scientific findings continue to affirm the value of human milk, such major health organizations as the American Academy of Pediatrics, the United Nations Children's Fund (UNICEF), the American Public Health Association, and WHO regularly issue strong statements urging virtually universal breastfeeding for at least the first year of life, and as long thereafter as mutually desired by mother and baby.

And the more people know about the importance of breastfeeding, the more babies are likely to be nursed. A 2007 media campaign in the small town of Herkimer, New York, sending the message "Babies are born to be breastfed," resulted in higher proportions of both men and women saying they would be comfortable with having their child breastfed in public. In Tennessee, billboards and transit signs get out the message that babies were born to be breastfed. And the British government has launched a breastfeeding help line to support new mothers. As of May 2008, more than half of U.S. states and territories were collecting data about breastfeeding, and others reported that they planned to do so soon. With this information, better health decisions are likely to be made.

Many hospitals and pediatric practices have hired lactation consultants to help new mothers, and breastfeeding is once again becoming the preferred way to feed babies. The first half of the twentieth century will probably go down in history as an aberration in its rejection of this age-old natural means of nurturing.

Still, even if you know you want to breastfeed, you may have many questions and concerns. Even after your questions are answered, you may decide that breastfeeding is not for you. You don't have to breastfeed to be a good mother. You shouldn't do something you are uncomfortable with to please your partner, your doctor, your mother, your next-door neighbor, or your best friend.

What Will You Do?

As you have seen, breastfeeding is both the most natural and the healthiest way of feeding a baby. However, a child raised in a loving home can grow up to be healthy and psychologically secure no matter how she receives nourishment. Although nursing is usually a beautiful, happy experience for both mother and child, the woman who nurses grudgingly, tight-lipped and stiff-armed, because she feels she should, may do more harm to her baby by communicating her feelings of resentment and unhappiness than she would if she were a relaxed, loving, formula-feeding mother.

Although breastfeeding is clearly the gold standard for feeding babies, ultimately, how you feel about your children is more important than how you feed them. A recent study compared six-year-olds who had been breastfed with six-year-olds who had not. The study showed no differences in problems with conduct, hyperactivity, and relationships with other children. And when psychologists from Harvard University followed up 78 people in their 30s whose mothers had been interviewed for a study 25 years earlier, they found that neither the fact nor the duration of breastfeeding, like many other specific child-rearing practices, had any discernible effect on the way these people turned out as adults. The one thing that did matter was whether the parents had truly loved their children—and had shown their children that love.

If you are unsure about whether you want to breastfeed, you will want to learn as much as you can about the importance of breastfeeding. And then you might ask the women in your family and your friends about their experiences with infant care—how they fed their babies, what the experience was like for them, and how they decided between breast and bottle. Also, you will learn a lot and get excellent support if you attend a nursing mothers' support group—like La Leche League International or one offered by your hospital or pediatrician—and hear about other women's experiences. Then, weighing all the evidence, you can make up your own mind.

As we said earlier, we urge you to give breastfeeding a try. Remember that thirty-day guarantee! If you never give it a chance, you may well look back on this time in later years and wonder whether you and your baby missed one of life's greatest gifts—the bond shared by the nursing pair. The regrets we have in life are less often for the things we have done than for missed opportunities that will never come again. This priceless chance to nurse your baby comes only once in each baby's lifetime. Make the most of it. You may count these nursing days among the most beautiful and fulfilling of your entire life.

CHAPTER TWO

Questions You May Have About Breastfeeding

"At the hospital I had to request a visit from the lactation consultant.
And even after speaking with her I had more questions.
Reading everything I could get my hands on really helped—
it made me feel better informed about my decision to breastfeed and
more confident that I would be able to successfully nurse my twin boys.
And if ever a new question arose, I always had something to refer to."

ELLEN Easton, Pennsylvania

As Alix, a mom from Boulder, Colorado, said, "I had so many questions and no one to go to with them. No one in my family ever breastfed, I had just moved to a new town where I didn't know anyone, and my doctor was so busy I was nervous about bothering her." Everyone has questions about something they haven't done before—and until you've had a baby, you haven't breastfed one. We know you must be wondering about many aspects of this new activity and how it will affect your life, so we'll address some of your concerns right away, even though most of them will also be answered somewhere else in this book. Consider this chapter a breastfeeding FAQ (frequently asked questions). The authors are both former nursing mothers, one is a physician, and both of us have researched the field of breastfeeding, so we can answer many of your questions. However, every woman is different and every baby is different, so when you have a question about your personal situation, you need to consult your own health care providers. Our answers to the following questions, like all the suggestions we offer in this book, are guidelines based on the latest research and expert opinions.

Q : **Will nursing make my breasts sag?**

A : No, it won't. A 2007 study by a plastic surgeon found that the shape of a woman's breasts bears no relation to whether she has breastfed or the length of time she nursed a child or children. Most women do find that their breasts become less firm and less erect after childbirth, but these changes are caused by pregnancy, not lactation. How much your breasts change will be determined by your genes, how old you are, how much weight you gained during pregnancy, and the size of your breasts before pregnancy. The larger they were then,

the more they'll droop later. And as women grow older, their breasts become less firm. Many pregnant and nursing mothers feel that wearing a good, well-fitting nursing bra, even during the night, not only makes them more comfortable but helps to maintain breast shape.

Your breasts will be larger during lactation, but if you're like most women, they will return to their former size after you wean your baby. Some women feel their breasts are smaller after nursing, some feel they are larger, but most find no change at all. In any case, the die is cast by the time your first child is born; the change occurs as a result of pregnancy, and whether you nurse this child or not will have no permanent effect on the size and shape of your breasts. One small-breasted woman told us with a grin, "My figure never looked so good as when I was nursing—I felt as if I were wearing a WonderBra!" Fuller-breasted women can also feel and look good during this time, with the help of a supportive bra and flattering clothing.

Q : **Will I gain weight if I nurse?**

A : No—on the contrary. Breast-feeding will help you return more quickly to your prepregnancy size. Many women have breastfed several children and ended up just as slim as they were before they became pregnant. Proper diet during pregnancy and lactation, combined with moderate exercise, will help you return to your prebaby size. In fact, there's some evidence that nursing helps women to regain their figures, since the fat stores developed during pregnancy are laid down specifically for lactation. Women who do not nurse may have a harder time working off this fat. Just think of it—you're burning about 500 calories a day through lactation, as many calories as you'd burn on a five-mile run. Some women do retain a few pounds of extra weight while they're nursing, which they often lose after weaning without doing anything special. Other women find that after weaning they need to cut calories and embark on an exercise program to lose this weight. (For suggestions on how to do this, see Chapter 8.)

Q: **If I nurse my baby, will I have to stay with him 24 hours a day? I can't bear the thought of being so tied down.**

A: Parenthood itself, like any major commitment, restricts your freedom. After the first few weeks, when your milk supply has been established, your baby has become an expert nurser, and her feeding times have become fairly regular, you'll be able to work out a schedule that allows you to be away from your baby for various periods of time. Many working moms breastfeed despite full-time work schedules. (For suggestions on combining working and nursing, see Chapter 12.)

The first couple of months after childbirth tend to be confining for most mothers, no matter how they feed their babies. You'll need to rest and you'll want to stay near your baby, so

you'll be staying close to home. Even if you plan to go back to work or to resume an active schedule that would make breastfeeding difficult, you can still nurse your baby in the early months and give him the benefits of colostrum, the antibody-rich early milk, as well as the mature milk, which will follow later.

Some women successfully combine breast- and bottle-feeding on a regular basis after the first six to eight weeks. The babies of working women may receive one or more bottles of formula or expressed or pumped breast milk while their mothers are on the job. Some fathers feed their babies bottled breast milk or formula in the middle of the night or in the early morning while the mothers catch up on sleep. And some mothers of twins regularly alternate breast and formula for each baby.

The course of breastfeeding almost always runs more smoothly when the mother provides almost all of her baby's nourishment herself, at the breast, and relies on only an occasional bottle. In most cases, it's best to wait until your milk supply is well established before combining the two forms of feeding— six to eight weeks after birth is best. Combining the two forms of feeding, however, works well for some women and prevents that tied-down feeling.

Q: **How long should I continue to breastfeed?**

A: There is no one best time to wean your baby from the breast. The American Academy of Pediatrics recommends breastfeeding for at least the

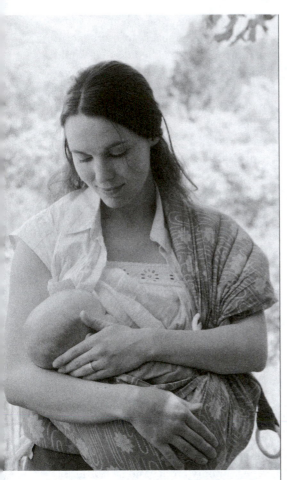

When the nearest store or refrigerator is far away, a nursing mom can still feed her baby.

first year of life—and longer, if both mother and baby want to continue. The academy states that exclusive breastfeeding (feeding nothing but breast milk) for the first six months provides ideal nutrition for your baby's growth and development. WHO advocates breastfeeding for at least two years. A recent study in Canada found that children who had been nursed exclusively for four months seemed to be as healthy as those nursed for six months. You will make your own decision about when to wean, based on many different factors in your life and the life of your baby.

Q: **Will weaning hurt?**

A: No, gradual weaning should not hurt and should not be traumatic for either you or your baby. For a detailed discussion of weaning, see Chapter 17.

Q: **I have to go back to work when my baby is three months old; is it still worth starting to breastfeed when I know I'll have to stop so early?**

A: Yes, it's well worth it. During those early weeks you will have given your baby a good start in life, providing antibodies and immunities in both your colostrum and your mature milk. Some breastfeeding is definitely better than no breastfeeding. Besides, you may find that after you return to work, it will be easier than you thought it would be to continue to breastfeed. For ways of doing this, see Chapter 12.

Q: **I like the idea of nursing, but won't it be embarrassing?**

A: It doesn't have to be. You don't have to bare your breasts to feed your baby; there are ways of nursing discreetly so that no one is even aware of what you are doing, and you can buy or make great-looking cover-ups (see Chapter 9). Even if people do realize that you're feeding your baby, there's nothing shameful about it.

Our society's erotic interest in women's breasts has generated a taboo against showing them in public, thus keeping many women from nursing. It's a pity that the nursing mother, one of the loveliest subjects in art or nature, should be such a rare sight in our society. If you were more accustomed to seeing breastfeeding women, you probably would not be so shy about doing it yourself.

You can deal with shyness in a number of ways. When you begin to nurse, insist on privacy. In the hospital, ask the nurse to draw a screen around your bed; at home, find a quiet nook where no one is likely to disturb you. Chances are that after you have nursed your baby a few times, you'll be so gratified by the experience that you won't find it embarrassing.

Furthermore, by being savvy about the clothes you wear, you can nurse in such public places as airplanes, department stores, or park benches without anyone being aware of what you're doing. For advice on nursing discreetly in front of friends or even delivery people who suddenly appear at the door, see Chapter 9.

Q: I hear so many stories about women who really wanted to nurse their babies but had to switch to the bottle because they didn't have enough milk or they couldn't nurse for some other reason. How can I be sure this won't happen to me?

A: Every healthy woman who has ever had a baby has had milk come into her breasts, and nearly all women can breastfeed when they receive encouragement, information, and support. Only about 2 percent of women are unable to breastfeed for physiological reasons. The first two to three weeks after delivery are the most crucial: It's important to build your support network and reach out for help. For suggestions on learning all you can and starting to build your support network while you're still pregnant, see Chapter 4. Chapter 5 takes you through the first few days of your new baby's life, and subsequent chapters hold your hand with many useful pointers. With this help, you can develop the attitude that you can overcome any problems that arise. With this viewpoint, you're virtually assured of a gratifying nursing experience.

Q: My mother didn't have enough milk to nurse me. Will I take after her?

A: Probably your mom didn't get enough encouragement or information. The ability to breastfeed is not inherited, nor is it completely instinctual. Women need to learn how to breastfeed. Almost all cases of insufficient milk supply are due to lack of information and lack of encouragement from doctors, hospitals, family, and friends. Today, with a renewed realization that this is the best way to feed an infant, we have relearned the old ways of building a mother's milk supply (see Chapter 7) and are constantly coming up with new ways to help mothers and babies.

Nursing is not instinctual for female primates, either. They, too, have to learn to nurse their babies. When Sue, a gibbon at a wildlife center in New Zealand, gave birth, she didn't know how to breastfeed, since she had been reared in captivity and had never seen another ape nurse her young. So the zoo used videos of other nursing gibbons—and real-life demonstrations from nursing human moms. Sue became very good at nursing.

Q: How can I tell whether I have enough milk for my baby?

A: If you have enough information and encouragement, and if you nurse your baby frequently, you are almost assured of having enough milk. There are ways to tell whether your baby is getting enough—one good way is to check your baby's diapers. For signs of adequate nourishment, see Chapter 6.

Q: I'm almost totally flat-chested. How could my breasts possibly hold enough milk to nourish a baby?

A: The size of your breasts has no relation at all to your ability to produce milk. Many small-breasted women breastfeed very successfully, and some have even donated extra milk for the benefit of sick or premature babies.

Your breast size depends on the amount of fatty tissue in your mammary glands. But the amount of milk you produce is determined by the milk-producing components in your breasts, which are independent of the fatty tissue (see Chapter 3 for a complete rundown of breast anatomy). Your bra size is completely irrelevant to your ability to nurse your baby.

However, breast size is relevant in two ways. Babies of women with large breasts sometimes have trouble latching on at first (for suggestions on dealing with this, see Chapter 6). At the other end of the spectrum, women with small breasts have smaller storage capacity, so that even if they produce as much milk, they may deliver less in a single feeding, and so they may need to nurse more frequently. But with the proper support and guidance, women with breasts of any size can provide all the nourishment their babies need.

Q: Does breastfeeding hurt?

A: It shouldn't, if your baby is nursing properly. Some women do feel tenderness, usually in the very beginning as the baby starts to latch on to the breasts. This initial discomfort usually goes away fairly quickly as the nursing mother becomes more expert in helping her baby feed. However, if you feel pain that lasts throughout a feeding and persists after the feeding is over, call your doctor or lactation consultant right away to diagnose and resolve the problem, which is usually one of nursing technique. It's important to deal with problems like this immediately before they get worse. For the right way to put the baby to the breast, see Chapter 6. And for help in preventing and treating sore nipples, engorgement, and other problems, see Chapter 15.

During the early nursing sessions—especially for second and subsequent babies—you will probably feel your uterus contract. These contractions feel like mild menstrual cramps and are a good sign—they mean that your uterus will soon be back to its prepregnancy size.

Q: **What happens when my baby gets teeth?**

A: Probably nothing. The baby who's nursing properly cannot bite the breast. Some teething babies may try to bite down toward the end of a feeding, after their initial hunger has been satisfied. As little as they are, these infants can be gently taught not to do this. See Chapter 7 for suggestions for teaching a baby that biting is a no-no.

Q: **Can I breastfeed if I have inverted nipples?**

A: Most nipples that seem inverted (pushed in) work themselves out during pregnancy so that they're able to function normally after the baby is born. Sometimes exercises during pregnancy will help to bring out such nipples. Other cases may be helped by wearing special breast shells. It's very rare that nipples don't respond to these measures, which we describe in more detail in Chapter 4. But even in these cases, your baby will probably be able

to nurse. Fortunately for the human race, we are born with strong survival skills.

Q: **How can I tell if my milk is rich enough for my baby?**

A: Your breast milk may look thin and watery, but if you are in reasonably good health and eating adequately, your milk will have enough of all the essential elements that your baby needs. Human milk normally has a bluish tint to it. See Chapter 8 for suggestions on how you should eat and take care of yourself.

Q: **Suppose my milk doesn't agree with my baby?**

A: Breast milk agrees with every baby. No baby is allergic to it. Some babies do react to certain foods that you eat. If you find that your baby is rejecting the breast or developing colicky symptoms (see Chapter 7), examine your diet for possible offenders (see Chapters 7 and 8).

Q: **I've always been the nervous type and I hear you have to be calm to breastfeed. Am I doomed to failure?**

A: Definitely not! A calm, relaxed mother may have an easier time breastfeeding than a tense, nervous one. But over the centuries, millions of women have nursed during wars, natural disasters, and other highly stressful events. During times of emotional upset, the flow of milk may be

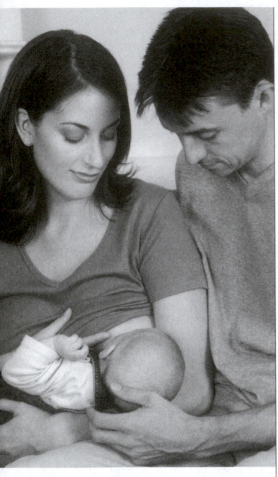

Partners in life, partners in breastfeeding.

Laboratory studies have shown that female rats fight less, maintain their body temperature better, and respond less to stressful situations when they're lactating. This moderation of the nursing mother's responses probably serves to protect babies from extreme changes in maternal behavior caused by outside stress. So you may be among the many nervous types who discover a new calmness through nursing.

Q ▪ **I want to breastfeed, but my husband doesn't like the idea. Is it worth making an issue about this?**

A ▪ Your husband or life partner may need both information and reassurance. You may want to point out some of the advantages nursing holds for him—like relieving him of the responsibility for those middle-of-the-night feedings! You can also reassure your partner that he can still play a major role in the baby's care; new babies need much more than food, as your partner will see by reading Chapter 14, which is addressed to fathers but is relevant to any life partner.

Many a partner who initially opposed breastfeeding goes on to become a mom's staunchest supporter. The help and reassurance of a supportive partner are a major factor in the success of breastfeeding, so it pays for you to make extra efforts to find out what his concerns are and to address them as well as you can. For ways to make your partner in life your partner in breastfeeding, see Chapter 14.

decreased because the let-down (the milk-ejection reflex) is inhibited, but the quality of the milk is unchanged. If you find it hard to relax when you start to nurse, you can help yourself by following some of the suggestions in Chapter 7.

For many women, the act of breastfeeding is a relaxer itself. This is probably due to prolactin, a hormone that's released by the process of lactation, as explained in Chapter 3.

Q. **Ever since I decided to breastfeed, everyone has been trying to talk me out of it. How can I deal with all this opposition?**

A. Opposition to breastfeeding is less common these days than it was a few years ago, but you may still sometimes hear put-downs like "Why can't you be like everyone else and do the natural thing—give the baby a bottle?" or "What are you trying to prove?" Or people may blame your baby's every crying spell on your milk (or what they diagnose as your lack of it). Or your doctor may suggest that you stop breastfeeding if you run into a minor problem.

When these situations arise, consider people's probable reasons for saying these things, and then respond accordingly. When friends have good intentions but poor information, you can enlighten them by pointing out the benefits of nursing to both mother and baby, as given in Chapter 1. When a trace of jealousy affects a grandmother (who sees you care for your baby so competently without her help) or a friend (who did not have a good nursing experience herself), you can be empathic, realizing that she may not have received the support she needed. And you can ask your partner to run interference and protect you from critical relatives. If a doctor seems to misinterpret your questions and thinks that you're asking for permission to stop nursing, while you're actually asking for support and information, you may need to think about looking for a doctor who is more supportive of breastfeeding. For more suggestions on dealing with criticism or surrounding yourself with people who will encourage you, see Chapters 4 and 17.

In any case, once you make your decision to breastfeed, stick with it. You may not be able to change other people's minds, but you don't have to let them change yours.

Q. **How will my older children react to my breastfeeding the baby?**

A. Research suggests that breastfeeding doesn't seem to add to the older children's stress. Most youngsters are fascinated and will respond to your own attitude. If you act as if you're doing the right thing, they'll accept this as the way things are. But if you feel guilty and afraid of making them jealous, they'll sense your vulnerability and will capitalize on it. For more about emphasizing the positive with the older brothers and sisters of a nursing baby, see Chapter 4.

Q. **When my baby is born, I'll be a single mother. Will it be too hard for me to take on the responsibilities of breastfeeding?**

A. You certainly will have your hands full, but if you're like many other single mothers, you may well find that breastfeeding actually makes your life easier by saving time and money—and is also more gratifying. In fact, some single nursing mothers find that they especially appreciate the activity of

nursing because of the relaxing properties of the high levels of prolactin in
their system. Breastfeeding has been
shown to decrease stress levels in both
mother and baby.

It's particularly important to take as
good care of yourself as you can and to
make special efforts to find people who
can become part of your support network. This is one time in your life when
you don't want to become isolated. You
may find help from an organization of
other single mothers, or from a local
breastfeeding or parenting group.
Some pediatricians offer groups where
mothers (and fathers, too) can come to
raise questions and receive answers,
from doctors, nurses, and other parents. Call upon your family and
friends—upon anyone who can offer
encouragement, as well as practical
help. You can find many helpful websites, chat rooms, and blogs about
breastfeeding on the Internet, so you
will never be alone. And try not to let
your day-to-day practical concerns
overshadow the pleasures you get from
this time in your life. It demands much
of you, but it also offers rich rewards.

Q: **I hate milk. Do I have to**
drink it to make it?

A: You don't have to drink milk at
all. Although milk is an excellent
source of protein, minerals (especially
calcium), and vitamins, it's not the
only source. You can either substitute
other foods or take a vitamin and mineral supplement. (See Chapter 8 for
suggestions on diet during lactation.)
Recent research has found, however,

that pregnant and nursing women do
not need calcium supplements if their
diet is adequate. The nursing mother
is especially efficient at absorbing calcium—one more piece of evidence
that nature intends women to nurse
their babies.

Q: **Do I have to eat or**
avoid special foods while
I'm nursing?

A: Probably not, but that depends
on what you've been eating up till
now. If you've been eating a variety of
healthful foods, you don't have to
change your eating habits—except to
take in about 500 extra calories a day
to make up for the ones you use in
making and giving milk. If your diet
has been deficient, however, both
pregnancy and lactation are good times
to make a change. For suggestions for a
well-balanced diet, see Chapter 8.

Some babies don't react to any
foods their mothers eat, but others do.
You may occasionally find that certain
foods in your diet may upset your
baby's stomach. Common offenders
are cow's milk and gas-producing foods
in the cabbage family, like broccoli and
cauliflower. Or your baby may seem
especially wakeful after you've been
drinking cup after caffeine-loaded cup
of coffee or soda. You can then cut
back on the foods in question while
you're nursing.

Be sensible—and moderate. Even
something as innocent as lemonade
in excess can cause problems. One
mother called her pediatrician to say
that her baby was fussy. "Do you think

it might be due to the fact that I ate chocolate last night?" she asked. When the doctor asked her what exactly she had eaten, she replied, "Half a cake." It's surprising she wasn't on the phone to her own doctor.

Q: **Can I have a glass of wine or beer while I'm breastfeeding?**

A: Yes. There's no evidence that moderate amounts of alcohol—a glass of beer or wine or one cocktail occasionally—will have any ill effects on your nursing baby. If your baby sleeps with you and your partner, however, neither of you should have any alcoholic drinks, since these often result in an adult's sleeping so heavily that you or your partner cannot be sufficiently aware of the baby in the bed. Furthermore, heavy drinking can be harmful: It can affect your ability to care for your baby, it can make her drowsy by depressing her nervous system, and it may diminish your let-down or milk-ejection reflex. For more information about alcohol, see Chapter 10.

Q: **Can I breastfeed if my baby is born by a cesarean delivery?**

A: Yes. A new mother's milk often comes in just as quickly after a surgical birth as it does after a vaginal delivery. If you have not had general anesthesia, you will be able to nurse immediately, just as if you had had a vaginal delivery. If you did have general anesthesia, you will be able to nurse as soon as you are awake and alert enough to hold your baby. You will probably need extra rest. And, at first, you will want to protect your incision with a pillow when you hold your baby. But these minor adjustments are only temporary. More information about postcesarean breastfeeding is in Chapters 5 and 6.

Q: **Can I breastfeed while I'm menstruating? I've heard that milk given at this time isn't good for the baby.**

A: Not true! Your milk is good. An occasional baby becomes fussy and may refuse his mother's milk during her period, possibly because the flavor may be different. (For suggestions to counter a baby's refusal to nurse, see Chapter 15.) And you may find you have less milk when you menstruate, but the simple solution to that is to nurse more frequently. In any case, only the quantity of your milk will be affected—not the quality.

You may not menstruate at all while you're nursing. But if you do, there's no reason not to nurse during your period.

Q: **I have heard that if you nurse babies for too long, they are at risk for tooth problems. Is this true?**

A: Although earlier reports have linked prolonged breastfeeding with dental cavities, recent research found that there is no increased risk.

(One factor that does increase the risk of developing dental problems is the mother's smoking). In any case, nursing mothers of babies with teeth should brush the babies' teeth frequently, since prolonged contact with milk can lead to decay.

Q: **Will my baby's suckling at my breasts arouse me sexually? Or will breastfeeding make my breasts seem less erotic during sex?**

A: Every woman is different. Most women do not experience sexual sensations from breastfeeding, but some do. Both responses are normal. Some women find that breastfeeding enhances their sense of themselves as sexual beings, whereas others feel that it seems to relegate their sexuality to the back burner.

The most important thing to remember is that you can enjoy nursing if you do become erotically aroused by breastfeeding—or if such feelings are the furthest thing from your mind. Female sexuality is a complex issue that involves many aspects of your history and self-image. To explore some of these aspects, you will want to read Chapter 13, which discusses the relationship between breastfeeding and sexuality.

Q: **Does breastfeeding prevent pregnancy?**

A: This is one of those questions to which the only answer is "Maybe." You have only a very slight chance of becoming pregnant if all of the following conditions are met: Your baby is under six months of age, your menstrual periods have not returned, you are breastfeeding frequently (no less than every four hours during the day and every six hours at night), and your baby is receiving your breast milk and nothing else. These criteria are the basis for the Lactational Amenorrhea Method (LAM), which we discuss in Chapter 13, along with other methods of birth control.

Generally, if your nursing baby is receiving no supplemental bottles of formula or solid food and is being nursed regularly during the night as well as the day, the hormonal balance in your body, with its low levels of estrogen, will prevent ovulation and therefore pregnancy for three to six months or even longer. Your first menstrual period after childbirth may be sterile; however, this period is a signal that you have either begun to ovulate or are about to do so.

Most women who breastfeed exclusively—and often—do not ovulate for at least the first two months after delivery. These women, then, can use the first months to think about the kind of birth control they'll start to use by the third or fourth month after giving birth. In some cases, LAM is effective even beyond six months. But—and this is a big but—some women have become pregnant while fully lactating and before their periods have resumed. If you want to be absolutely, positively sure not to become pregnant, you will want to use contraception as soon as you resume sexual intercourse. You have to look closely at your own situation and make your contraceptive decisions accordingly. For more information about birth control choices, see Chapter 13.

Q: If I do become pregnant, can I continue to nurse my first baby?

A: You can continue to breastfeed, but many women choose not to. It's probable that your milk supply will diminish somewhat after the first few months of your new pregnancy. Some women nurse one child right through pregnancy and then nurse both the first and the second (known as tandem nursing); others choose not to. Lactation and pregnancy both demand energy from the mother; the two of them together may take too much of a toll. Also, you need to be sure that the infant gets the colostrum she needs and an adequate supply of milk, which may be difficult if you're also nursing a toddler. Most women around the world wean a nursling as soon as they learn that they're pregnant. It is up to you to decide what is best in your circumstance.

Q: Can I breastfeed a premature baby who has to stay in the hospital for several weeks?

A: Yes, and giving your milk to your baby is one of the very best things you can do for him. Providing milk for a premature baby is something that only a mother can do. The milk of women who have delivered prema-
turely has higher percentages of protein and fat, and a lower percentage of lactose (milk sugar) than does the milk of women who have had full-term babies. Because this milk's higher caloric density meets the special growth needs of preterm infants, it's better for them to get their own mothers' milk than to receive formula or even human milk from a milk bank. Therefore, many women feel it's well worth the extra effort to maintain their supply of milk until the baby comes home.

Although you may not be able to actually feed your preterm or very small baby at your breast, you can express your milk and take it to the hospital until he is big enough and strong enough to suckle at your breast. More about this in Chapters 11 and 16.

Q: Can I still breastfeed after breast surgery?

A: You may be able to, depending on the kind of surgery you had. In recent years, more surgeons have tried to perform breast operations in ways that would permit future breastfeeding. If you had implants inserted to make your breasts larger and if the incision did not cut the nerves around the areola (the dark area surrounding the nipple), you can probably breastfeed, at least partially. If you had surgery to make your breasts smaller and if the nipple/areola complex is still attached to the breast tissue beneath it, most likely you will be able to breastfeed. Even if you had one breast removed because of cancer, your baby can nurse from your other breast. Your milk will be fine for your baby, and breastfeeding will not increase your risk of cancer recurrence. You will want to discuss your surgical history with your obstetrician during your prenatal examination, and you will also want to consult the surgeon who operated on your breasts. For more on this topic, see Chapter 16.

Q : **Shouldn't breastfeeding come naturally? Why has it become so complicated that whole library shelves are stocked with books about it, a whole new profession (lactation consultant) has developed, and so many organizations focus on it?**

A : Human beings do very little by instinct alone. Practically everything we do has to be learned. If your mother and other women in your family and perhaps your neighbors breastfed their children, you probably learned from them, just as women across the globe learn from their own mothers. But some women did not grow up in families or communities where breastfeeding was the norm. In fact, the late 1960s and early 1970s had the lowest rate of breastfeeding in U.S. history, so many women don't have the know-how to pass on to their daughters and granddaughters. New mothers need to find other ways to learn how to nurse their babies.

With this book, we aim to offer a wide range of the information you need to have a happy, fulfilling breastfeeding experience. However, there is no way any book can cover every possible situation or advise from a distance. For specific advice on your baby's and your individual situation, you need to talk to your doctor. Meanwhile, you can learn more about breastfeeding. If you're reading these words while you're pregnant, you have a head start. You're in a good position to get the name of a lactation consultant to call once you give birth. After you have begun to breastfeed, she can hook you up with other nursing mothers to "talk shop" with, either individually or in breastfeeding support groups. And one day, you'll be such an expert that you'll be able to help other new mothers.

Q : **Will I be able to exclusively breastfeed twins?**

A : Yes. That's why we have two "feeding stations." Many mothers of twins give them no food other than breast milk for the first six months of their lives. One set of quadruplets was even reported to have been breastfed exclusively for one year. Most breastfeeding mothers of triplets or quadruplets do alternate breast milk and formula, as do some nursing mothers of twins.

An interesting biological fact is the "one-half rule," that is, that the number of young that mammals bear is typically one half the number of mammary glands, and the maximum litter size is equal to the number of mammary glands. Of course, some human mothers—even without fertility drugs—bear three or more babies, but these events are unusual. Scientists who have studied mammals believe that the extra mammary glands are designed to keep sharing and fighting among the babies to a minimum.

Q: **I've heard that environmental chemicals like DDT and dieldrin (insecticides banned from use in the U.S.), dioxins, PCBs (polychlorinated biphenyls), perchlorate, and other chemical contaminants are in breast milk. How harmful are they to babies?**

A: There is absolutely no medical evidence that breastfed babies suffer any ill effects from such chemicals—except for a few rare cases of heavy occupational or accidental contamination. Scientists who have studied the levels of such substances in milk have stated repeatedly that the advantages of breastfeeding far outweigh the risk from these chemicals. No baby has been known to fall sick or become injured because of chemicals in human milk. As Cheston M. Berlin Jr., MD, a professor of pediatrics and pharmacology, has said, "The mere presence of an environmental chemical in human milk does not indicate that a health risk exists for breastfed infants."

Human milk does contain some pollutants, as does the milk of every mammalian species. But the water in formula contains contaminants, too. For suggestions on protecting yourself and your baby from environmental chemicals, see Chapter 8.

CHAPTER THREE

The Miracle of Lactation

*"The human breast reaches its full
functional capacity during lactation with the
production of breast milk."*

DONNA T. GEDDES, PH.D. University of Western Australia

I f you're curious about just how breastfeeding works, this chapter is for you. The explanations here reflect some of the most innovative research in the field of lactation, which has completely changed what we thought we knew about the physiology of breasts and breastfeeding, rendering obsolete practically every textbook and book for lay readers published up to the last few years.

Some of the material here may tell you more than you want to know at this point, so you may want to skim through this chapter and read only those parts that answer your questions, then look back later as new questions arise. If you do read the whole chapter, we're sure you'll agree that lactation, the process by which a mother feeds her newborn baby with the milk produced by her own body, is truly a miracle of biological design.

Along with other information, this chapter reveals:

❖ How your breasts make milk and get it to your baby.

❖ How lactation can sometimes postpone menstruation and pregnancy.

❖ How human milk differs from cow's milk, the base of many infant formulas.

❖ How breastfeeding works and what is happening in your body.

The Development of Your Breasts

You probably remember when you first noticed your breasts beginning to grow. In fact, your breasts began to develop long before that momentous day.

Your mammary glands began to develop when you were a six-week-old embryo in your mother's womb. By the time you were born, the main milk ducts (small tubular canals that carry the milk) in your breasts were already formed.

Right after birth, your breasts may even have swollen and excreted a small amount of milk, often called "witch's milk." This very common phenomenon among both boy and girl infants is caused by the stimulation of the infant's mammary glands by the same hormones produced by the placenta to prepare the mother's breasts for lactation. This milk is actually colostrum (more about this later) and, after a few days, no longer appears in the newborn.

The parts of the human body that develop secretions are called glands. Your breasts are powerful and important parts of your body's glandular system. The endocrine glands (*endo* means "within") secrete hormones, powerful chemical substances that pass directly into the bloodstream and then travel to other parts of the body. These hormones influence such basic processes as growth, sexual development, and even the formation of personality. The exocrine glands (*exo* means "outside") secrete substances into ducts that carry them elsewhere in the body.

The breasts are exocrine glands, which are stimulated, both in their development and in their production of milk, by the hormones of the endocrine glands. Your mammary glands were inactive from shortly after birth until shortly before the onset of puberty, when hormones began to flood your body.

Changes in Your Breasts at Puberty

Your body then took its first step toward changing from that of a girl to that of a woman when your pituitary gland, the master gland of the endocrine system, sent a message to your ovaries, directing them to make estrogen in sharply increased amounts.

Estrogen is the principal female hormone, the substance responsible for the growth of a woman's body hair, for the sexual maturation of the genital organs, and for the development of a feminine shape, including the swelling of the breasts that led you to the bra department for the first time. The pituitary gland also stimulated the manufacture of other female hormones, most notably progesterone, a hormone that actively prepares the body for pregnancy.

A combination of growth hormones and female sex hormones spurred the development of your breasts throughout your adolescence, until you reached your full body growth sometime in your late teens or early twenties.

Changes in Your Breasts During Your Menstrual Cycle

Although your breasts do not begin to produce milk until after the birth of your baby and the delivery of the placenta, they have been preparing for this process for many years. From the time you reach menarche (your first menstrual period) until you arrive at menopause (the end of your menstrual periods), a rhythmic cycle regulates your body.

Every month, your body produces a series of hormones that prepare you to bear children, thickening the lining of your uterus and increasing the blood supply to it. In the months when you do not conceive, the blood, secretions, and tissue debris are discharged during your menstrual period. Ever optimistic, however, your body begins the entire cycle anew the next month.

Estrogen and progesterone produce changes in your breasts every month, in case this will be the month in which sperm and egg unite to create a new being. Just before you menstruate, your breasts may enlarge and may also feel tender. This is because the high levels of estrogen in your body make the blood vessels and glands in the breasts increase somewhat in size during this premenstrual phase, in preparation for a possible pregnancy. While estrogen stimulates growth, it inhibits the production of milk. This is why your breasts will not begin to produce milk until after you have a baby.

With the beginning of each menstrual period, your breasts quickly return to their previous state. If, however, you become pregnant, the heightened levels of estrogen and progesterone in your body produce many changes in your breasts. These changes often alert a woman to the fact that she is pregnant.

Changes in Your Breasts During Pregnancy

To confirm your pregnancy, your doctor will perform a pelvic examination and will closely examine your breasts. Some of the signs that appear by the fifth or sixth week of pregnancy include a persistent fullness and tenderness of your breasts similar to premenstrual sensations, the sudden prominence of the Montgomery's glands (little bumps located on the areola) and the enlargement and darkening of both your nipples and your areolae.

The complete duct system in your breasts develops only now, when you are pregnant, stimulated in large part by the hormones from your placenta. The duct system is completed sometime during the middle trimester of your pregnancy. Thus milk is available for your baby even if you should deliver prematurely.

Glandular tissue replaces much of the fatty tissue in your breasts. The development of this glandular tissue increases the size of your breasts during pregnancy and lactation. By the time of your baby's birth, you will probably have about twice as much glandular tissue as fatty tissue in your breasts, although this varies from woman to woman. Each breast will gain about one and a half pounds of tissue. They will stay about this size during the early months of lactation and then will probably revert to their previous size once you revert to your prepregnancy weight. (But don't worry—they will continue to produce milk.) In a very small percentage of women (only about 2 percent), not enough glandular tissue develops, their breasts don't have enough milk-producing cells, and they cannot prduce enough milk to completely nourish their babies. However, they can often partially breastfeed, with supplementation of formula. This glandular insufficiency is very rare.

The placenta, the organ that transmits nourishment and oxygen from your system to your unborn baby's, also has another function. It serves as a chemical factory: In early pregnancy, it takes over from your ovaries the job of producing large amounts of hormones.

Somewhere around the fifth month of your pregnancy, the placenta begins to produce a new hormone, human placental lactogen. This hormone contributes to the growth of the breasts and also stimulates the development of the alveoli, the little rounded sacs where the milk is made. Once these are formed, your breasts begin to produce colostrum, a sticky colorless or slightly yellowish liquid that may occasionally drip from your nipples during the latter part of your pregnancy. (More about this "liquid gold" later.)

During pregnancy, your body experiences rising levels of prolactin, a hormone that's very important for lactation. Your pituitary gland has been producing prolactin all your life, but when you are not pregnant or nursing, its release is usually blocked by a hormone known as prolactin-release inhibiting factor (PIF). During pregnancy, prolactin levels are high, but its action is inhibited by the high levels of estrogen in your system.

Changes in Your Breasts After Childbirth

Once your baby has been born and the placenta has been delivered, the estrogen and progesterone levels in your body drop sharply. No longer inhibited by estrogen, your prolactin level rises dramatically, enabling the full-scale production of milk within 24 to 48 hours after childbirth. (Of course, you can put your baby to the breast immediately after birth. She'll receive your colostrum, which provides her with essential antibodies.) Your baby's suckling stimulates your pituitary gland to inhibit the secretion of prolactin-release inhibiting factor (PIF) and to permit the production and release of high levels of prolactin.

Besides producing milk, prolactin has psychological effects. It has been dubbed "the mothering hormone," since laboratory experiments have shown that injecting it into a virgin animal induces maternal behavior. Other hormones also trigger motherly impulses. The painkilling proteins called endorphins prepare the mother for the discomfort of childbirth, make her feel good, and draw her to her baby.

The changed hormonal balance in your body sets in motion a chain of events necessary for lactation to occur. Extra blood is pumped into the small blood vessels of the alveoli, causing these vessels to enlarge and become visible beneath the skin, and making the breasts firmer and fuller. The manufacture of milk and the vascular expansion of the ducts and the alveoli are responsible for the engorgement experienced by many—but not all—women. This engorgement (swelling caused by the pressure of the newly produced milk), and the temporary discomfort associated with it, is almost always relieved by the baby's early and frequent nursing. (See Chapters 6 and 15 for more detail.)

Immediately after birth, the cells in the center of the alveoli dissolve and are extruded into the first milk as colostrum. This high-protein, low-fat, and low-lactose substance contains so many protective elements that it constitutes your baby's first immunization at this most vulnerable stage of life. Colostrum, then, is the first milk.

At approximately three days after birth to the end of the first week, the breasts gradually produce the much more plentiful transitional milk. By about ten days to two weeks postpartum, the mature milk has replaced the transitional milk. However, colostrum remains, in diminishing amounts, until six weeks postpartum. This change to mature milk that no longer contains colostrum has an effect on the baby's bowel movements, so that instead of passing several stools a day, she now has one a day or fewer.

The sooner and more frequently you put your baby to your breast, the sooner your transitional milk will replace the colostrum. (The baby will still receive enough colostrum to get the benefit of the antibodies it contains.) If you have nursed a baby before, your milk will come in earlier—typically as much as a day sooner—since your breasts have previously been conditioned for breast-feeding. Women who have nursed a baby previously seem to have a greater number of mammary gland receptors for prolactin. Therefore, they seem to produce more milk in the beginning, explaining why later-born infants begin gaining weight a little faster than firstborns.

When a New Mother Does Not Breastfeed

The woman who does not breastfeed is apt to experience a great deal of discomfort from engorgement, which in her case may last from 24 to 36 hours. She may develop fever, headache, and throbbing pains in her breasts and under her arms. A firm bra; a mild pain reliever like aspirin, ibuprofen, or acet-aminophen; and the application of cold packs usually help to relieve discomfort until her breasts stop producing milk. In the absence of a suckling baby, this should happen within a few days. While medication used to be given to a non-nursing mother to dry up her milk, this is no longer done. The strongest factor in drying up the milk is the lack of stimulation to the breasts. If a baby does not nurse and the milk is not otherwise removed from the breasts manually or with a pump, the alveoli get the message that they are not needed and they stop producing milk.

The Anatomy of Your Breasts

For some 160 years, scientists explained the anatomy of the lactating breast the same way the physician Sir Astley Cooper had described it in 1840. With the development toward the end of the twentieth century of a computerized breast measurement system using ultrasound imaging, researchers have radically revised our knowledge of the anatomy and physiology of the breast. This book reflects the cutting-edge and widely accepted findings of researchers working with Dr. Peter E. Hartmann at the University of Western Australia.

No matter what the size and shape of your breasts, you can have a gratifying breastfeeding experience. Whether your breasts are broad or narrow, high or sloping, small or large, round or tubular, you can happily nurse your baby. Just as women differ in height, general body build, and facial features, they vary considerably with regard to the size and shape of their breasts. Furthermore, most women have one breast that's larger than the other, and it's not uncommon for one breast to produce more milk than the other. None of these characteristics affects feeding a baby.

This is because the milk-producing glands are just one of the four types of tissue that make up the breasts. These four types are the glands that secrete milk, the ducts that carry it, the fibrous connective tissue that supports and attaches the breasts to the muscles of the chest, and the fatty tissue that encases and protects these other structures.

Breast size is determined mostly by the amount of fatty tissue, and since the only purpose of this tissue appears to be to encase and protect the more functional elements, it has no bearing at all on your ability to produce and give milk. Breast size does, however, influence how much milk a woman's breasts can store at any one time, and since small breasts have less storage capacity, small-breasted women usually have to nurse more frequently than women with larger breasts. Still, the bottom line is that you can be an excellent breastfeeder, whatever your bra size is.

The Nipple

Let's look at the breasts with a baby's-eye view. The nipple is the bull's-eye and also the spout through which he receives his milk.

Nipples come in different shapes. They are cylindrical in some women and conical in others. Although the size of the nipple is usually as unimportant for nursing as is the size of the breast itself, sometimes a mother with large nipples who has a baby with a small mouth needs to help her baby learn how to attach to the breast (see Chapter 6).

You have probably noticed that your nipples become erect when they're cold or when you become sexually aroused. The erect nipple becomes two to three times longer than in its softer state. The same thing happens when your baby nurses.

Each of your nipples has several tiny openings through which milk is secreted. The average number of openings, which reflect the number of ducts in the breast, is 9, with a range, found so far, of 4 to 18. The nursing baby stimulates the nerve endings in the nipple, which causes uterine contractions that help return the uterus to its prepregnancy size.

The nipples of some women look flat or folded in and do not become erect when cold or when stimulated. Most often, however, by the end of pregnancy such "pseudo-inverted" nipples protrude normally and come out fully when the baby starts to suckle. In very rare cases, a woman has truly inverted nipples, which do not protrude enough for the baby's mouth to close around them and which do not protrude with the baby's suckling. Fortunately, this condition is almost always correctable during pregnancy by the measures described in Chapter 4.

The Areola

Surrounding the nipple is a darker-colored circle called the areola. In most women, the areola is between 1 and 2 inches in diameter, but it can be considerably larger. The areola and nipple are darker than the rest of the breast, ranging from a light pink in very fair-skinned women to a very dark brown in others.

The areolar coloring deepens in pregnancy and remains darker during lactation, after which the color fades somewhat; it never reverts, however, to the lighter shade it was before pregnancy.

The darker color of the areola may be some sort of visual signal to newborns (Hey, Baby, here it is!), since they have to close their mouth upon the areola, not upon the nipple alone, if they are to obtain milk.

The Montgomery's glands, those little bumps on your areola, become enlarged and quite noticeable while you're pregnant and nursing as they secrete a substance that cleanses, lubricates, and protects the nipple during nursing. The antibacterial properties in this substance help prevent infection in both you and your baby. Some women have secreted milk from their Montgomery's glands, and there is some evidence that they are primitive or simple milk glands.

These glands may also send scent signals to the nursing baby, directing her to the breast. Like other animals, babies' ability to recognize and prefer their own mothers' natural perfume may help to establish breastfeeding. (New mothers also seem to have enhanced sensory abilities, which enables them to recognize their own babies' odors and sounds.)

One study has found that higher numbers of the Montgomery's glands (which range from 1 to 15) are associated with infants' higher weight gains in the first three days after birth. After lactation, these glands recede to their former unobtrusive state.

How Your Body Makes and Delivers Milk

Branches of the milk ducts drain milk from the glandular tissue in the breast and merge into main collecting ducts very close to the nipple. During the let-down, milk is ejected into the ducts, which widen so they can better carry the milk to the nipple, where the baby can get at it. The ducts are intertwined like the roots of a tree.

Each of your breasts has an average of nine ducts, each of which ends at the tip of the nipple. These ducts carry the milk to the baby through tiny holes in the nipple corresponding to the number of ducts.

Within the breast, the ducts branch off into other canals of gradually reduced size toward the chest wall; these canals are called ductules. At the end of each ductule is a grapelike cluster of alveoli. The milk is made in the alveoli. Each cluster of alveoli and branch of ducts is referred to as a lobule (a small rounded complex); a cluster of lobules is called a lobe. The lobes, each of which is a miniature gland, are situated at the base of the breast next to the chest wall. Each lobe is connected to one duct, which empties into one nipple opening, or milk pore.

Some researchers describe the milk ducts of nursing women as being larger than those of women who are not breastfeeding. Also, studies have shown that women with larger ducts express more milk and have longer milk ejections than women with smaller ducts.

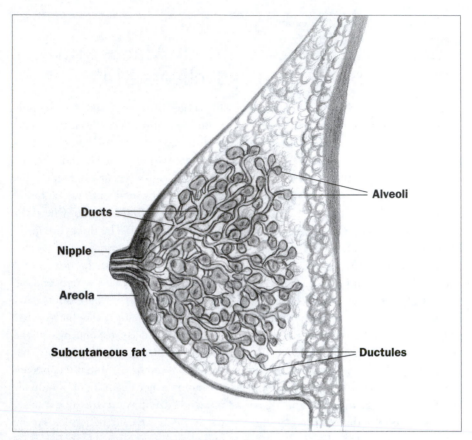

This cross-section of the lactating breast reflects the latest research.

So the anatomy of your ductal system may influence the rate at which you can deliver milk to your baby, thus partly explaining why babies feed differently. Typically, ducts dilate to about twice their original diameter during the let-down.

Both the ducts and alveoli are covered with smooth-muscle cells. Under the influence of the hormone oxytocin (more about this important hormone later), these smooth-muscle cells squeeze the milk out from the alveoli into the duct system. The milk released at the beginning of a feeding when the breasts are full, called the fore milk, has relatively little fat. The fat cells stick to the walls of the alveoli and are expelled toward the end of the feeding as the breast empties. This fatty milk is called the hind milk (the milk released at the end of a feeding session).

A full breast has lower-fat milk and a nearly empty one has high-fat milk. However, when the fat content of the breast milk is measured over 24 hours, the baby normally receives enough calories, and therefore energy, from the fat in the milk.

The Supporting Structure

In some cultures, women deliberately pull at their breasts to make them longer, so that it will be easier to nurse a baby strapped to their backs. Since this is probably not your aim, you'll want to give your breasts as much support as possible.

Nature provides some support—through the muscles attached to the ribs, the collarbone, and the bones of the upper arm near the shoulder. You can help Mother Nature along by wearing a good, supportive bra, even during sleep, during the latter part of your pregnancy and while you are lactating.

Although wearing a bra or going without one has no effect at all upon the breastfeeding function, the force of gravity tends to pull down the heavier breasts of the pregnant or nursing woman. A supportive bra helps to prevent undue stretching of the suspensory ligaments of the upper part of the breast, called Cooper's ligaments. This is why some doctors recommend wearing a good sports bra during jogging and other strenuous exercise (to avoid getting "Cooper's droopers"). Other doctors feel that a woman whose breasts are wide at the base will retain their shape, whether or not she wears a bra.

As we pointed out in Chapter 2, a woman's likelihood of developing ptosis (the medical term for drooping) of the breasts is not related to whether she has breastfed or how long she nursed. The latest research attributes this to prepregnancy bra size; to pregnancy, and especially a greater number of pregnancies; to smoking, since this can weaken the elasticity of the skin; and to age.

How Your Baby Gets Your Milk: The Let-Down Reflex

When your let-down reflex is operating well, more than likely you're overjoyed, not let down in the sense of feeling disappointed. Also known as the milk-ejection reflex (MER) and, in England, the draught (pronounced "draft"), the let-down reflex allows your milk to reach the ducts near the nipple. This reflex is automatic, and in almost all cases it operates very well, as it has for millions of years for almost all women.

In the early stage of lactation, it takes anywhere from several seconds to several minutes of your baby's suckling to produce a let-down reflex. After lactation is well established, hearing your baby cry or even just thinking about your baby will often bring it on.

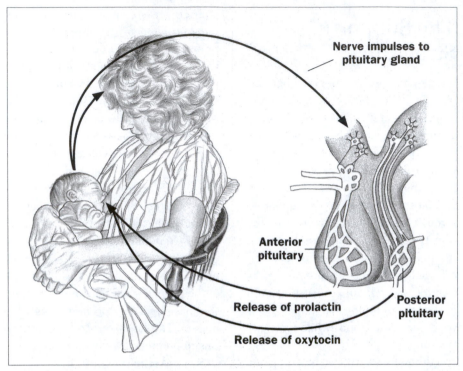

The baby's suckling initiates nerve impulses that direct the endocrine system to produce the hormones prolactin (which helps make the milk) and oxytocin (which causes contractions that send the milk down the duct system).

Before the let-down reflex occurs, only small amounts of milk are available to the baby—or to expression by a breast pump. If not enough milk is removed, milk production decreases. If the milk is adequately removed, there may be up to nine separate let-downs, or ejections of milk, in a single feeding, and the more let-downs that occur, the more milk the baby takes in. Meanwhile, the baby is doing his vital part in this transaction: He extracts your milk by moving his tongue downward in such a way that he creates a vacuum. As the vacuum increases, milk flows from the ducts to the nipple,

making it available to the baby, who can then suck the milk into his mouth.

How can you tell when your let-down reflex is working to get your milk to your baby? The box on page 56 lists the usual signals, from the mother's point of view. To judge whether your baby is getting milk, which is a clear indication that your let-down reflex is working, see "Is My Baby Getting Enough Milk?" on page 124.

As your baby suckles, he stimulates the nerve endings in your nipples, which then send signals to your pituitary gland, directing it to produce more of the hormone prolactin. The prolactin stimulates the alveoli to produce milk. The most important thing you can do to ensure a plentiful supply of milk is to nurse your baby as soon as possible after birth and frequently in the early weeks of life. This will serve to remove the milk from your breasts as thoroughly as possible, and thus stimulate the production of more milk. As long as your breasts are suckled or otherwise stimulated (as with a breast pump or with manual expression), they will continue to make milk.

Your baby's suckling also causes your pituitary to release oxytocin, another very important hormone for lactation. Oxytocin travels through your bloodstream to your breast, where it causes the smooth-muscle cells surrounding the alveoli to contract. As they contract, they squeeze the milk from the alveoli into the ducts. The walls of these ducts also contract, sending the milk out to the ducts near the nipple.

Prolactin helps to make the milk, and oxytocin makes it available to your baby. Animal research suggests that oxytocin also plays a part in stimulating the release of prolactin. In addition, oxytocin released into the brain promotes calming and positive social behaviors. Oxytocin has been called "the quintessential mammalian hormone," "the satisfactional hormone," and the "hormone of love." Besides its role in fostering bonds between parents and offspring, it also causes the uterus to contract during childbirth, orgasm, and lactation. And recent research using brain scans has found that oxytocin helps to regulate fear and

has given rise to theories that oxytocin evolved eons ago to aid in mating and breastfeeding.

The Renaissance artist Tintoretto portrayed a beautiful representation of the let-down reflex in his work *The Origin of the Milky Way*. The painting tells the story of Hercules, Zeus' son by a mortal woman, whom Zeus put to the breast of the sleeping goddess Hera to make him immortal. After the infant had stopped nursing, Hera's milk continued to flow from the goddess's breasts. Some went up into the sky, forming the galaxy, and the rest dropped to the ground, forming a garden of lilies.

The British scientist S. J. Folley points out that this picture illustrates two important attributes of the milk-ejection reflex: first, that the stimulus of suckling creates an increased pressure of the milk inside the breasts, causing it to spurt from the nipples, and second, that even though only one breast may be suckled, milk will flow from both.

Although the let-down reflex operates like clockwork in almost all women, occasionally some women need a little help to "oil the mechanism." Problems can usually be resolved quite easily. The let-down reflex has a strong psychological basis. The pituitary gland, which controls the release of oxytocin, is itself controlled by the hypothalamus. This walnut-size organ in the brain is often referred to as the seat of emotion, since it receives messages about the individual's psychological state and, acting on these messages, sends its own orders to the glands, translating emotions into

Signs of an Active Let-Down Reflex

Some of the most common signs that your let-down reflex is functioning are:

❖ A tingling pins-and-needles sensation in your breasts

❖ A feeling of warmth and/or fullness in your breasts

❖ Dripping of milk before your baby starts to nurse

❖ Release of milk from the nipple other than the one your baby is suckling

❖ Feeling thirsty

❖ Pressure or pain in your breasts

❖ Abdominal cramps (like menstrual cramps) caused by the contractions of your uterus

❖ The relief of nipple or breast discomfort as your baby nurses

Some women with very powerful let-downs do not experience many of these sensations, and some feel a brief period of pain in the early days when their milk lets down. Even women who do feel the signs of initial let-down often do not feel additional let-downs in the feeding. One way to check your let-down reflex is to look at your baby for signs of active swallowing (listed in the box on page 113); if she's swallowing, you're getting milk to her.

---

physiological reactions. The emotions, therefore, exert a powerful influence on such hormone-regulated functions as the menstrual cycle, childbirth, and lactation.

When you have the confidence that you will have milk for your baby, even major stresses like war or natural disasters will not dam up the flow. But when you live in a society like ours, in which women often worry about their ability to provide milk, the slightest of emotions can interfere with your milk production. Pain, embarrassment, fear, fatigue, illness, or distraction can inhibit the let-down reflex and hold your milk back from your baby. If your nipples hurt, your let-down may not

work right. If you are distressed by the disparaging remarks of relatives and friends, your let-down may let you down. If you overtire yourself, don't eat properly, don't respect your own needs for privacy and for relaxation, your let-down reflex may be affected.

This is why it's important to prepare yourself for breastfeeding, both emotionally and intellectually. Chances are that even if you did nothing and knew nothing, you would probably still be blessed with good milk production and an active milk-ejection reflex. But the more you know and the better you can manage the course of breastfeeding, the better your experience is likely to be.

Menstruation, Ovulation, and Pregnancy

Women who do not breastfeed usually begin to menstruate and ovulate within one to three months after childbirth, while nursing mothers may not resume their cycles for more than a year. Your baby's suckling at your breast maintains high levels of prolactin in your system for at least the first few months of exclusive breastfeeding. These quantities of prolactin tend to suppress the action of your ovaries, preventing them from producing the hormones that trigger ovulation, the periodic release of ova (eggs).

Most women do not ovulate or menstruate at all while their babies are receiving no food other than breast milk and are suckling frequently, day and night, especially in the first few months after birth. If you are not releasing eggs, you cannot become pregnant. When you do begin to menstruate, more frequent breastfeeding will not suppress your periods. Once the process has started, there's no stopping it.

Nursing mothers who give their babies no water, no solid foods, no pacifier, and no milk other than their own breast milk in the first six months; who continue breastfeeding frequently (going no longer than five or six hours without nursing); and who have not yet resumed menstruating have only a very small likelihood of ovulating during this time. The Lactational Amenorrhea Method (LAM) of birth control is based on this premise. LAM is no longer effective once your baby is more than six months old or if any of these other conditions have not been met.

However, as soon as your baby takes any supplementary bottles or solid foods, the baby's suckling becomes less vigorous and the prolactin level in your system drops. When your baby doesn't nurse for long stretches of time (during the night, or during the day for working mothers), your prolactin levels also drop. Pumping or expressing milk does not stimulate your breasts to the same extent that a baby's suckling does, and so while these measures may produce enough milk for your baby, they don't produce prolactin at the same levels. When there is not enough prolactin in your body to inhibit your ovaries from functioning normally, you will again resume your regular ovulatory and menstrual cycles. And you will be fertile.

There's a great deal of variability among women. One woman may have one sterile menstrual period before ovulation begins; that is, she may begin to menstruate but not yet be able to conceive. Another is fertile with her first menstrual period after childbirth. Some women don't begin to ovulate and menstruate for several months after their babies are completely weaned from the breast. (Some don't menstruate for up to a year after childbirth.) Others ovulate even while they're fully lactating and before their periods resume.

So while you are less likely to conceive when your baby is totally breastfed, there's still a chance that you can become pregnant. Some fascinating research suggests that in traditional societies where lactation was often the only birth control used, the pheromones (chemical compounds produced by an individual that affect others around them) from nursing mothers seem to have reduced the fertility of the women around them. However, this is not a reliable means of birth control for any individual woman. It's possible that this mechanism may have developed as an evolutionary protection so that women could help one another—and also to maintain populations at a level that could be supported by the available food supply.

Since it's impossible to tell when any particular woman will begin to ovulate, if you want to be sure to space your children, you'll want to use some kind of contraception. (For a discussion of birth control for nursing mothers, see Chapter 13.)

Human Milk: The Ultimate Health Food

One of the most exciting results of new technology has been the discovery of human milk cells that look like stem cells. This finding alone shows the vast difference between breast milk and formula. Breast milk is bioactive, that is, it has an effect on living tissue in both mother and baby, whereas formula is not. If further research shows that these cells can *act* like stem cells, they could be harvested from pumped breast milk, be reprogrammed to form other types of human tissue, and lead to far-reaching developments. (Dolly, the famous sheep, was cloned from a mammary cell.) Mammary stem cells could be harvested from pumped breast milk, without causing problems for the lactating woman.

Colostrum, the Early Milk

"One of the dumbest things I was told in the hospital," one mother told us, "was that I shouldn't bother nursing for the first few days after my baby was born, since I wouldn't have any milk anyway."

Yes, this advice was truly unfortunate, since this mother's baby could have begun receiving the many benefits of colostrum right from birth instead of having to wait for this good food. Throughout history and in various cultures around the world, mothers have often been discouraged from nursing their babies immediately after birth, which deprives both mother and baby of important benefits. Even though colostrum is produced in quite small amounts (only about 1 tablespoon a day, compared to the quart or more a day of mature milk produced by the typical woman), it packs a lot of goodness into a small portion that's perfect for a newborn's tiny stomach.

As we said earlier, probably from as early as the beginning of the second trimester of your pregnancy, your breasts have been producing colostrum, a wonderfully protective fluid that will give your child a head start toward a healthy life. For the better part of the first week after giving birth, your breasts will be providing colostrum for your baby.

This clear or golden fluid is an ideal first food for your baby for several reasons. While it's similar to mature milk, it's easier to digest and richer in disease-fighting antibodies, growth-promoting substances, and living immune cells.

Over the past three decades, a great number of additional components have been identified in human colostrum, thirteen of which are unique to breast milk. The composition of colostrum is different from mature milk in a number of ways. Colostrum contains more protein, minerals, salt, vitamin A, nitrogen, and complex carbohydrates (mostly oligosaccharides). It contains nearly three times the amount of protein as mature milk; it has several amino acids and antibody-containing proteins that are not found in mature milk.

Colostrum has higher levels of immunoglobulin A (IgA) proteins, which ward off disease. Secretory IgA, the most prevalent antibody in colostrum, coats the baby's intestinal and respiratory tracts. This coating action seals the tiny spaces between the cells lining the gut and inhibits foreign proteins from entering the baby's system. It kills bacteria and viruses, preventing them from damaging body tissues and entering the bloodstream. Colostrum also contains higher numbers of white blood cells than milk does. And it's lower in calories, since it has lower levels of fat and sugar.

The fat that colostrum does have is, however, higher in cholesterol than the fat in mature milk, which, in turn, has higher levels of cholesterol than formula. This seems to confer an advantage on breastfed babies, who have higher cholesterol levels than formula-fed children during the first year of life. These higher cholesterol levels may reflect a natural programming that helps breastfed babies handle cholesterol later in life, and may explain why babies who have been breastfed are apt to have lower cholesterol levels later on and to have a lower risk of heart disease as adults.

The main function of colostrum seems to be to protect the newborn against infection, but it may also provide important nutrients. It is especially beneficial for sick and premature infants. It also performs a valuable laxative function by cleaning out the meconium from the baby's bowels. This greenish-black waste matter, formed in the baby's intestinal tract before birth, decreases the likelihood of jaundice in the baby by carrying a substance called bilirubin out of the baby's body. (For more about jaundice and bilirubin, see Chapter 6.)

Colostrum is very important to most animals because it provides many essential immunities in the early weeks. Antibodies from colostrum have been found in the stools of breastfed babies, showing that the babies received these antibodies through their mothers' milk and that they are not destroyed by the digestive enzymes. These antibodies are not present in the intestines of babies who receive formula exclusively. It seems probable that the breastfed baby's superior resistance to disease is due in part to these early antibodies, and in part to the oligosaccharides (carbohydrates consisting of simple sugars) in human milk, the presence of which is highly correlated with resistance to disease. Formula is often sweetened with sugar, which does not provide the same nutritional and growth-producing benefits.

Therefore, providing infants with this valuable fluid is a prime argument for feeding newborns as soon and as frequently as possible. It's also an important reason for beginning to breastfeed even if you feel you can do it for only a short time.

The Mature Milk

The mature milk itself is another magical elixir. You custom-make your baby's fare especially for him at each stage of his development. Breastfeeding provides everything your baby needs—appetizer, main course, and dessert, all wrapped up into one delicious food.

First, as we said, comes the colostrum, which is usually a yellowish color, but may also be clear, brown, green, or red. Then, from about four or five days to two weeks after birth, the breasts produce what's known as transitional milk; it contains high levels of fat, which helps your baby regain any weight lost after birth. And finally, from about six weeks on, they produce a more mature milk. What is this true milk like?

First of all, it looks different—from colostrum and also from cow's milk. Human milk looks like skim milk, with either a bluish or yellow-gray tint to it. It's not surprising that it looks different from cow's milk. It *is* different. Although the cow's milk used in many infant formulas has been modified to make it more like human milk, this base is still the milk of a nonhuman animal. The milk of every mammal has the same basic structure, but there are striking differences in chemical composition and proportion among the milks of various species. It seems reasonable to suppose that the milk of each species is especially suited to the needs of its young.

The whale, for example, gives milk that's very rich in fats and calories—elements important for survival in cold water. Cow's milk is high in protein, calcium, and phosphate, ingredients that are important for the rapid growth of young calves. While human babies usually require about six months to double their birth weight, calves do this in a month and a half. It stands to reason that the higher protein and mineral levels in cow's milk (which are four times greater than those in human milk) foster this rapid growth, whereas the lower levels in human milk are more suited to the human growth timetable.

Even though we're constantly learning more about the unique structure of human milk, we'll probably never be able to identify every single one of its more than one hundred different components. Over the last fifty years, hundreds of scientific papers have been published on the biochemical properties of human milk, and ongoing research continues to find new substances in it.

Like the milk of other species, human milk is mostly water—88 percent. Its nutrient portion—the other 12 percent—is made up mostly of fat, carbohydrate in the form of lactose (milk sugar), undigestible complex carbohydrates (mostly oligosaccharides, or simple sugars), and protein. While this ratio is fairly constant, there is some variation among women, as well as in the same woman at different times. Some of this variation stems from what you eat. The vitamins and minerals you take in are reflected in your milk, as is the kind of fats you eat. As you'll see in Chapter 8, it's important for you to eat a variety of foods.

As discussed on page 52, milk composition also varies during a single feeding session. It also seems to vary from one feeding to another, although research is somewhat conflicting on this. Some studies have shown breast milk to be richest in fat in the morning and leaner as the day goes on, while others have shown it to be fattiest in the afternoon, leanest in the morning.

One study found that the breast milk of women who had nursed for twelve to thirty-nine months had more than three times the amount of fat that is present in milk from women who had been nursing for only two to six months. This study indicates that the nutrient value of breast milk continues even beyond a year, and that the implications for cholesterol levels in children breastfed beyond a year should be studied.

The protein content of milk also varies, with slight differences sometimes recorded even between the left and right breasts. Substantial change takes place over the course of nursing. The very high protein level in the colostrum drops sharply in the first week, then drops gradually throughout lactation. After about eight to ten months, babies generally need additional sources of protein.

The Uniqueness of Human Milk

It's most probable that, even with all our scientific know-how, no one will ever be able to isolate, identify, and copy all the constituents of human milk—the best food for the human baby.

Manufacturers of formula products do try. Aware of the differences between human milk and raw cow's milk, they use the latest scientific knowledge as a guideline for the preparation of nutritionally sound baby formulas. They use tables of recommended minimum daily requirements—and all their ingenuity. For a detailed comparison of cow's milk and human milk, see Appendix IV, page 405.

Most formulas, for example, replace the butterfat in cow's milk with some combination of oleo, soy oil, corn oil, coconut oil, palm oil, or olive oil. They experiment with various types of sugar, add substances to help the baby's body synthesize fatty acids, and in other ways try to copy breast milk.

From time to time, however, scientists discover new compounds in breast milk, requiring new modifications in formulas made from cow's milk.

One of the most exciting discoveries was the finding that the composition of the milk secreted by women who have given birth prematurely is different from that of women who have borne a full-term baby. Nature's design is so elegant that each mother of a preterm baby produces milk that has the specific constituents needed by her own baby. This preterm milk is higher in protein, fats, and the salts sodium, nitrogen, and chloride. Thus it's better constituted to meet the needs of the preterm baby (the tiniest preterm babies may need additional supplementation).

As in so many cases, human milk is a sterling example of the inability of human invention to equal the creativity of nature.

CHAPTER FOUR

Before Your Baby Comes

"I always assumed I would breastfeed because it would be healthier for my babies. What I never anticipated was how profound the experience of breastfeeding would be on so many levels. The idea that my body was sustaining my babies, that there was nothing they needed but me: *This idea continues to amaze me even years later."*

LAUREN Westport, Connecticut

Even before you feel your baby's first stirrings inside your womb, you can prepare for your happy breastfeeding experience. You're already doing your baby and yourself a favor by reading this book and getting answers to some of your many questions.

During the months before your baby's birth, you'll have many decisions to make. Of course, the questions you have before your baby is born are probably different from the ones you'll have later. In this chapter, we'll answer questions like: What kind of medical and birth practitioners will you want?

Where will you want to have your baby? What kind of delivery will you want?

Other questions will be answered in later chapters. For suggestions on diet during pregnancy and after childbirth, see Chapter 8. And in Chapter 12, we talk about issues that concern the breastfeeding working mother, such as how soon you'll be going back to work, what kind of maternity leave you'll ask for, and what kind of child care you'll arrange for.

Choosing Your Health Care Providers

Because the kind of medical and nursing care you and your baby receive before, during, and after the birth has such far-reaching impact on your health, as well as your baby's, you want to be sure that the people you consult are knowledgeable and skilled. And because how you feel about pregnancy, childbirth, and your family relationship has such a major influence on the emotional well-being of everyone in your family, you want to feel comfortable and happy with your helpers.

These days, you have many options, and you should be able to find caregivers who match your needs and your preferences. The kind of practitioner you choose will depend on many factors—the community you live in, your philosophy about childbearing, child rearing, and medical care in general, your physical condition, your finances, your health plan, and your personality. You may want a well-established, older parent-figure type, or you might be happier with someone close to your own age. You may prefer a woman rather than a man. The practitioner's location and the medical facility she or he is affiliated with may be important factors as well.

For help in choosing a specific practitioner, see "Finding a Practitioner You Trust" later in this chapter. Also consult the Resource Appendix.

To clarify your thinking and help you decide, talk to friends, as well as representatives of childbirth education organizations. You can also consult books about pregnancy to find out more about the specialties described in the following section.

Types of Health Care Provider

Obstetrician-Gynecologist (ob/gyn): Most women in America have their babies with the help of a physician who specializes in treating women and in delivering babies. Such a doctor will see you throughout your pregnancy, monitor the progress of your baby while he or she is still in the uterus, deliver your baby, examine you after childbirth, and then see you throughout your life for routine checkups and care of your reproductive organs and your breasts. Women whose medical histories or present circumstances put them in the high-risk category are especially likely to seek the services of an obstetrician.

You want to feel that your obstetrician is knowledgeable about and supportive of breastfeeding and gives you enough time to ask questions. (Your ob/gyn is unlikely to have learned much about breastfeeding in medical school; however, many physicians have educated themselves.) Your doctor should record your medical history, including any breast surgery you have had, and should examine your breasts and nipples to either identify possible problems or reassure you that they are normal and that you should have a good breastfeeding experience.

If your obstetrician thinks that you may be at a higher-than-normal risk for complications, you may be advised to consult a *perinatologist,* who will care for you and your baby before and immediately after birth.

Family Physician: This up-to-date version of the doctor who takes care of everyone in the family is a far cry from the old-fashioned GP (general practitioner) who made house calls in a horse and buggy. Family practice is a recognized medical specialty, and family physicians receive certification after passing rigorous examinations enabling them to be the doctor of first contact. Family physicians can provide a continuity of medical care born from long years of treating family members. Many family doctors undergo special training to deliver babies, after which they continue to care for the new baby, as well as for the rest of the family. One advantage to this kind of care shows up when either mother or baby is ill and the treatment affects the other half of the nursing couple.

Midwife: The tradition of women who are not trained as physicians but who assist women giving birth is an old and respected one. Today, such practitioners generally care for women with low-risk pregnancies and uncomplicated births. They usually devote a great deal of time to their patients and offer emotional, as well as physical, support. They help both before and after childbirth, lending a hand when needed, and offering experience-based advice. Midwives assist at both hospital and home births.

Midwives differ considerably in terms of training and accreditation, from certified nurse-midwives to lay midwives, as described below. Before engaging a midwife, learn her qualifications, talk to other women who have used her services, and discuss with her in what circumstances she would call in a physician who could respond quickly in case of a medical emergency. Ask who her medical backup is and if you can meet this doctor to get acquainted during your pregnancy, just in case. To find a midwife, see the Resource Appendix.

A *certified nurse-midwife* (CNM) is a registered nurse who has completed a course in midwifery training and passed a written examination and skills assessment given by the American College of Nurse Midwives Accreditation Commission for Midwifery Education (ACME). Certified nurse-midwives generally work together with physicians in private practice, in maternity or birth centers, and in some hospitals. CNMs are legal in all fifty states and the District of Columbia. In thirty-three states, private insurance must reimburse for CNM services, and in all states Medicaid mandates this. Ninety-eight percent of CNM births take place in hospitals. The percentage of CNM-assisted births has risen nearly every year since 1975, when statistics were first recorded.

Other midwives, who are not nurses, are known as *lay* or *direct-entry midwives*. Many are licensed and legally permitted to practice in most states. Some have served as apprentices to experienced midwives and/or studied at private or college-affiliated midwifery schools. They usually do home or clinic births. Some midwives practice independently (legal status varies by state) with neither certification nor license.

Pediatrician: These physicians are specially trained and certified to take care of children from birth through adolescence, although some pediatricians continue to see their patients into young adulthood. Since they usually see at least one parent, and often both, when they see a child, they come to know the entire family and often serve as the doctor of first resort for everyone.

If you plan to consult a pediatrician for your child, it's a good idea to choose one at least three months before your due date. While this doctor will not care for the developing fetus, she or he should examine your baby within twenty-four hours after birth. If you deliver prematurely or if any complications arise with your baby's health, you'll feel more confident placing your baby's care in the hands of someone you have already met rather than having to deal with a complete stranger.

If your baby needs special care after birth, a *neonatologist* may be called in. Doctors in this specialty care for premature and seriously ill infants and those with injuries or birth defects. Their care is given primarily in the hospital.

Lactation Consultant (LC): This kind of health care professional specializes in promoting, protecting, and supporting breastfeeding, largely by person-to-person contact with a nursing mother and baby. Such consultants can give telephone or in-person counseling for breastfeeding problems, either in private practice or in affiliation with a pediatrician, a hospital, or a maternity center. LCs come from many different backgrounds; some started out as nurses, midwives, or physical therapists, while others come from completely different fields, including lay breastfeeding support organizations. If you have had breast surgery, have inverted nipples, or have other concerns about breastfeeding, you may want to consult an LC before you have your baby.

After watching you nurse your baby, an LC can evaluate a breastfeeding problem, come up with a treatment plan, and then report to you and your doctor. There are different levels of LC, including a person with no training who calls herself a lactation consultant; a person who has taken a week's training and can put CLC (Certified Lactation Consultant) after her name; and the most highly qualified LC, someone who has passed an examination given by the International Board of Lactation Consultant Examiners (IBLCE) and can use the letters I.B.C.L.C. (International Board Certified Lactation Consultant) after her name. To sit for the IBLCE exam, candidates have to show that they've had the required minimum of lactation education and hundreds of hours of practice consulting. To find a lactation consultant, see the Resource Appendix.

Volunteer Breastfeeding Consultant: The women who lead local chapters of La Leche League International are experienced nursing mothers who have undergone training to become accredited leaders. They hold monthly meetings for pregnant and nursing women; the first meeting is free and, after that, women who want to continue attending meetings are asked to become League members for a modest fee. The leaders provide answers to breastfeeding questions, either over the phone or in person, and also refer women to professional sources of information. In some communities, similar groups help nursing mothers in this way. La Leche League International publishes many helpful materials and offers a help line for questions. (See the Resource Appendix.)

By attending meetings during your pregnancy, you can get a preview of what to expect after your baby arrives, establish a relationship with people knowledgeable about breastfeeding, and meet other nursing mothers. Going to these meetings before your baby is born is especially helpful if you have never seen a baby nursing. Some meetings are also open to fathers, and it's a good idea to take your mother or mother-in-law to them also, to help her understand how breastfeeding has changed since she did it (or didn't). To find the closest La Leche League group, look in your local telephone directory, or contact the League; see the Resource Appendix.

Doula: Anthropologist Dana Raphael gave a new definition to the Greek word *doula* when she used it to describe a woman who "mothers the mother." DONA International, a doula membership group, uses the word to mean "wise woman of birth."

A doula provides nonmedical emotional and practical support before, during, or after delivery—or at all three times. Her most important job is usually during labor and childbirth, when she stays with the mother and strives to make her more comfortable and to ease delivery. This may involve massage, positioning suggestions, hot compresses, and helping the mother to begin breastfeeding. Research has found that the support of a birth doula results in shorter labors, less use of childbirth medication, fewer forceps and cesarean deliveries, and more positive breastfeeding outcomes. Some doulas make postpartum home visits, which may center around infant care, breastfeeding, and other postpartum needs like cooking, laundry, and caring for older siblings.

In traditional societies, and sometimes in our own, a new mother's doula is often her own mother or another woman in the community who offers her help for no pay. Professional doulas often (but not always) receive special training, register with agencies, and are paid by the hiring family. Before you hire a doula, you will want to know about her training, experience, references, and fees. Although this service can be costly, if you have no one else who can help you and if your budget will allow it, it is often well worth the expense. Furthermore, some insurance plans pay for doula help. To find a doula, see the Resource Appendix.

Baby Nurse: Some new mothers hire someone whose principal duty is to care for the new baby. The baby nurse is often a licensed practical nurse (LPN) or a personal care aide (PCA) rather than the more highly trained registered nurse (RN); or she may be a woman who has had no further training beyond her experience in raising her own children. Typically a baby nurse diapers, bathes, and comforts the baby. She also launders the baby's clothes and bed linens. In the case of a breastfed baby,

she takes the baby to the mother for feedings. Often, the nurse will also prepare simple meals for the family and do light housework.

This service is also costly. If your pregnancy and delivery have been uncomplicated and you feel good, you would probably be better served by a doula or by someone who comes in to do household chores, so that you can be your baby's principal caregiver. However, if you are not feeling well, have no family members who can help you, and can afford it, you may want to hire a baby nurse for the first week or two of your child's life. You should interview baby nurses with particular emphasis on their attitudes toward breastfeeding.

In addition to personal recommendations from other women, you can find a baby nurse (or a housekeeper) through local employment agencies that specialize in home health care. They are listed in the Yellow Pages under Home Health Services or under Nurses. You can also search online.

Visiting Nurse: Some hospitals offer home visits by nurses during the first ten days of your baby's life, and these visits are often covered by medical insurance plans. The nurses can assess a baby's condition and can help the mother with breastfeeding. A 2004 study found that babies who had been visited at home were less likely to be readmitted to the hospital or to require emergency room care.

Family Member: To get the maximum help from your mother, mother-in-law, or other relative, it's good to discuss your breastfeeding plans with her ahead of time to get her on your side and bring her up to speed on current recommendations for nursing. While she may not help you birth your baby, she can be a source of valuable help both in preparing for your delivery and in mothering you after your baby is born.

Finding a Practitioner You Trust

It's not always easy to find the right person or people for you—someone who is skilled, who shares your philosophy about childbearing and child care, and who is both knowledgeable and enthusiastic about breastfeeding.

To find the most suitable doctors and other practitioners, you can:

❖ Ask friends who have recently had babies.

❖ Ask your family doctor or gynecologist.

❖ Call your local medical society and ask for referrals.

❖ Call a local hospital or birthing center and ask for a recommendation to one or more people on their staff.

❖ If you want to give birth at a particular hospital, check to be sure that the obstetrician and pediatrician you want to go to are on staff there. If you do decide to choose a pediatrician who is not on the hospital staff, ask that

doctor or your obstetrician to recommend a pediatrician with staff privileges (the ability to admit and treat patients) who can do the first postbirth examination of your baby. Once you have the names of one or more practitioners in the categories you're looking for, you can make your selection based on a number of criteria.

❖ Find out if the practitioner is a member of a professional organization. Contact one of the organizations listed in the Resource Appendix to find out. Or ask the practitioner or his/her office staff about the practitioner's degrees, accreditation, and certification.

❖ For information about a physician, go to www.abms.org, the website of the American Board of Medical Specialties. After you register on the site, you can learn whether your physician is board-certified in a particular specialty. For additional information, including when and where doctors were educated, and which hospitals and insurance plans they're affiliated with, consult your library's copy of *The Directory of Medical Specialties,* which is updated yearly. The directory comes either as bound books or in searchable CD-ROM format.

❖ Find out if the practitioner is knowledgeable and enthusiastic about breastfeeding. Some pediatricians are certified as lactation consultants themselves, and many have one or more lactation consultants on their office staff. You can consult the LCs by phone or in the office.

Questions to Ask Health Practitioners

Although you do want answers to your questions about a practitioner's philosophy and practice, the most important consideration in choosing a birth attendant—or any other helper—once you have satisfied yourself as to the person's professional qualifications, is the feeling of comfort you get from this person.

You need to feel as if you can ask any question and get a reasoned, thoughtful answer; you need to feel comfortable giving your personal information to your practitioner; and you need to feel you are good partners in this important endeavor. The helper has to fulfill his or her professional duties—but in the end, this is your body and your baby.

Says Dr. Laura Marks, "I want the parents who come to me to feel comfortable with me, since that sense of comfort gets transmitted to their children. Their feelings about health care will last throughout their lives—and so it makes me feel good to hear that my young patients love to come to see me!"

Questions for an Obstetrician or Midwife

❖ How do you feel about anesthesia during labor and delivery? (See the discussion of childbirth medication in Chapter 10, which can help you talk to your doctor about this.)

❖ Under what circumstances would you use forceps to deliver a baby?

❖ How frequently do you perform an episiotomy on the mother?

❖ What circumstances would call for induction of labor?

❖ What conditions do you feel warrant a cesarean delivery?

❖ What circumstances would call for a birth before 38 weeks' gestation? (See discussion of late preterm and near-term babies on page 345.)

❖ Do you encourage mothers to breastfeed within an hour of birth?

❖ Ask to make an appointment for a consultation, and ask what the fee for a consultation is compared to a complete examination. Ask your partner to go with you. If the practitioner does not offer consultations, ask if there is another way for you to get to know him or her.

❖ Make a list of your questions ahead of time, with the most important ones first so you'll be sure to ask them. Write down the practitioner's answers.

❖ Ask whether the practitioner is affiliated with an accredited hospital or center whose maternity policies are at least close to those in the Baby-Friendly Hospital Initiative described in this chapter.

❖ When do you recommend rooming-in for mother and baby? (Rooming-in is an arrangement whereby the newborn stays in the mother's room instead of the nursery. See box on page 76.)

❖ Do you recommend circumcising newborn boys?

❖ If I go into labor at a time when you are not available, what is your backup coverage?

❖ What provisions do you have for childbirth emergencies?

Questions for a Pediatrician or Family Doctor

❖ Are you on staff at the hospital where I'll give birth?

❖ Will you examine my baby right after birth?

❖ How many breastfed babies are in your practice?

❖ How long is a typical office visit?

❖ Whay topics are covered in a typical office visit?

❖ About how long do the mothers in your practice breastfeed?

❖ At what age do you think babies should begin to eat solid foods?

❖ What are your office hours and when can I reach you by phone during the day, at night, and on weekends?

❖ If I have a nonemergency question, how can I reach you?

❖ Do you charge for telephone consultations? (Many doctors do these days, and these consultations are often covered by health insurance.)

❖ Do you routinely order sugar water, formula, or pacifiers for newborns?

❖ How soon after birth should I bring my baby to your office? (A breastfed baby should be seen in the first week.)

❖ How do you help breastfeeding mothers?

❖ If the practitioner is part of a group practice, ask whether it would be possible to meet the other members of the practice in case you or your baby will need to see them someday.

❖ Find out how a prospective birth attendant or other health care practitioner feels about issues like those covered in the box above and any other child-birth and child care issues that are important to you. If you go in with a fair, nonbelligerent attitude, you should get a friendly and open-minded reception.

If, however, the practitioner wants to impose his or her views on you, you will have learned something valuable right at the beginning, and you may want to continue your search for a more compatible caregiver.

❖ Actions sometimes speak louder than words. If, for example, you have already consulted an obstetrician, ask yourself: Did she or he examine your breasts at your first prenatal visit; assure you that there is no reason why you cannot breastfeed, or else pick up on problems that need to be taken care of; point out the benefits breastfeeding confers on both mother and baby; and answer your questions patiently and knowledgeably?

❖ Especially for doulas and midwives: Ask your prospective candidate whether she provides prenatal and/or postpartum visits to your home, and what she will do in these visits; how many births she has attended; what her training has been; what references she can provide; what kind of backup arrangements she has in case of emergency; and how she defines her role during labor, birth, and the postpartum period.

❖ Fees. Ask the practitioner directly, or talk to the office receptionist. Find out which insurance plans she or he accepts. Ask whether a sliding scale or an extended payment plan is available.

❖ Check out the office setting: Is the staff welcoming? Is the office clean and attractive? An absence of coupons for formula and pictures of baby bottles suggests that the practitioner may be helpful to breastfeeding mothers.

If you emerge from your consultation feeling confident that you made the right choice, your shopping is over. If you're not completely convinced, you don't have to say anything yet. Meet the other people on your list and then make up your mind.

You may find that you're not 100 percent happy with any of the practitioners you meet. Few matches are perfect, whether you're talking about a spouse or a doctor. When you're searching for the right health care provider, it all comes down to finding the right fit for you. You should feel comfortable asking questions. After all, medical questions—and those involving breastfeeding—can sometimes feel intensely personal. So when you choose your physician or other health care provider, take into account bedside manner, training, experience, reputation, and any other factor that's important to you.

And remember, no decision is etched in stone. As you read this, you may be well along in your pregnancy— and uncomfortable with your practitioner. Or maybe your baby has been born already and you're not completely at ease with the doctor you've been seeing. Changing birth attendants or doctors is not a decision to be undertaken lightly, but it is possible, and sometimes advisable. If at any time you feel that the fit is not right for you or your family, it's okay to switch to another provider. You may want to tell your doctor that you think it would be better for you to see someone who might be a better match. Most doctors will be happy to refer you to a colleague. Their primary responsibility is to make sure you and your baby receive the best care possible, and they know that sometimes that is best provided by another physician.

Who is the expert here? You are. No matter how knowledgeable and experienced a professional person is, you are the expert on your own life. This is your pregnancy, your labor, your birth experience, and your baby. While the practitioner may be an expert in his or her field, you are an expert on your body and your child. You need to have enough faith in yourself and in your good judgment to know when to follow advice and when not to.

Yes, of course, you will follow your doctor's advice in medical matters and your lactation consultant's in breastfeeding matters—but when they express their beliefs about parenting (like what constitutes "spoiling" a baby, when he should be sleeping through the night, or at what age you should wean your child from the breast), you need to remember that such beliefs are only opinions, nothing more. No one has all the answers on what is right for you and your baby, but everyone has advice for new mothers. So you need to treat all advice, including this book, as a smorgasbord from which you take what seems to make sense for you and leave the rest.

Your Health Insurance

Often we have little or no say over which insurance plan will cover our medical care. We take what we can get from our employer or our spouse's employer—and feel lucky to be insured at all in these days of soaring medical costs. However, if you are in a position to choose your health insurance provider, you will want to choose the plan that offers the most benefits to you as a breastfeeding mother.

If you have a managed care plan, it probably stipulates that you get your services only from the providers included in the plan network (or else pay extra for your care) and that you be assigned to a primary care physician who makes all referrals to specialists.

If you or your partner is covered by an employer's health plan, you want to contact the appropriate person for details on eligibility and rules for adding your baby to your present policy. You should make this contact before your baby is born, since you usually have to enroll the baby very soon after birth; if you don't, you may not be able to cover the baby.

If you are exploring different plans, you will want to ask the following questions:

❖ Do you cover the services of a nurse, midwife, or lactation consultant?

❖ If so, how many visits is a midwife or lactation consultant allowed under the plan? (Many plans will pay all or part of the cost for initial and follow-up visits.)

❖ If you don't pay all the costs, what percentage do you pay?

❖ If lactation consultants are not covered under the basic plan, do I have the option to upgrade my policy?

❖ If I have a breastfeeding problem, do you offer a free follow-up visit on the second or third day after birth with a physician, a nurse, or a lactation consultant?

Even if you do not have a choice of plans, it is worth raising these questions about the plan you have. If consumer demand is great enough, your employer or other organization that contracts for your plan can sometimes negotiate a special rate for special services.

A powerful argument for including lactation consultants in a health plan is its cost-effectiveness. According to the cost analysis prepared by Miriam H. Labbok, MD, director of WHO Collaborating Center on Breastfeeding, if insurance companies spent money to provide lactation consultants, more babies would be breastfed, so fewer would get sick. If infants nursed for 12 weeks, the insurance companies would save 57 cents for every dollar currently spent for care of the illnesses that would not occur among these babies. Nationwide, over the next ten years, public and private insurers and HMOs would save about two billion dollars.

If your health insurance does not cover the services of a lactation consultant, some LC agencies will give you the opportunity to self-insure. You may be able to sign up before your baby is born and pay a flat rate that covers one prenatal breastfeeding class, an initial visit in hospital or home, and as many follow-up visits as are necessary. This is an option that might be well worth the money if you have received glowing recommendations for a particular LC or agency, and especially if you do not have other knowledgeable resource people to help you. For information about submitting claims, appealing denied claims, and getting assistance from your employer, health care provider, and lactation consultant, go to www.breastfeedinginsurance.com.

Choosing Where You'll Give Birth

At about the same time that you choose your birth attendant, you'll be deciding where you want to have your baby. There are three basic options:

Hospital: While many hospitals are big and impersonal, with rigid rules that often seem designed for the smooth functioning of the institution rather than the individual, others are run with the comfort and well-being of the patient in mind.

As more has been learned about the optimal conditions for successful breastfeeding, more hospitals have implemented at least some of the policies of the Baby-Friendly Hospital Initiative, launched in 1991 by UNICEF and WHO. According to this program, every facility providing maternity services and care for newborn infants should follow ten steps to support the breastfeeding mother and baby. Although these steps represent the ideal, as of this writing the United States has only 73 certified Baby-Friendly Hospitals. So the odds are that your hospital won't be practicing all ten steps listed in the box on page 76. In fact, a recent U.S. government study that analyzed responses from nearly 2,700 birth facilities found that seven in ten hospitals still give nursing mothers gift bags with baby formula.

However, the policies in the initiative have been gaining ground. For one thing, as hospitals have needed to compete for fewer maternity cases, they have become more responsive to the desires of patients. Many now have rooming-in policies, permit fathers or other labor coaches to remain with the mother during labor and birth (including cesarean births), and offer such other aspects of family-centered maternity care as birthing rooms and family rooms that let siblings be present during childbirth. (Some even have queen-size beds for fathers who want to spend the night.) Another policy that benefits nursing mothers and babies is not distributing discharge packs of infant formula (or coupons for them) to nursing mothers. Research has shown that mothers breastfeed for a longer time when they have rooming-in and when they do not receive formula when they leave the hospital.

Hospitals can change and be more humane in response to demands from patients and medical and nursing

Sharing prenatal and birth experiences with a supportive partner helps cement family bonds.

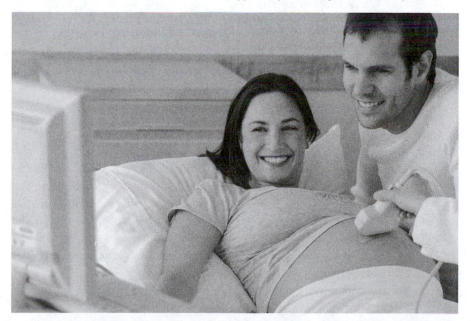

The Ten Steps to Successful Breastfeeding in a Baby-Friendly Hospital

A baby-friendly hospital should:

1. Have a written breastfeeding policy and routinely communicate it to all health care staff. (The policy should assume that breastfeeding is the standard method of feeding.)

2. Train all health care staff in skills necessary to put the policy into practice.

3. Inform all pregnant women about the benefits and management of breastfeeding. (Ideally, the hospital should offer prenatal classes for couples.)

4. Help mothers begin to nurse within about an hour of birth.

5. Show mothers how to nurse, and how to maintain lactation even if they should be separated from their infants.

6. Give newborns no food or drink (including water) other than breast milk, unless there is a medical reason.

7. Establish rooming-in: Allow mothers and babies to remain together, twenty-four hours a day. A major advantage of rooming-in is that, by being with her baby, the new mother can learn to recognize signals of hunger—like rooting (moving his head around in search of the breast), sucking on his fist, or making small sounds—before he starts to cry vigorously. He is likely to nurse better if he can be fed before he gets very hungry and frustrated.

8. Encourage breastfeeding "on cue"; that is, whenever the baby seems to want to nurse, as shown by rooting, sucking on his fist, or crying.

9. Give no pacifiers to newborn nursing babies.

10. Help to establish breastfeeding support groups and refer mothers to them when they leave the hospital.

professionals. If you have a choice of hospitals in your community, ask about their regulations and policies. Ask whether the hospital provides breast-feeding education for its nurses and residents. After the Children's Hospital of Philadelphia held education and training programs, one nurse said, "It used to be that breastfeeding was invisible in our hospital—you knew it occurred, but everyone ignored it."

This program and a similar one for residents at the University Health Systems of Eastern Carolina emphasized the benefits of breastfeeding and helped the health care professionals provide more help to mothers. The more often patients ask for family-centered services, the more hospitals will offer them.

The big plus of a hospital birth is that, should any complications occur, you will have an array of modern technology and professionals available immediately. If your pregnancy is considered high-risk, you'll certainly want to give birth in the hospital. According to a federal law enacted in 1998, neither your hospital nor your insurance company can demand that you leave the hospital earlier than 48 hours after a vaginal delivery and 96 hours after a cesarean birth. If, as usually happens, your vaginal birth proceeds smoothly and your baby is healthy—and if you have helpful resources at home—you may elect to go home within 8 to 24 hours.

Even if your hospital's policies are good ones, it is still a good idea to have a specific birth plan and a doula who can advocate for you and help you. If you have a choice about when to deliver your baby (as for an elective cesarean delivery), try not to schedule the birth on the day before or after a major holiday, when the hospital is likely to be short-staffed, the lactation consultant may not be on duty, and no "baby and me" classes are scheduled.

And even if your hospital does not have ideal family-centered policies, you can still have a good birth experience. Ask your doctor to leave written instructions for the staff: to help you nurse your baby within one hour of birth; to have your baby brought to you whenever she seems hungry, including the middle of the night (if you do not have rooming-in); not to give her any bottles of water or formula or pacifiers; and to follow any other procedures that will help launch a successful course of breastfeeding.

And you need to remember one very important thing: Even if your hospital stay does not go the way you'd like it to, remember that you'll be there for only a short time and that many women have overcome less than ideal hospital practices to go home and embark upon long and happy breastfeeding experiences. As one mother told us after reading an earlier edition of this book: "When I was crying in the hospital because I was getting such conflicting advice, I read what you said about trying to nurse in less than an ideal situation, and I felt so much better. I had almost gone to bottle-feeding, but I stayed with the breastfeeding, and once I got home everything worked out fine."

Maternity Center/Birthing Center: These freestanding centers offer a happy compromise between the comfort of home and the security of a well-equipped medical facility. They're usually staffed principally by nurse-midwives, with one or more physicians and nurse assistants. They are designed for low-risk, uncomplicated births, and offer prenatal care, birth in a homelike setting, and discharge the same day. Should complications arise, patients are transferred to a hospital. Before making your decision about a birthing center, ask about its staff and its provision of emergency backup services, including its contract with an ambulance service, agreement with a nearby reputable hospital, and on-premises emergency equipment.

Home Birth: Some women choose to have their babies at home. They prefer

Packing Your Bag

About six weeks before your due date, pack a small bag to take with you to the hospital or birth center. Among those items you may want to include:

❖ **A nursing bra.** Buy one or two in your eighth month of pregnancy. By then, your breasts will be the same size or close to the size that they'll be during breastfeeding. For suggestions on choosing a nursing bra, see Chapter 9. Some hospitals supply halter-type tops. Ask if yours does. Although your own bras are more attractive, the hospital launders its supplies but not your personal items. Which do you want: beauty or convenience?

❖ **A nursing nightgown.** This will have hidden side slits on the bodice. You'll feel more comfortable in a nightgown you choose than in a one-size-fits-all hospital gown. Or you may prefer a large T-shirt or a robe that opens in the front.

❖ **A few pairs of panties.** Whatever you wore while you were pregnant—bikini or maternity panties—will still fit, since it takes a while to regain the waistline you once knew. Some hospitals provide panties, which you might find more convenient; they all provide you with sanitary napkins.

❖ **Telephone numbers.** These should include your childbirth educator, your doctor or midwife, your pediatrician or family doctor (so you can call your doctor in the office, instead of trying to catch him or her in the hospital), your lactation consultant, and a local La Leche League leader, so you can reach them easily if you have questions. And, of course, the friends and family members you'll most want to talk to. You might want to program your lactation consultant's number into your phone for easier access.

❖ **This book,** and any others you like about pregnancy, childbirth, and breastfeeding. Questions will arise and it's good to have something to refer to.

to be in familiar surroundings, with family and friends and any older children, and to treat the birth as a normal family event. These births are often staffed by certified nurse-midwives or lay midwives (also known as direct-entry midwives), but are sometimes attended by physicians. If the pregnancy is low-risk and the birth uncomplicated, this usually works fine.

However, if you are considering a home birth, be sure that you have no reason to think that your baby's birth will be at all complicated. You should not have heart disease or diabetes, there should be no family history of genetic disorders, you should not be expecting a multiple birth, the fetus should not be in the breech position, and your pregnancy should have gone to full term.

Because it's often impossible to foresee a crisis during childbirth when all signs have been normal up to the time of delivery, it's vital to have backup plans in case of emergency so you and your baby can get to a hospital quickly. Your home should be no more than ten minutes away from the hospital, and previous arrangements should have been made with physician and hospital in case their services are needed. It's especially important to check the qualifications of your birth attendant if you're planning to have your baby at home.

Choosing When You'll Give Birth

Traditionally and historically, babies were the ones who "decided" when to be born. Today, though, some mothers and their doctors are scheduling deliveries, often cesarean, to coincide with a convenient time for either or both of them. Although in some cases there is an important medical reason to schedule an early delivery, in ambiguous or convenience-based cases, it's best to let the baby remain the decision-maker. Humans have a 40-week gestation period because human babies need all the womb time they can get. In recent years, we have seen an increase in near-term and late preterm babies (born at 34 to 38 weeks' gestation), who very often need extra care in the days after birth to keep them healthy, and who usually need extra attention to initiate and maintain breastfeeding. (See the discussion about nursing these babies in Chapter 16.) In most cases, then, we're best off trusting our bodies to do what they're designed to do. This is an important issue to discuss with your obstetrician.

Your Maternity Leave

Fairly early in your pregnancy, you'll want to think about your plans for returning to work (or not) after your baby is born. For suggestions about this important issue and for other employment concerns, see Chapter 12.

Prenatal Classes

Whoever your choice of practitioner and wherever you bring your baby into the world, both you and your partner will benefit from enrolling in a prenatal education course. After reviewing twenty-two studies of efforts to help women breastfeed, a federal panel found that a class was more effective than any other program—even classes that were only one hour long. If you're a single parent or if your husband or partner cannot or chooses not to attend, another supportive person (like a mother, sister, or friend) can go with you to learn how to coach you during labor and delivery. Ideally, you should begin attending classes during your second trimester, because if you wait for the last trimester, you might miss some of the most important sessions if your baby comes early.

Besides teaching techniques to help you during the birth, these classes help you plan your delivery, familiarize you with hospital procedures, and teach you how to get started with breastfeeding. Some hospitals also give courses to prepare children for the birth of a new sibling, to prepare grandparents for the birth of their grandchildren, and to educate couples expecting a second cesarean birth.

As a bonus, it's fun to attend classes with other expectant parents, and you may well meet someone with whom you'll develop a friendship that will continue many years after the births of your babies. To accommodate the needs of prospective parents who cannot schedule eight consecutive weekly classes, some childbirth educators have developed weekend cram classes. To find out what's available in your community, you can call the obstetric department of a local hospital or contact Lamaze International or the International Childbirth Education Association (see the Resource Appendix).

Preparing Your Breasts

You don't have to do anything to prepare your breasts for nursing. Mother Nature does it for you. Most women around the world do nothing at all to their breasts before their babies are born, yet they breastfeed with hardly any problems. Although a number of routines are often recommended in our country, some actually hinder successful nursing and most don't make much difference one way or the other.

One pregnancy manual from the 1940s advised women to throw open the windows every morning and stand topless before them, while giving themselves a good brisk nipple scrub with a nailbrush. Ouch! This and other, milder measures that have sometimes been recommended in the past are very harmful. They irritate the nipples and predispose them to cracking and pain. Among the biggest no-nos:

❧ Do not rub your nipples to toughen them.

❧ Do not apply alcohol, witch hazel, or tincture of benzoin to harden the nipples. These drying agents irritate the nipples and predispose them to cracking and pain.

❧ In fact, during the last two or three months of pregnancy and while you're nursing, you don't need soap on your nipples—and it's best to avoid using it on them. When you're soaping up in the bath or shower, just skip your nipples. The glands on and around them will be secreting substances to keep them clean, so there's no need for soap, which can dry them out.

✤ Do not engage in prenatal hand-expression of colostrum. At one time, this was thought to open the milk ducts and prevent engorgement, but there's no evidence that it makes any difference. Also, since no one yet knows whether there's a fixed amount of colostrum in the breasts or whether it replaces itself, there's a chance that you might waste this "liquid gold" through hand-expression.

✤ Do not massage your breasts. This has sometimes been recommended to bring the colostrum from the alveoli to the milk ducts, to stretch and prevent clogging of the milk ducts, to improve circulation and help prevent engorgement of the breasts after birth, and to help women get used to handling their breasts. However, there's no evidence that it's helpful, and it might stimulate uterine contractions, so don't do it.

Inverted Nipples

Inverted nipples constitute the one condition for which prenatal preparation may be of value. These are nipples that may look normal, but when pressure is applied near their bases or when they're cold or stimulated, they retract into the breast tissue instead of becoming erect and protruding.

To test for inverted nipples, hold your breast at the edge of the areola between your thumb and forefinger and press in firmly but gently about an inch behind the base of your nipple. If the nipple seems to disappear within the flesh of the breast, it is inverted.

Usually nipples like these protrude normally by the end of pregnancy, and in almost all cases they come out fully when the baby starts to nurse. Slightly inverted nipples do not affect breastfeeding. Occasionally, however, they remain severely inverted and pose a real problem to the baby, who cannot grasp the nipple with her mouth. If your nipples are inverted after your baby is born, you should seek help from a lactation consultant as soon as possible.

Although not all professionals agree with the wisdom of screening for inverted nipples or the effectiveness of the following measures to draw them out, many women feel they are helpful.

Exercise: The Hoffman technique was once recommended for use during pregnancy but is no longer suggested until after delivery. This exercise aims to break any adhesions at the base of the nipple that keep it inverted. Place the thumbs of both hands, opposing each other, at the base of the nipple (where it meets the areola) and gently but firmly pull the thumbs away from each other. Do this both up and down and sideways. You can do these exercises twice a day at first, and increase to five times a day during early lactation.

Breast Shells: Another common treatment for inverted nipples is the wearing

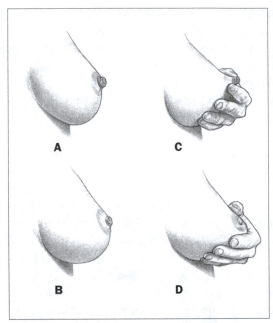

Breast A has a normally protruding nipple. Breast B is flat. To tell whether your breast is inverted, hold the edge of the areola between your thumb and forefinger. Press back firmly but gently, while at the same time pulling your fingers away from each other. This will make your nipple either protrude (C) or invert (D).

of special plastic breast shells during pregnancy. These shells, also known as shields or milk cups, exert a constant gentle and painless pressure that gradually draws out a flat or inverted nipple. You can find them through your childbirth or breastfeeding education organization, through a catalog, or online. They are different from the rubbery nipple shields that are sometimes advised for sore nipples (which should not be used at all).

Check with your lactation consultant about using these shells. They come in two parts, fit easily into a bra (preferably one a cup size larger than what you would ordinarily wear), and are easy to wash with soap and water. If you use them, start to wear them in the last trimester of your pregnancy, beginning with an hour a day and gradually increasing the length of time, according to your comfort. If the shells fill up with colostrum, empty them frequently and wash them every day, since warm moisture is an ideal setting for the growth of infection-causing microorganisms.

If your nipples are still inverted after your baby's birth, wear the shells for about half an hour before feedings, again being sure to empty them often. Do not feed any trapped milk to your baby.

You won't need to wear these shells forever—only until your nipples protrude enough for effective nursing. Your baby's suckling will help, and your nipples may protrude well enough in your baby's mouth even though they may still look flat and inverted when you're not nursing. Since your baby will become more expert at grasping the breast, you'll probably be able to do away with the shells after the early stages of nursing. Once breastfeeding is well established, you can start to wean yourself from the shells by going without them for a couple of hours before one of the midday feedings, not one for which your baby is apt to be frantically hungry. If the baby seems to have trouble nursing, go back to them for a while longer.

Breast Pump: If your nipples are still inverted after your baby's birth, it's sometimes helpful to use a breast pump to draw them out just before nursing your baby. Don't use it during pregnancy.

Who Will Mother You?

In many countries around the world, mothering the new mother is taken for granted. There are plenty of women nearby to help her recover from childbirth and care for her baby. In fact, anthropologists now theorize that in prehistoric days the only reason that families survived was the availability of older female relatives, who could help new mothers and take over their work while they were busy nursing their babies.

In the United States today, however, such help is often not available. A harried mother in Boston confided to us, "When I push my baby in his carriage, I keep wishing that I were the one being pushed and rocked and taken care of."

The key word for most Western women today is independence. You may live far away from the relatives and friends who would ordinarily help you. Or you may feel that you need to prove your adulthood, your womanhood, or your maternal competence by doing everything yourself. Or the most likely candidates—a mother, mother-in-law, or sister—may not be knowledgeable or supportive of breastfeeding. This puts a tremendous amount of pressure on you at a time when you need all the help you can get. So look out for yourself, and before your baby is born, look for the person or persons who will be your special helpers.

What Kind of Help Will You Need?

You'll need several kinds of helpers. First, although you'll be excited about your baby's arrival, you'll also be tired. The biggest surprise for many new mothers, no matter how they feed their babies, is the constant fatigue they feel for the first few weeks. Aside from your body's reaction to the delivery itself (it's called "labor" for a reason!), the lack of a full night's sleep, night after night, makes you long for someone who can help you with household chores, at least for the first week or two. Meanwhile, you'll have dozens of questions, including: Why is the baby fussing? How can I organize the diaper-changing area? Is my baby getting enough nourishment?

Here are some options for people who may be able to help you:

❖ If your partner can take time off from work for the first week or two after your baby's birth, or if your mother or mother-in-law can stay with you (and if you get along well), either of these might be a lifesaver.

❖ A doula who can care for you and the baby, and perform some household chores. (To find one, see the Resource Appendix.)

❖ A high school or college student or an older person who can come in for a few hours every afternoon, straighten up the house, take your older children out, and cook and clean up after dinner.

❖ A neighbor who can come in for just an hour or so every afternoon to run the washing machine or put away the clean laundry, hang up clothes, take out the garbage, and wash whatever dishes are piled up in the sink.

❖ Another helpful—and inexpensive—option is to hire a youngster (age 9 to 14) to be a "limited-responsibility" sitter. You wouldn't leave a baby or even an older child alone in the house with a sitter this young, but children this age often love babies and small children and would almost pay you to let them stay with your youngsters.

Such a sitter can play an important role. She or he can, for example, play with an older child while you're busy with your baby. During the "witching hour," that hour or two before dinner or bedtime when babies are often fussy, she can hold your baby while you're fixing dinner or reading to your older children.

As one mother who took this route said, "The young neighbor I hired to be a 'big sister' to my three-year-old was more mature and useful as a sitter when she was nine than she turned out

to be when she hit her teen years!"

❖ A friend or family member who can help out and for whom you can reciprocate in the future.

❖ People, including partners, sometimes ask "What can I do?" They genuinely want to help but may not know just what you want or need. You're more likely to get the help you want if you can be as specific as possible with requests like: "Please fold the laundry," "Take the baby's brother out for two hours," or "Take this list and go to the store."

❖ Keeping a running list on your refrigerator with tasks that need to be done will help your helpers help you better.

Finding Help and Support

Becoming a mother often fosters new connections between you and your own mother or your mother-in-law. It's good to develop a close relationship with your baby's grandparents—good for your children, for you, and, of course, for the older generation.

You will understand them as you never could before you had children of your own! But if neither of your baby's grandmothers is supportive or knowledgeable about breastfeeding, if they live far away, or if for some other reason they would not be your best helpers, you can reach out to develop a larger support network.

To Grandmas: How You Can Help

Of course, you're excited about your new grandbaby. And you want to help as much as you can. Even though you can't feed the baby or expect her to miss a feeding by staying at your home without her mom, there is so much you can do that will earn the gratitude of the proud—but tired and stressed—new parents. Ask them what they would like you to do to help. If they don't come up with specifics, here are some great ideas.

If you can spend time at the baby's house:

❧ Protect the mother's privacy by answering the door and telephone and keeping visitors at bay until Mom is ready for them.

❧ Spend special Grandma time with any older children, who are likely to feel left out of the new-baby excitement.

❧ Offer to drive or accompany baby and mother to the doctor's office and anywhere else she wants to go.

❧ Cook some meals, do some dishes, or straighten up some corners.

❧ Learn as much as you can about contemporary breastfeeding—maybe by attending a La Leche League meeting with mother and baby.

❧ Bite your tongue when you disagree with such parenting issues as bed-sharing, feeding on demand, and the like. You had your turn bringing up babies; now your job is to support, not to question.

❧ If you breastfed your child(ren), tactfully offer suggestions, but back off if they're not wanted.

For Grandmas near and far:

❧ Coordinate with the other grandparents so you won't be visiting at the same time.

❧ Consider giving the family a few months' worth of housekeeping service. Or ask them what they would like that would make life easier.

Over the next few months, part of your mothering experience will include "talking shop" with other new mothers, expanding many of your relationships in new baby-oriented ways, and developing new ties. Possibly the most important step you can take to make the course of breastfeeding go more smoothly is to build your breastfeeding support network. There are scores of websites and blogs where you can go for answers to questions, help with problems, and supportive understanding. (Some of these sites are listed in the back of this book.)

You might find a great source of support in your husband or life partner, your sister, your parents, a friend or neighbor, your midwife, your doctor, a lactation consultant, a member of a breastfeeding support group like La Leche League International, your childbirth educator, a professional doula, and/or someone you hire to help out with food shopping, other errands, and household chores.

A great deal of help and emotional support can come from another new mother or a more experienced mother, whom you may meet at your doctor's office, at the hospital, in a prenatal class or workshop for new parents (given in many communities by hospitals, family service agencies, or other social welfare organizations), or in a babysitting co-op. Some pediatric practices (like the one coauthor Dr. Laura Marks belongs to) hold regular meetings for new moms where they can bring their questions and get answers from a lactation consultant or a physician. If you're planning to go back to work, try to find another working mother. Raise your questions about breastfeeding and parenthood with the people who might be able to help you. Find out which ones you'll be able to count on for support and how much each is able and willing to give. You'll also find out the ones to stay away from—anyone who's negative and discouraging about breastfeeding. Some friends and relatives may want to be helpful but may know so little that they're too ready to urge you to switch to formula. So acknowledge their good intentions, but don't take their bad advice! Take advantage of their interest in helping by asking them to bring you lunches or

dinners, so they'll focus on feeding you instead of telling you how to feed your baby.

You'll need the most help in the first few weeks after your baby is born, the time period that's most crucial for the success of breastfeeding. Many early problems can be resolved with the right kind of help. If you can't find anyone to count on, you can be your own doula with the help of books to give you basic information and your telephone and computer to contact resources. Whatever your situation, when questions come up, don't stew over them privately. Seek help. And seek it right away. The sooner you ask the questions, the sooner you'll be able to come up with answers.

Your Older Children

If you have other children, you may wonder about their reactions to your nursing their baby brother or sister. You may be afraid that feeding your new baby in such an intimate way will make your other children especially jealous. Actually, your older children, especially the child closest in age to the new baby, are likely to have ambivalent feelings toward the baby—loving the baby and feeling jealous of him—no matter how you feed him. This is normal.

If you breastfed your older children, you can tell them that you fed them this way when they were babies and that now it's the new baby's turn. If you did not breastfeed them, there's no need to volunteer this information, but neither do you want to be dishonest by implying that you did. If they ask whether you nursed them as babies, explain that when they were little you didn't know how good breastfeeding was for the baby and the mother. Now that you know that this is the healthiest way to feed a baby, you want to be as good a mother as you can to the new baby, just as you want to be a good mother to all your children. Most youngsters accept a simple explanation like this and are happy to hear that even adults keep learning new things.

You can expect your older children to be on your lap or by your side as your baby nurses. (We're not talking here about toddlers whom you nursed throughout a subsequent pregnancy and are still tandem nursing—which we'll say more about in Chapter 16—but about those who were never nursed or were weaned some time back.) Embrace this as an opportunity to nurture the older children, who need your attention more than ever, and make feeding times family times.

When you breastfeed, you have a free arm to draw your toddler close to you or to turn the pages of her favorite book. While the infant has your breast, your older child has your attention in another way. Show your other children in many ways that the new baby has not displaced them in your affection, but don't let them feel that you'll discontinue nursing just because they express unhappiness about it.

One way to keep your older child busy while you're nursing your baby is to set aside special toys or books that can be played with only while you're nursing, or to turn on a special DVD or CD as a nursing-time-only treat.

Occasionally, toddlers ask whether they can nurse, too. If you let your child try, she'll probably laugh and forget about it or may even put her mouth to your breast and then not know what to do about it. The suckling movements that come so naturally to a newborn seem to be easily forgotten. Many babies forget how to do it as soon as a month after they have been weaned. If your toddler is different, though, and does want to go back to nursing, you can point out to her that this is something that only little babies do—and you can follow this by giving her a treat that is only for "big kids." Or you can tandem nurse both children.

Your older children can probably offer more help to you than you realize. Take advantage of their interest in being eager baby-amusers, willing fetch-and-carriers, and pleasant companions to you as they help you fold the laundry, set the table, or push the baby carriage. Some of the happiest family times occur in such everyday activities. At the same time, you don't want to put your older children in the position of being the baby's caretaker or give them too much responsibility so they end up resenting the baby.

As a breastfeeding mother, you have a lovely opportunity to provide some elementary sex education in an easy, natural way. The child who sees his little brother or sister at the breast learns some of the biological differences between men and women and gains a sense of the function and beauty of the human body. Your young daughter may be especially inspired by the thought that she will be able to care for her babies in this special way when she grows up. Your little boy may think he'll be able to do it, too—but will probably accept your explanation that he'll have other ways to love his babies.

Now you're ready to meet someone you will love forever. And you're about to embark upon one of the most exciting—and challenging—adventures of your entire life. It will be full of everything: questions, worries, and anxieties, yes—but also thrills and joy, and gratification like nothing else. Sound like a roller coaster? Hold on—and enjoy the ride!

CHAPTER FIVE

Your Baby Is Here

"I will never forget when my newborn latched on to my breast for the first time on the delivery table. I knew right then and there that breastfeeding was going to go okay. Even though I wasn't quite sure what to do, my baby certainly did! We stared into each other's eyes and a bond was forged."

BETTY Hemet, California

Finally, you set eyes upon that squalling, squirming bit of humanity whose arrival you have so eagerly awaited all these months. You marvel at the wonder of tiny fingers and toes. You are amazed to realize that this small person actually grew in your body. You draw the little body close to you, to cuddle and love.

And then, if you are a first-time mother, the questions rush through your mind. How will you be able to care for such a dependent little creature? How will you know what to do? And when and how to do it? It may buoy up your confidence to stop for a minute and consider that women have been having first babies since the beginning of humankind and have somehow coped well enough so that each succeeding generation has survived to bear its own progeny.

Like every other new mother, you have questions about every aspect of child care—how to diaper, burp, bathe, and dress your infant. Or you may already have other children but are now breastfeeding for the first time, or wanting to refresh yourself on the many aspects of feeding your baby. In this chapter, we talk about the first few days after birth, when you and your baby take your initial steps toward bonding as a nursing duo.

Surprising as this may seem, human beings are not born knowing how to breastfeed; both mother and baby need to learn how to do it. Actually, other animals do, too—like that gibbon mom whose story we told in Chapter 2. If you know what to expect and what to do, you'll be better prepared for these first few weeks. You can make the beginning of breastfeeding easier if you arm yourself with information and seek any needed help early. You'll need the most help in the first few weeks after your baby is born, the time period that's most crucial for the success of breastfeeding. Getting help early is vital, since many problems that women encounter in the early weeks can be resolved in a short time with the right kind of help.

Meanwhile, you may need to be patient to give the two of you time to develop your relationship. You may have a love-at-first-sight relationship, with nothing but good experiences right from the start. Or you may have a longer courtship, taking a few weeks to establish a smooth and mutually satisfying bond. Not all new mothers bond with their babies immediately—but happily, almost all do within a short time.

The Ideal Beginning

In the best of all possible worlds, every baby would be born healthy, after the full gestation period. Every mother would have an easy, fast, unmedicated delivery. Both mother and baby would be alert and feeling good. Right after birth, the mother would put her baby to the breast. The baby would latch on and nurse eagerly. Mother and baby would then spend their time together in the same room, where the mother would rest, nursing her baby every time he wanted to feed. She would have supportive health care professionals to go to with her questions, as well as helpful friends and relatives.

In the real world, this scenario sometimes unfolds exactly as it's written here. Too often, however, one or more of the elements just described are not present. Some babies are born prematurely; some mothers have long, difficult deliveries or cesarean

Breastfeeding i Hospital or Bir

ng

The emergence of modern hospitals as places for babies to be born coincided with the popularity of feeding babies with artificial milk. So it's not surprising that many hospital routines were developed to fit the patterns of formula-fed babies—and the convenience of hospital staff. Some of these routines have included separating mother and baby, feeding infants on strict four-hour schedules, and limiting the length of feeding sessions.

As we pointed out in the previous chapter, in recent years many hospital administrators have recognized that breastfed babies thrive best according to very different practices. An unexpected bonus is that many of the changes fought for by nursing mothers have improved the physical and emotional health of formula-fed babies, too.

The box on page 91 lists the most recent research-based recommendations from the American Academy of Pediatrics for providing ideal nutrition to babies through a happy breastfeeding experience. Although the academy recommends that, ideally, breastfeeding continue through a baby's first year, if for any reason you cannot nurse for this long, be assured that for whatever length of time you do breastfeed, you will be giving your baby the best start in life. Remember, some breastfeeding is better than no breastfeeding. Also although the academy recommend

mother and have a healthy baby. We'll talk specifically about postcesarean breastfeeding later in this chapter, and we'll talk about nursing premature babies in Chapter 16.

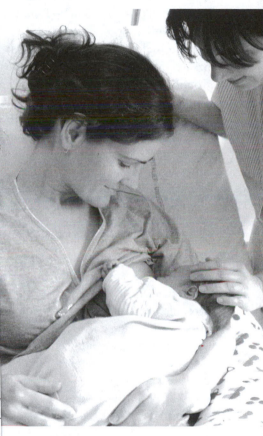

Mom and baby can get help from a nurse, a lactation consultant, or an experienced nursing mom.

up from her belly, where he was placed immediately after birth (often even before the placenta has been expelled), and reach the breast, to which he attaches himself with no help at all.

Many other babies need help in finding the breast. You can help your baby latch on (see the section "Latching On" in Chapter 6), and if you need help, the attending nurse should be able to assist you.

You'll both be more comfortable if a blanket is put over your baby's body so his back will be warm and his front will get warmth from your bare skin.

The only times that immediate breastfeeding might not be a good idea would be in such rare circumstances as these: if the mother is ill or very drowsy from heavy medication or if the baby is very premature, tiny, ill, or fragile for some other reason. If you cannot nurse right away, either because of hospital regulations, your condition, or your baby's, don't worry. Immediate is best, but most women who have not been able to nurse right away have gone on to have satisfying, gratifying breastfeeding experiences.

Immediate breastfeeding is one of those issues that you may have discussed with your doctor and hospital staff before you gave birth, letting everyone involved know that you wanted to do this. If not, as soon as you go into the hospital or birthing center, ask your doctor to leave orders accordingly.

Why You'll Want to Breastfeed Right Away

Recent research has confirmed the value of doing what most mothers intuitively want to do—nurse their babies as soon as they're born. Even though the mature milk has not yet come into your breasts, they have, from the last weeks of pregnancy, had a rich supply of colostrum, that fluid that provides such a good start to an infant's life (see Chapter 3).

Also, while your baby is getting the benefits of colostrum, she is also helping to "prime the pump," to establish her future food supply. Your milk will become more plentiful if you begin to nurse early and then nurse often. Women who do this and women who have given birth previously often get their transitional milk on the second day after birth, while those who begin to nurse later and keep to rigid schedules don't get theirs till the third day, or later. The best way to produce an abundance of milk is to allow a hungry infant to suck vigorously and frequently soon after birth. The more she sucks, the more milk you will produce.

Babies fed within one hour of birth pass their first stool earlier, expel meconium earlier, and have lower levels of bilirubin. This waste product is formed by the breaking down of red blood cells; high levels of bilirubin in the blood cause jaundice (most often a harmless condition, which we'll talk about in Chapter 6). This early nursing when there is just a small amount of colostrum helps a newborn, with her tiny stomach, to learn the technique before having to deal with a large volume of milk.

Early nursing helps you, too. Since stimulation of the breasts causes the uterus to contract, your baby's imme-

A Gift That You Don't Want

Many hospitals present every new mother—even those who are breastfeeding—with a free six-pack of formula, or coupons for free formula, when she leaves the hospital with her baby. This is usually the result of formula manufacturers' aggressive promotion practices. Hospitals that have discontinued this practice find that breastfeeding rates rise accordingly. In fact, the guidelines for the Baby-Friendly Hospital Initiative (described in Chapter 4) and the regulations from some state departments of health specifically mandate that formula should be given out *only* upon special request by a doctor or mother.

If your hospital offers you free formula, tell them you don't want it. Show your confidence in your body's ability to produce the milk that your baby needs. If you do decide to use formula for an occasional supplemental bottle later on, it's better to buy it then, after your own milk is established, than to have it sitting on your pantry shelf during these vulnerable first days at home when you might encounter a problem and be tempted to feed formula to your baby, thus making breastfeeding more difficult.

diate suckling can speed delivery of the placenta. The contractions of the uterus also shut off the maternal blood vessels that fed your baby in the womb and, thus, help to discourage excessive bleeding. They also serve as the first steps to your regaining your prepregnancy figure.

No Bottles, No Pacifiers

Your healthy newborn should not be receiving any bottles or pacifiers. In the past, some hospitals have insisted on giving newborns bottles of water to make sure they could swallow correctly. However, this is not necessary, and breastfed babies do not need water since they get enough fluid in Mom's milk. Furthermore, the bottle itself may sabotage breastfeeding. While some infants are adaptable enough to go back and forth between bottle and breast with hardly a break in rhythm, about one baby in four becomes temporarily confused when made to alternate between nursing and sucking on a rubber nipple or pacifier. And you don't know ahead of time which category your baby will fall into.

As we pointed out in Chapters 1 and 3, the two forms of feeding require different mouth and tongue movements. Furthermore, since milk flows more rapidly from the rubber nipple, babies fed bottles too early in their lives sometimes get used to this and are less willing to expend the effort required for nursing. Although this nipple confusion (or "suck confusion") is probably temporary, it can lead to sucking problems, so it's best to avoid giving your baby a bottle or pacifier until breastfeeding is well established, which may take six to eight weeks. This, of course, is the ideal scenario. However, if you have to supplement your baby's diet with formula for medical reasons or you have to feed him your pumped breast milk, you may need to use bottles before this time. (If you plan to give your baby bottles before one year of age, it's best to introduce them by three months. Many breastfed babies refuse to take a bottle if it's presented for the first time later than this.) For suggestions for introducing bottles, see Chapters 6 and 12.

Cesarean Birth

"I was so disappointed to need a cesarean delivery," one mother told us. "I'd been looking forward to the experience of childbirth and learned only at the last minute that I wasn't going to have it the way I'd expected to. I felt my body had let me down—it had failed to do its job. So I found breastfeeding very healing and reassuring. It was proof that my body could function properly, after all."

If your baby was born by cesarean delivery (also called C-section), your breastfeeding experience can be just as happy and complete as if you had delivered vaginally. Your breasts probably filled up just as soon, and you may be able to nurse right after delivery. But if you need to rest and recover from the surgery for a few hours or even a day, this will not interfere with the course of nursing. Keep in mind that the sooner you begin, the better you're likely to feel, and so the faster you'll recover from your surgery.

Be sure to tell your own doctor ahead of time, as well as the hospital anesthesiologist, that you plan to

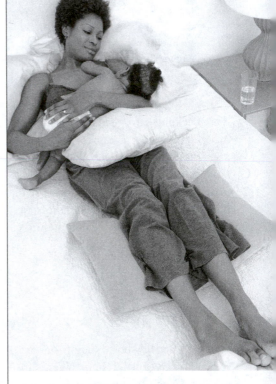

A mom who had a cesarean delivery appreciates lots of pillows to support her back, knees, and feet and to bring her baby up to breast level. If your hospital cannot supply enough, ask someone to bring them from home. Be sure to keep the baby's face away from pillows.

breastfeed your baby, and that you want medication and treatment compatible with your baby's well-being, as well as your own. After the surgery, it's okay to get relief from pain through medication that may be administered by injection or pills and that is compatible with breastfeeding (see the discussion of childbirth anesthesia and pain medication in Chapter 10). Normally, very little of this medication comes through your milk. And even if it does affect your baby temporarily, the American Academy of Pediatrics has stated that the benefits of breastfeeding outweigh the possible mild lethargy your baby might experience after you have received pain medication. You don't have to suffer to breastfeed!

You'll probably stay in the hospital a couple of days longer than women who deliver vaginally. And you'll need more rest, both in the hospital and at home. Because of your abdominal incision, you'll want to make special efforts to find comfortable positions for breastfeeding. Ask the hospital nurses for help, and experiment with different positions until you find the one that you like best. You'll need to position your baby so she isn't lying across or kicking the site of your incision. The most popular postcesarean nursing positions are (1) sitting up, with pillows on your lap to bring your baby up to breast level, (2) the clutch position, and (3) lying down. (See the section on positioning in Chapter 6.)

Mother-Baby Contact

All other things being equal, mothers and babies usually bond best when they're close to each other. This is easy to achieve at a birthing center or at home, and in those hospitals that have rooming-in. This policy lets you keep your baby in your own room rather than in the newborn nursery, either around the clock or during daytime hours only. It's comforting for both mother and baby, and it provides an opportunity for both you and your partner to get to know your baby and learn his natural eating and sleeping rhythms.

Being together makes the beginning of breastfeeding that much easier, since you can nurse your baby when he's awake and hungry without having to depend on his being brought to you on a set schedule or when it's convenient for the nurse in the newborn nursery. Also, you can feed him when he shows the first signs of wanting to nurse (see Chapter 6 for these cues)—before he becomes so hungry that he gets frustrated and has trouble latching on. Only through living with your baby can you adjust your milk supply to his needs.

All other things are not always equal, of course. If your baby needs special care, he may have to be in another room. If you're exhausted from a hard labor and delivery, you may not yet feel up to having your baby with you all day long. If you and your baby are in for a longer than typical hospital

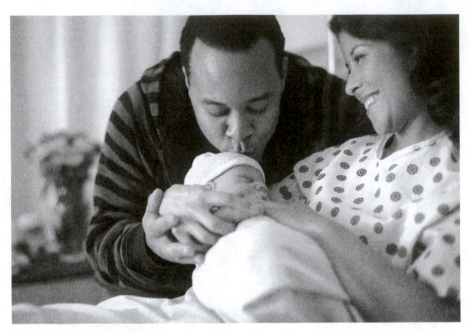

With rooming-in, mom and baby—and dad, too—can get acquainted sooner, and mom can learn baby's cues that signal readiness to nurse.

stay and are not roommates for the first few days of his life, ask to have him brought to you as soon and as often as possible. You will, of course, be "rooming in" as soon as you get home. Human beings are remarkably resilient, and babies can overcome much more traumatic early experiences than brief separations from their mothers to grow up to be healthy and well adjusted.

Hospital Help

If your doctor, midwife, and nurses are knowledgeable and supportive of breastfeeding, don't hesitate to take your questions to them. They have probably heard most of them before and will be able to advise and reassure you. Often you can call on them with questions after you go home with your baby. If not, refer to "Who Will Mother You?" in Chapter 4.

While you and your baby are in the hospital, a lactation expert should come by twice a day to assess your baby's position while nursing, his latch-on, and the frequency of feedings. He should be weighed once a day. Then, when your baby is three to five days old, or 48 to 72 hours after hospital discharge, you should visit his doctor for a follow-up evaluation that includes weighing the baby. If he has lost 7 percent of his birth weight or more, breastfeeding should be evaluated again, and any needed corrections should be put in place.

You can do a great deal to help yourself in the hospital. Most important, you need to be both informed and assertive. You are only one patient among many. Busy hospital personnel, who have other concerns on their minds, may not be as closely attuned to your wishes as you would like. Don't be shy about asking or reminding them about aspects of care that are important for you and your baby. If you're polite and pleasant, no one is likely to take offense. Some of the points you may want to bring up are listed in the box on page 100.

Hospital Hindrance

Suppose you meet with resistance in every quarter. Or you're in an unsupportive hospital with outdated regulations (such as four-hour feeding schedules and giving bottles of water to nursing babies). If you have a full-term, healthy baby and someone to help you at home, it may be possible—and advisable—for you to leave the hospital within 24 hours of giving birth. You will then want to take your nursing baby to the pediatrician for a "look-see" the day after you go home, as well as breastfeeding support. If you go home after two days, you will want to see the doctor three to five days after birth.

Another problem with staying in the hospital is the typically high rate of interruptions. As La Leche League leader Melissa Clark Vickers, IBCLC, has written, "Imagine you have a new job that requires some serious on-the-job training. You need to really focus on what you are doing so you can learn the basics efficiently. Now imagine on your first day that every few minutes someone opens your office door and enters. Some of the visits are short, some are long; some visitors are welcome, some are intrusive. Is it any wonder that you might find it challenging to learn much of anything with all those interruptions?"

One study of new mothers during their first day after childbirth in a large Midwestern university hospital found that from 8:00 A.M. until 8:00 P.M. the average mother-baby pair had an average of fifty-four interruptions. Very often the minute the mother would put her baby to the breast someone would come into the room or the telephone would ring and the baby would be taken off the breast.

Interrupters on the hospital staff included the mother's primary nurse, dietitians, physicians, midwives, janitors, and various others. Then there were the grandparents and family friends. Obviously, some of these interruptions are necessary, but what can a new mom do to assure her baby and herself of a more peaceful learning environment? With a little preparation

Speak Up in the Hospital

❖ Ask your doctor to leave written orders for hospital personnel at the time of your baby's delivery, specifying that your baby is not to receive any pacifiers or bottles of formula or water. (You may want to put a sign on your baby's bassinet that says NO, THANK YOU—NO PACIFIERS, NO BOTTLES.)

❖ If you have not already made arrangements to have your baby room in with you, ask for this when you enter the hospital. Ideally, you will either have a private room or be able to room with another breastfeeding mother. In any case, you may be able to have rooming-in in a private or semiprivate room with one or more other mothers and their babies, even if the other babies are formula-fed. (See page 76, "The Ten Steps to Successful Breastfeeding in a Baby-Friendly Hospital," for the advantages of rooming-in.)

❖ If your baby cannot be in your room, ask your doctor to leave orders for her to be brought to you whenever she cries or seems hungry, at least every three hours, around the clock.

❖ Communicate your wishes personally to the nursery staff when you first go into the hospital. Remind your baby's doctor and any nurses who come to you that you are breastfeeding.

❖ Remind your doctor and nurses that you want to feed your baby during the night, as well as during the day. Your breasts need the stimulation, and your baby needs your milk. If you are modest about breastfeeding in front of your roommate or visitors, pull the curtain around your bed. Don't be afraid to ask for assistance.

❖ If you need help positioning your baby at the breast, or are having any other kind of trouble getting started with breastfeeding, ask the nurse or hospital lactation specialist to help you.

❖ If your baby is not rooming-in with you and your breasts are filling up uncomfortably between feedings (which is not likely to happen during the first couple of days after birth), ask a nurse to bring your baby to you so you can breastfeed. If you and your baby cannot be together, the nurse should be able to help you hand-express or pump some of your milk. Ask for an electric breast pump. (For information about pumping, see Chapter 11.)

❖ If the hospital nurse asks you to wash your nipples with sterile water before each feeding, you can go ahead and do it. It's not necessary, but it doesn't have any ill effects. But if you're told to wash with a drying agent (like soap), do not do it just to be a "good" patient. You can always say your doctor told you not to.

❖ If you're uncomfortable for any reason at all, tell your doctor, nurse, or lactation consultant.

❖ If you have any questions at all, ask them.

and thought you may be able to stem the flood.

✤ Ask your friends and family to wait a few days before visiting to let you get some rest. Of course, the grandparents and siblings have to have one visit—and then even they can wait until you and your baby are at home.

✤ Ask the baby's father or some other support person (maybe the grandmother) to run interference—to answer the phone and eliminate as many interruptions as possible.

✤ Ask your nurses to perform several tasks at one time, whenever they can, to avoid making multiple visits to the room.

Even if you have to stay the full time in the hospital (usually only one or two days for a vaginal delivery, four days for a cesarean) in a less-than-ideal setting, take heart. You'll be home in only a short time. Many other women have borne babies in much more

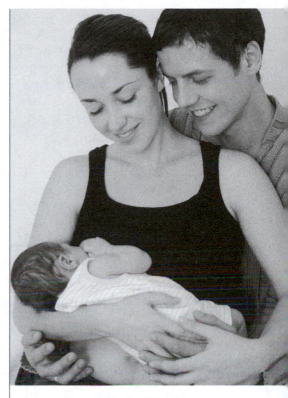

A couple becomes a nursing family.

restrictive circumstances and have gone on to nurse them long and happily. You can, too.

Newborn Health Measures

Immediately after birth your baby should receive a shot of vitamin K, which is essential for improving her immature blood-clotting ability and for preventing a rare bleeding disease of the newborn. While the intestines will produce vitamin K within a few days of birth, infants are born without this necessary vitamin, which is present at insufficiently low levels in breast milk. Thus all babies need to have vitamin K administered, and most receive it as a matter of routine. If your baby is born in a hospital or birthing center, both vitamin K (to prevent bleeding) and eye drops (to prevent infection) will be administered as preventive health measures. If she is born at home, your birth attendant should take care of these important procedures.

All 50 U.S. state health departments mandate that your baby must be tested 24 to 72 hours after birth for a few rare birth disorders that can now be easily identified and treated. One important test is performed to screen for PKU (phenylketonuria), a disease caused by an enzyme deficiency. If untreated, PKU can have serious effects, but if caught early it can be treated by a special diet. These screening tests are performed on a tiny sample of blood obtained from your baby's heel. (A recent study found that if a mother holds her diaper-clad baby between her breasts, maintaining skin-to-skin contact before and during the procedure, the baby will feel less pain afterward.)

Your doctor may also order a hearing test. And she or he will undoubtedly prescribe drops of a multivitamin solution that contains vitamin D for the baby. (For more about vitamin recommendations, see Chapter 17.)

If your baby is born in a hospital, you'll be informed about the testing procedures. If for any reason they are not performed during your hospital stay, you should take her back to the hospital for them as soon as possible, and definitely within the first week of life. If you leave the hospital within 24 hours of your baby's birth, talk to your doctor to make arrangements for any testing that was not done earlier. The doctor may be able to perform these simple procedures in his or her office. If you give birth in a nonhospital setting, call your local department of health to find out how to have the screenings performed.

Your Baby's First Doctor's Appointment

Of course, your baby will be examined immediately after birth as the first in a long series of well-baby visits to be sure that he is developing normally. The next medical assessment should take place during the first 24 to 48 hours after delivery, when a doctor or other lactation expert should evaluate how your baby is doing at latching on and suckling. A follow-up visit should then take place at three to five days of age, or within 48 to 72 hours after discharge from the hospital. This visit should take place sooner if you have not established effective breastfeeding.

Now you will go on to nurture your baby in the best way possible—at your breast. What you as a mother have looked forward to for so long has really begun. We talk about the first days of breastfeeding at home, the beginning of the unique relationship between a nursing mother and her infant, in Chapter 6.

CHAPTER SIX

Breastfeeding Begins

*"When Benjamin was born, I wanted to do
everything I could to nurture and protect him. Breastfeeding
became a special quiet time for me to be with my baby—
to gaze at his adorable eyes, cheeks, nose, and fingers, and feel
the ultimate pride and delight of being a mommy."*

RACHEL   New Hyde Park, New York

T his is the moment you have been anticipating so eagerly—the beginning of nursing. It's exciting and wonderful—and probably a little scary, too. It may comfort you to remember that your normal full-term infant was born with enough reserves to keep him healthy even if he goes without eating much for the first day or two. In fact, most babies lose weight after birth, often up to 7 percent of their birth weight. They typically start to gain weight within four or five days, and by two weeks are back to their birth weight.

Aside from the healthy colostrum your newborn receives, the first few feeding sessions are more for education—yours and his—than for nourishment. This is why these early nursings are sometimes called practice feeds. During the first couple of days, while your milk supply is becoming established, you learn how to nurse and your baby learns how to suckle.

Of course, it's easier for both parties if your baby is an eager pupil. But if not—if he keeps yawning or snoozing or can't get the nipple in his mouth or keeps letting go of it—ask a lactation specialist to observe your feeding sessions and help your baby nurse. The sooner you get help, the better off you and your baby will be.

Bringing Your Baby to the Breast: Positive Positioning

Whether you get to cuddle your baby right after birth or not until later, she may not at first show a great interest in nursing. Many babies do not nurse well at all for their first few days. They have to learn what it's all about. One study of 600 newborns found that 40 percent of them had to be actively helped to suck. Some infants start out by licking their mothers' nipples, which is a fine get-acquainted maneuver and also serves the practical function of making the nipples erect. Eventually, with the help you give your baby, her inborn reflexes assert themselves and she begins to nurse.

If your baby is sleepy the first time or two, offer your breast and try to rouse her by using the techniques listed in the box on page 116. If none of these techniques work at first, don't worry about it. Even if she sleeps through her first meal or two, she'll wake up when she's ready.

Most new mothers feel awkward the first few times they put their babies to the breast. No matter how much you've read or how many other nursing babies you've seen, it's very different when you're actually doing it. So be patient at the beginning, and be reassured that before long you and your baby will both be experts. And like riding a bicycle, once you learn, it's easy—and you never forget.

It's sometimes hard to find the best position. At first, your hand or her arm may feel like it's in the way; then when you zig, she zags; but before long it will feel as if you're fitting together like two pieces in a jigsaw puzzle.

There is no single best position for everyone. You'll probably find several that are comfortable and efficient. As you experiment, you'll develop your own favorites, and when you find two or three that work for you, alternate them. This will serve to stimulate different milk ducts and thus prevent the ducts from getting clogged. It will also help to prevent sore nipples by spreading out the pressure on different parts of your breast. (If your nipples do become sore, see Chapter 15 for treatment suggestions.)

In Chapter 16, we discuss various situations related to either mother or baby that present special challenges to breastfeeding. However, since one particular issue—the overweight mom—is especially relevant to positioning the nursing baby, it's pertinent to talk about it here.

If you're very overweight, you may have difficulty getting started breastfeeding, for several reasons. You may not have enough of a lap to rest your baby on; if your breasts are large, it may be hard for your baby to get into a good position and to latch on; you may not be able to see how she is nursing; and you may have trouble finding a comfortable position yourself. Also, because you are likely to have a lower prolactin response to your baby's suckling, you may experience delays in the onset of copious milk secretion. The good news, however, is that you can breastfeed successfully if you get assistance from a lactation consultant as soon as possible after your baby's birth. For helpful suggestions, see the Resource Appendix.

Here are some good positions for nursing, whether you're sitting up or lying down.

SITTING UP: Sit up in bed, or on a comfortable chair or couch, with your back and head supported by one or more big pillows and your arms supported by an armrest or pillow. Put your

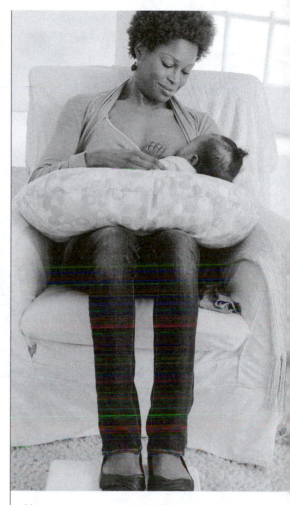

Nursing in a sitting position is most comfortable when mom's arm is supported by an armrest and her feet rest on a stool or other footrest. During the nursing session, baby's tummy should face mom's body.

baby on a pillow on your lap, with your arms resting on the pillow. This will make it easier to bring his mouth to nipple level, so you won't have to strain your arm, shoulder, neck, or back muscles. Some mothers swear by pillows made specifically for breastfeeding.

One popular model, shaped like a sideways letter U, fits comfortably around the mother's waist and has built-in armrests.

Raise one or both knees to bring your baby closer to your body. If you are in a chair, rest your foot on a chair rung, a footstool, or a large book like an unabridged dictionary (in these busy postpartum days, that's probably all you'll find time to use the dictionary for).

If your breasts are large, you may be more comfortable if you rest the nursing breast on a rolled-up washcloth or cloth diaper. This will lift the breast to let your baby latch on more easily, and will take the strain off your hands and arms.

Sitting Up Position One—The Cross-cradle, Cross-over, Transitional Hold: This is a good position for newborns, since it lets you see what's going on at the breast, and makes it easy to move the baby to your breast. When the baby gets bigger, it's harder to use this hold effectively, so you may want to switch to the cradle hold (see the next section).

In the cross-cradle position, the arm on the side opposite the breast your baby is nursing from goes under his back, and his neck rests on that hand. His abdomen is against the center of your midriff or below your other breast (depending on his length), facing you. His face, chest, and knees also face you. Hold his knees against you sideways; don't let them dangle. When nursing from your right breast, use your left hand to support the base of your baby's head, shoulders, and neck. Use your right hand to support

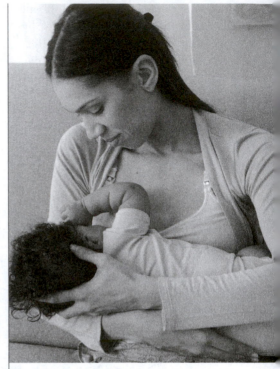

This mom is using the cross-cradle, cross-over, or transitional hold, which is especially good for newborns. Mom's arm opposite the nursing breast goes under baby's back, and her neck rests on mom's hand.

your right breast if necessary. Switch arms when you switch breasts.

Sitting Up Position Two—The Cradle Hold: While you are sitting, hold your baby close to your body so that she does not have to turn her head to reach your nipple. She should be horizontal, not diagonal. Her face, abdomen, and knees should all be facing your body. If her head is turned to the side, she will not be able to swallow.

Your baby's pelvis will be up against your abdomen; her lower arm should be under your arm and around your

What Makes a Good Position for Breastfeeding?

You'll know a position is good because:

❖ You're supported in such a way that you are comfortable and can hold the position for some time without feeling cramped or stiff.

❖ You're not hunched over, trying to bring the breast to your baby; instead, you bring your baby to the breast.

❖ Your baby's body and face are facing your body and pressed against you; neither his head nor his body is turned sideways.

❖ Your baby is close enough to take a mouthful of breast (at least one-half inch back from the base of the nipple) into his mouth while nursing.

❖ Your nipple is far enough back in the baby's mouth so that it touches the soft part of the roof of his mouth.

❖ You may feel your nipples being tugged or a brief feeling of pain that goes away very quickly. If feeding really hurts, something is wrong! Most cases of women with sore nipples and babies who fail to gain weight can be traced to incorrect positioning at the breast or incorrect suckling technique on the baby's part. By readjusting nursing positions, both these problems often clear up quickly and dramatically.

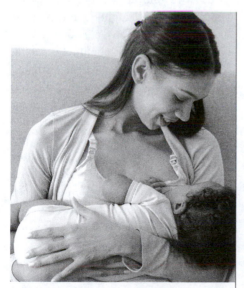

This mother is using the cradle hold.

waist, tucked out of her way. Your arm on the side of the breast she's nursing from should support her head as it rests in the crook of your elbow. Your arm should be extended as far down your baby's back as possible, with your hand holding her bottom or lower thigh, keeping her as close to your body as you can. Hold her knees against you; don't leave them hanging down. Meanwhile, your other hand can support your breast if necessary.

Sitting Up Position Three—The Clutch Hold (also known as the football hold): For this position, you tuck your baby under your arm as you would a favorite

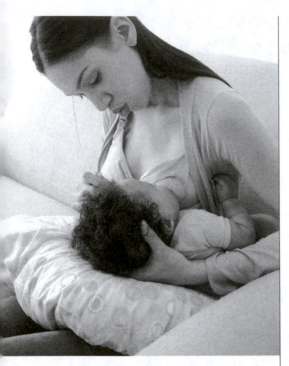

The clutch (or "football") hold is especially good for nursing babies born by cesarean delivery, twins, and babies who need special help with suckling technique. Mom's hand supports the back of the baby's neck, and the baby's feet are close to the mother's body, facing back.

evening bag, with her head at your breast and her torso and legs tucked against your body. Her head rests on a firm pillow on your lap. She may be slightly bent at the waist so that her body better fits around yours. Your hand is at the back of your baby's neck, lightly supporting the back of her head but not pressing it.

This position is especially good for mothers who had a cesarean delivery, since the baby's legs cannot kick or put pressure on the incision. It's also good for twins, since you can put one

on each side and nurse both babies at the same time. And some babies who don't suckle easily in other positions do fine this way.

LYING DOWN: For the first few days after your baby's birth and for night feedings afterward, you may find it most restful to lie down to nurse.

If you had a C-section, ask your nurse to help get you comfortable. (Being a good patient means doing whatever you can to feel good and taking the best care you can of your baby; it does not mean "not bothering the nurses.") Keep your legs bent. Ask the nurse to place something firm, such as a tightly folded blanket, at the bottom of your bed to push your feet against.

There are two basic lying-down positions.

Lying Down Position One: Lie on your side with one or two pillows behind your back for support, under your head, and between your knees. Your baby's entire body should be facing you, as you support his head with the hand opposite the breast he is nursing from. Your bottom arm can be bent under your head, so it is out of the way, or under his head, cradling him. You may find it helpful to place a flat pillow (made of folded cloth diapers, a receiving blanket, or a towel) under your baby's head; this will put his mouth at breast level and make it easier for him to reach the nipple.

There is more than one way to shift positions from nursing on one side to the other. One way is to nurse your

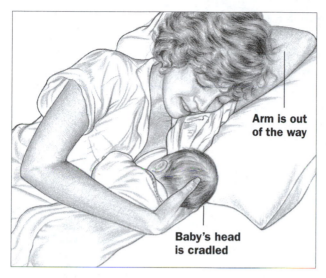

Arm is out of the way

Baby's head is cradled

In this position, the baby's entire body is facing mom, who can comfortably rest her head on her arm. Some moms like having a pillow under their head. The baby's head should not be on the pillow.

baby on one side, then pull him over onto your stomach and roll both you and baby over to your other side, using the guard rail on the side of the bed to help (if you're still in the hospital). Ask

the nurse to show you how. Another way of changing, which some women (especially small-breasted women) find comfortable, involves nursing on the bottom breast, then tucking your bottom arm over that breast, leaning over your baby, and nursing with the top breast. At the next feeding, you switch sides.

Lying Down Position Two: Lie flat on your back or semireclining in a bed or armchair, supported by pillows. If you like, set a pillow under your bent knees. Lay your baby tummy-down on top of your body. The baby's head is at your breast and her body lies on yours, either parallel or on a slight diagonal. One study

In this position mom lies on her back or semireclines, supported by pillows. Baby lies tummy-down on top of mom's body, either in a straight line or diagonally, with her head at mom's breast.

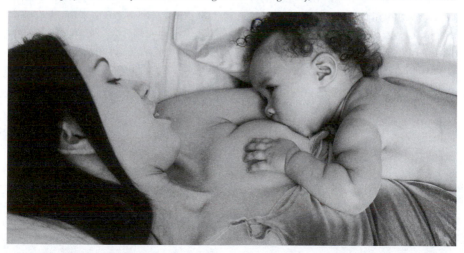

of mothers breastfeeding in different positions found that this position was most comfortable for the mothers, and midwife Suzanne Colson, who developed a technique called biological nurturing, maintains that this position helps to trigger an infant's primitive reflexes in a way that stimulates breastfeeding. In this position, she says, babies find the breast and attach themselves more easily, and continue to nurse in their sleep.

Latching On

When you and your baby are in position, you're ready to "plug him in," as one five-year-old said of his baby brother. Many babies find the nipple easily, latch onto the breast right away, and take off as if they were born knowing what to do. (Apparently they were.) Others need a lesson or two (or more).

Briefly, your baby needs to have a good firm hold on the breast between her upper gum and her tongue (which remains over the lower gum throughout the nursing session) and then needs to suck on the nipple and much of the areola to extract the milk from it. You'll know that your baby is latched on successfully if you feel a gentle pulling sensation on your breast, not a pinching feeling on your nipple. If she does not seem to be latched on correctly, insert your finger in the side of her mouth to break the suction. Detach her from your breast, as described on page 114, and then bring her back.

Correct latch-on is crucial to your baby's nourishment and to your comfort. When your baby is not latched on

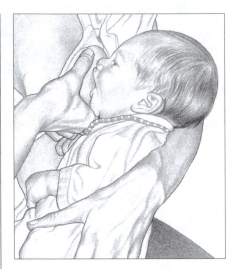

It helps a baby to latch on when the mom supports her breast with her hand, especially if she has large breasts. The baby nurses best when his top lip is open and curled upward and his bottom lip is open and curled downward.

the right way, she cannot remove enough milk from your breast, and you can develop sore nipples, a plugged duct, or even mastitis (infection of the breast). If you have problems with the latch-on or you're unsure if your baby is fully latched on, get help immediately. The most common reasons for early weaning are a mother's concern that her baby is not getting enough milk or the mother's development of breast problems. The box on page 111 offers a detailed description of how your baby gets your milk.

No matter which hold you use or which position you're in, hold your breast in the C hold like this: Slide your free hand under your breast. Support it underneath with your four fingers and put your thumb on top of it. Your hand thus makes the shape of

How Your Baby Gets Your Milk

With the help of ultrasound imaging, we now have a more complete picture of the process by which your baby extracts milk from your breast. He starts to suckle by curving up the front of his tongue and then closing his mouth around your breast, raising his lower jaw. He holds the breast between his upper gum and his tongue (which remains over the lower gum throughout the nursing session) and stretches the nipple to at least twice its resting length. (Fortunately, nipples are elastic!) As he moves the back of his tongue downward, he creates a vacuum inside his mouth. Through the suction created by this negative pressure, he is able to extract milk. This longer nipple extends far into his mouth but moves only a little as he sucks. His tongue still covers his lower gum. The sides of his tongue fold around your nipple, forming a trough; your nipple lies in this trough, like a hot dog inside a bun.

As the baby sucks on the nipple and much of the areola, the vacuum inside his mouth increases. As the vacuum increases, milk flows from the ducts inside the breast to the nipple, making it available to the baby, who then sucks the milk into his mouth. The milk is carried along inside the baby's mouth by a rollerlike wave along the top of his tongue, which is underneath your elongated nipple. After the milk exits from the milk pores at the tip of your nipple, it goes to the back of your baby's mouth. For the first five or ten minutes of nursing, your baby will be suckling forcefully, usually at the rate of one swallow to no more than one or two sucks. After this initial period, the rate may slow down, which may signal the need to change him to the second breast. However, if he is still nursing vigorously, he may benefit from continuing to nurse at the first breast, thus getting more of the rich hind milk.

the letter C. Your fingers should not touch your areola. If they do, they will be in your baby's way, preventing her from taking it into her mouth properly. Do not use the "cigarette" or "scissors" hold (the one most often shown in Renaissance paintings—maybe breasts were different then!), in which your index finger is on top of the areola, since this sometimes interferes with a baby's grasp of the nipple.

Moving your breast with your hand, tease your baby's mouth open by tickling her lip with your nipple. When your baby opens her mouth wide (like a yawn), quickly draw her body even closer to you while putting your breast in her mouth. This will guide your baby's head onto your breast, rather than inserting your breast into her mouth. If she does not open her mouth wide at first, repeat the tickling procedure on the lower lip, and wait until she does open wide before you gently guide her mouth over your breast. Another way to entice your baby to the breast is to gently stroke one of her cheeks, which will make her turn toward that

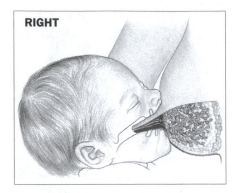

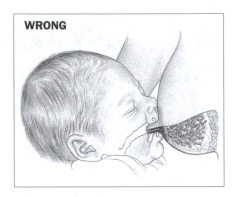

Baby A (left) is latched on correctly, with the entire areola in her mouth. The tip of her nose and her chin are both touching, but not depressed into, the breast. Baby B (right) is sucking only on the nipple, with her chin away from the breast, so that her nose is pushed into the mother's breast. This would make it hard for her to breathe easily and would make mom's nipples sore. Baby B should be gently taken off the breast and put back on again until she is properly latched on.

side. Opening your mouth wide may help, since newborn infants sometimes imitate adults' mouth movements.

Continue to support your breast with your hand until your baby is able to support the weight of your breast while nursing—unless you are full-breasted, in which case you should always support your breast in your baby's mouth.

Do not try to open your baby's mouth by pressing in on both cheeks. Her natural tendency is to turn toward the side being touched. If both cheeks are touched at once, she will become confused and move her mouth frantically from side to side. Do not push her head onto the breast. She may become frightened as her nose is pushed into your flesh and be more likely to wail her frustration than to seize the opportunity to nurse.

An easy way to help a baby latch on to the breast is to focus on bringing her to the breast in an off-center way. This approach is known as the "asymmetric latch." Instead of aligning your baby so

that her mouth is directly across from your nipple, line her nose up with your nipple and tilt her head back slightly. She'll be leading with her chin, her lower jaw will drop naturally when she opens her mouth, and she'll be able to swallow easily.

Sometimes latching on is difficult for a baby with a small mouth, especially if the mother's nipples are large. If your baby seems to be having problems because of this, talk to a lactation consultant.

When properly positioned, your baby's lips will be sealed tightly over your areola. Her jaws will go beyond your nipple to come together on your areola, about an inch and a half in, not on the nipple itself. (It's not called "nipple feeding" for a good reason.) This is very important for the prevention of sore nipples.

If nipple discomfort occurs, it's most apt to happen when your baby is first latching on to your breast. If your nipples hurt after your baby has begun to nurse, she has not latched on properly. If taking her off your breast and repositioning her does not relieve your discomfort, seek help as soon as possible from a hospital staffer, a lactation consultant, or a La Leche League leader. You should not be grimacing in pain, dreading the next feeding, or suffering cracked or bloody nipples. Remember: If it hurts, it's wrong.

If your baby takes only your nipple into her mouth, put your finger into the side of her mouth to break the suction, take her off your breast, and start over again. If you let her mouth the nipple alone, not only will you get sore nipples, but she won't be able to get any milk. It's important for her to take enough of the areola into her mouth to enable her to compress the breast with the gums. It is the up-and-down pressure of the infant's jaw and tongue that propels the milk into her mouth.

Your baby's chin should be dug into your breast, and her nose will probably be touching it. If she's facing you squarely, she will be able to breathe. Babies' noses are very flat (probably for just this purpose). If your breasts are large or engorged (so full of milk that they are hard), gently press your thumb on your breast to keep it away from your baby's nose. Or lift your breast from below to angle your baby's head slightly away from your breast. Or pull your baby's bottom more closely to your body; this will cause the baby's head to tip back slightly.

If your breast is so engorged that your baby cannot get a good grip, express a little bit of milk by hand and then bring her back to the breast. Or exert firm pressure on the tissue around the nipple to temporarily force the extra milk back into the breast and allow the baby to get a good grip on the nipple and now softer

How to Tell When a Baby Is Actively Suckling

❖ You can feel a strong suction, especially at the beginning of a feeding.

❖ You can hear him swallowing and feel him sucking, in a ratio of no more than one or two sucks per swallow. When your milk first lets down, he will swallow milk after every suck. As he begins to slow down, he will swallow after every two sucks. When he is swallowing only after three or more sucks or comes off your breast spontaneously, it's time to switch to the other breast, or to end the feeding.

❖ You can see and feel his jaws and temples working.

❖ You do not see dimples by the sides of his mouth, or lips sucked in. If you do see dimples, it means that the baby is not properly latched on. He's sucking but not obtaining milk.

❖ He pauses between sucks, indicating that he got a substantial amount of milk into his mouth. He is able to coordinate sucking, swallowing, and breathing.

areola. (For suggestions on relieving engorgement, see Chapter 15.) Be sure that she can breathe through her nose, since most babies won't open their mouths to breathe unless they're forced to. This is why babies are so distressed when they catch a cold and have difficulty nursing. Call your doctor if your baby is having trouble breathing through her nose. The doctor may suggest suctioning out the nasal mucus with an infant bulb syringe. Or the doctor may want to see the baby.

If your baby pushes your breast out with her tongue, start over again. Keep doing this until she gets it right. Both you and your baby have to learn how breastfeeding functions, and like any other learning process, this takes time and patience. It often takes some weeks for mother and baby to work together efficiently at every feeding.

dripping or spurting from the other breast, fullness of the breasts before a feeding and their softer feeling afterward, and signs of your baby's active swallowing. Eventually, you'll experience let-down at various times throughout the day, sometimes when you just think about your baby. You may not be aware of these let-downs.

You may also feel afterpains, abdominal pains similar to menstrual cramps. Afterpains tell you that your uterus is contracting and shrinking back to its prepregnancy state (another advantage to you as a nursing mother). They're also another sign that your let-down reflex is operating. If you're really uncomfortable, your doctor may prescribe a mild pain reliever. In any case, these pains are short-lived. Although your uterus will continue to shrink for about six weeks, you'll be aware of its contractions only for the first few days after childbirth.

Feeling Your Let-Down Reflex

About the third day after delivery (or sooner if this is not your first baby), you may feel a tingling pins-and-needles sensation in your breasts within minutes after you begin to nurse. It may occur within the first minute of nursing, not for several minutes, or not at all. Most women feel this sign of the let-down reflex, which is also known as the milk-ejection reflex. Some, however, don't feel it (but still produce abundant milk).

The let-down is one sign that your milk is flowing. Other signs include

Taking Your Baby Off the Breast

How do you know when it's time to end a feeding session? The clearest signal is when your baby has fallen asleep after a good nursing or comes off your breast spontaneously. Another way to tell she has stopped suckling actively is to count the suck-and-swallow ratio. If you hear only one swallow for every three sucks, and/or her temples have stopped wiggling, she has clearly slowed down.

If she is still on the first breast, you might detach her as suggested below, then burp her and put her on the other

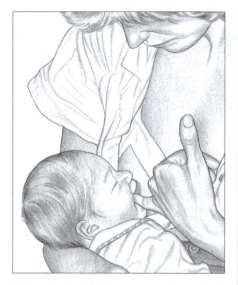

Taking the baby off the breast is easy and painless when you break the suction by inserting your finger deeply on the side of her mouth (not just at the edge of her lips, which does no good).

breast. If she has nursed on both breasts, you can assume that this meal is over, unless you are trying to increase your milk production, in which case you may want to put her back on the first breast.

To take her off your breast, insert your finger deeply into the side of her mouth, between the gums (not just at the edge of her lips), to break the suction between her mouth and your breast. If you try to pull her off the nipple, she will automatically tighten her mouth; and aside from the immediate pain you'll feel, this can contribute to sore nipples.

One Breast or Two?

There are two schools of thought on this, with reasons for each approach. We recommend that you offer both breasts at each feeding, especially during the early weeks of nursing, until a dependable milk supply has been established. After that time, some mothers and babies prefer alternating breasts from feeding to feeding. Once you have settled into a breastfeeding pattern, you can decide which feels more comfortable. As long as your baby thrives, you can stick with your own preference.

Most women have one breast that is larger than the other, and often one breast will produce more milk than the other. And sometimes a baby will prefer one breast over the other. Occasionally, a refusal to nurse from one breast may indicate that Mom has a medical problem. This is not common, but you should still have your obstetrician check so she can reassure you that everything is all right—and that you just have a baby with particular preferences.

Both Breasts: Offer both breasts at each feeding. This will give your baby more milk at each nursing session; will increase your prolactin production, which will increase your milk supply; and will help to prevent engorgement. Don't take your baby away from the first breast while he's actively nursing. Wait until he stops to rest and his active suckling on that breast has decreased or stopped; then make the change.

If your baby falls asleep on the first breast, changing his diaper or burping him may wake him up enough to interest him in the second breast. If not, he may want to eat again soon, so you can offer him the other breast in about an

Waking a Sleepy Baby

One or more of the following actions will sometimes rouse a sleepy baby enough to interest her in nursing.

❖ Speak softly and slowly to your baby, explaining what you're going to do. She won't understand your words, but may respond to your voice.

❖ If the room isn't cold, take off all your baby's clothing but the diaper. The feel of the air may do the trick.

❖ Hold her upright between your breasts, her bare chest against your bare chest. (This is kangaroo care, discussed in Chapter 16.)

❖ Change her diaper.

❖ Use the "doll's eyes" technique: Place the baby on her back on a firm surface and slowly raise her by holding your hands under her shoulders while supporting her head. Raise her until she is slightly bent forward, gently lay her down again, and repeat until she wakes.

❖ Lay your baby on her back on a thinly padded hard surface and rock her gently from side to side.

❖ Sit your baby on your lap and lean her forward slightly—not to a jackknife position. Then walk your fingers up the back of her spine, or rub her back between the shoulder blades.

❖ Gently massage her legs and arms.

❖ Give her a sponge bath.

❖ Dab her on the forehead with a sponge dampened with cool water.

❖ Express a little milk into her mouth.

❖ Lightly rub your nipple on her lip. This will elicit the rooting reflex, one of the many reflexes human beings are born with that help us to survive. The rooting reflex prompts a baby to respond to a touch on her lip by opening her mouth and making sucking movements. If her head is turned away from your breast, lightly touching the near cheek will make her turn her head toward the touch and then open her mouth and suck.

❖ Sometimes you don't have to wake a baby to feed her. Some babies will take the breast and actively suckle even while they're in a light sleep. In this case, you may see her eyes moving under her eyelids and her lips starting to smack before she latches on.

❖ Do not flick your baby's feet with your fingers. This used to be recommended, but babies do not like it. You don't want to irritate her into wakefulness. (Think about how you feel when you're abruptly awakened by the sound of screeching brakes outside your window.)

hour or so even if he hasn't shown any signs of wanting to nurse. Or you can pump milk from the second breast and save it for a future feeding. (See Chapter 11 for advice on pumping and storing breast milk.)

Since the first breast is usually drained more completely, alternate first choice at each feeding, starting on the side that was not suckled or was suckled last at the previous feeding. To keep track of first and second servings, pin a safety pin to your bra on the side that was offered first; switch the pin at every feeding. Or you can switch a ring, bracelet, or rubber band from hand to hand. Soon you won't need these aids. You'll be able to tell which side to start nursing from, since the breast suckled last or not at all at the previous feeding will be firmer than the other breast.

If you want to stimulate milk production and increase the amount your baby takes, you might even want to offer both breasts more than once at a single feeding, switching between the two.

One Breast: Offer only one breast at each feeding, and let your baby nurse as long as he wants to. Remember to alternate at each feeding. The advantage of this approach is that your baby will be sure to suckle long enough to get the fattier hind milk, which is produced toward the end of a feeding. Also, although the lactating breast is never emptied completely, suckling only one at a feeding may extract more milk from that one than might be the case if your baby nursed at both breasts.

The disadvantage of this approach is that during the first days or weeks of nursing, the unsuckled breast may become uncomfortably full, resulting in engorgement, but you won't know whether this will occur until you try the one-breast option. If you do get uncomfortably full, you can hand-express or pump a little milk to relieve your fullness (see Chapter 11 for instructions on pumping and hand expressing). You probably won't need to keep track of the breast last suckled, but if you do, you can use the same methods described above.

How Frequently Should You Nurse Your New Baby?

In many societies around the world, mothers and their nursing infants are constantly together, and mothers nurse their babies every time the baby fidgets, squirms, or makes a sound. Among the !Kung people, who live in the Kalahari Desert in Botswana, babies nurse several times an hour, day and night. This may involve 48 short feedings in one day! Not surprisingly, the babies gain weight well.

As a way of protecting their nipples, women in our society are often cautioned not to feed their babies too frequently. (!Kung women would be surprised to hear this, since they don't develop sore nipples even after their 48 daily nursings!) But nipples do not become sore from frequent nursing; they become sore from a baby's not latching on properly, not suckling well, or being improperly positioned.

At the beginning—when you're establishing your milk supply and your baby is learning how to nurse—it's better for both of you to nurse very frequently. Many new mothers are surprised at how often they have to nurse their babies, especially early on. Mothers and babies do best when feedings average between 10 and 14 times in a 24-hour period during the first couple of weeks (an average of every two hours). Some infants may nurse even more often over 24 hours.

One study compared mothers who fed their new babies 10 times in a 24-hour period with mothers who nursed only 7 times. Even though the total number of minutes of nursing was almost the same in each group, the more frequently nursed babies had a much larger weight gain than the other babies.

Frequent nursings carry another benefit, too. Newborns who are nursed often are less likely to become jaundiced. (See the discussion of jaundice later in this chapter.) In sum, more frequent nursings result in a more bounteous milk supply and greater gains in a baby's length, weight, and overall health.

Babies nurse more enthusiastically at the beginning of a feeding, stimulating the breasts to a greater degree. Since they get most of the milk from a breast in the first 4 to 5 minutes of suckling, it's common for them to nurse for 5 to 8 minutes, then doze off for 10 or 15 minutes, wake up, and want to nurse more. (Meanwhile, your breasts have been making more milk.) So while the average might be one nursing every two to three hours, this might work out into a regular pattern by which your baby nurses three separate times within an hour, then sleeps for four to five hours, then groups together another couple of feedings, followed by another nap. During the first few weeks, it's best to nurse at least once every three hours, and probably more often. It's important to feed your infant *at least* eight to ten times in 24 hours.

Fortunately for mothers, this pattern holds true only for the first few weeks of nursing. You don't have to commit yourself to doing nothing but breastfeeding over the next several months. In fact, although breastfeeding may involve more work than formula-feeding for the first few weeks (while you and your baby learn together), the time and effort you put into nursing your baby drops sharply, so that sometime between five and eight weeks, it becomes more trouble to formula-feed than to breastfeed.

Moms who have trouble getting started can take comfort from the experience of an English mom, Julie, who said, "My daughter is nine weeks old and we had a very rough time at the beginning. I was very sore, bruised, and uncomfortable. I also broke every rule! But now she is a fantastic feeder, and I'm so glad I persevered."

As we saw in Chapter 3, your baby's stimulation of your nipples causes your prolactin levels to rise, and the higher your prolactin, the more milk you produce. More prolactin is produced at night, with the highest levels between one and five A.M., which helps to explain why for at least the first three weeks, most infants are night owls who don't know that most human beings (including parents) like to be awake by day and asleep by night.

Perhaps the fact that babies are born with their days and nights mixed up explains why prolactin levels are up at night. During pregnancy, the mother's activity during the day rocks the fetus to sleep; then when she lies down to sleep at night her baby's kicking becomes more energetic. After the baby is born, nighttime still indicates "party time": the baby wants to feed more, and the more the mom nurses at night, the higher her prolactin levels rise. It's kind of a chicken-and-egg scenario.

It's possible that for the first six to eight weeks and maybe longer, you may have to feed your baby around the clock. Few things are as exhausting as having to "sleep like a baby" (meaning getting up every couple of hours), but try to think of this as an investment of your time and your energy that will pay off in a dependable and rich milk supply and a healthy baby.

More important than counting feedings per day or hours between feedings, however, is paying attention to your new baby. When he shows any signs of hunger, like putting his hand in his mouth, rooting and looking for the nipple, moving around, or looking more alert, nurse him. Don't wait for him to cry, since by the time he cries for a feeding, he's probably been hungry for a while.

With frequent feedings, your baby is getting good practice in suckling and you're building up your milk supply. He's being comforted and you're not going crazy trying to figure out a way to stop his crying. (For help with long bouts of crying, known as colic, see Chapter 7.) He's gaining weight and you're gaining confidence. In Chapter 7, we'll talk more about the way feeding on cue works after the newborn period.

How Long Should Early Nursing Periods Last?

Early nursing periods should last as long as your baby is actively suckling. You can tell when a baby is actively nursing by the signs listed in the box on page 113. When your baby stops suckling, take her off the breast. If she falls asleep at the breast, burp her after one breast and put her to the other.

The big problem with very short nursing periods is that they don't give the let-down reflex a chance to work. It may take several minutes of nursing for the let-down reflex of a new mother to take effect. Taking a baby from the breast before the milk lets down is frustrating for the baby who doesn't get the milk and for the mother who is left with full breasts. This situation can lead to painful engorgement, clogged ducts, or infection.

Other advice that is sometimes given is to let the baby "empty" the breast. However, your breasts are never empty. Even though they may feel soft after a feeding, they are constantly producing milk. In fact, some women who want to build up their milk supply switch breasts more than once during the same feeding session, and their babies obtain more milk that way.

Every baby is different, and yours may want to nurse for either shorter or longer periods of time. However, you want to watch out for extremes in either direction. Although some babies can get most of the milk from the breast in the first 5 minutes of nursing, at least 10 to 15 minutes per breast provides more of a safety margin, and will go a long way to ensure that your baby ingests the calorie-rich hind milk necessary for adequate weight gain. If, in the very early weeks, your infant nurses less than 10 minutes or more than 50 minutes in one nursing session, she may not be getting enough milk.

As your baby gets older, she'll become more efficient and may get all the nutrients she needs in only 5 to 7 minutes per breast. In Chapter 7, we'll talk more about nursing sessions after the newborn period and about how to tell whether your baby is getting enough to eat.

Burping Your Baby

The loud burps that erupt from the mouth of a tiny baby can be startling. They signal that your baby has emitted gas or air swallowed during a feeding. If he can bring this up in the form of a hearty burp, he'll be more comfortable and ready to nurse some more to fill the space that had been occupied by the air brought up in the burp.

When to Burp Your Baby

After your baby has finished suckling from one breast it's time to burp her.

Breastfed babies usually swallow less air than do bottle-fed infants, and some nurslings hardly ever burp after a feeding. Others invariably do, especially if you produce a great deal of milk so that your baby has to gulp to keep up with the supply and thus takes in a lot of air. If this is happening with your baby, see "If You Have 'Too Much' Milk" on page 148.

Babies often spit up milk when they burp. This is normal. However, if your baby vomits two or more times in one week with the milk spurting forcefully out of her mouth for some distance (known as projectile vomiting), call your doctor, since this may indicate a problem. Projectile vomiting is sometimes a symptom of pyloric stenosis, a serious condition that tends to occur suddenly between two weeks and two months of age, and needs to be treated immediately. Gastroesophageal reflux (GER, otherwise known as acid reflux, which we discuss in Chapter 7) is another fairly common problem. It comes on more gradually and it may or may not involve projectile vomiting.

How to Burp Your Baby

Here are three equally effective burping positions:

1. Holding him vertically with his head over your shoulder

2. Sitting him on your lap, supporting his head with one hand

3. Laying him on his stomach across your knees

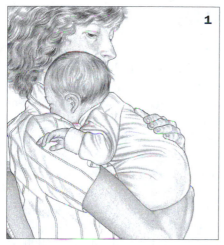

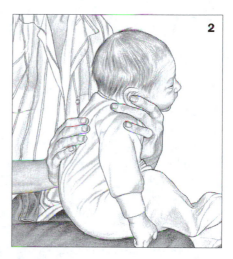

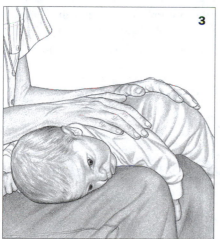

These pictures show the three best ways to burp your baby. Babies feel much better after they bring up air bubbles after feedings. Sometimes these burps are very loud. This mom is taking a risk by not having a cloth diaper or other burp cloth under baby's mouth to catch any spit-up.

Place a diaper loosely under your baby's mouth to catch any spit-up milk and then gently rub or pat his back. Don't pound! He won't like it, and he won't bring up his burps any faster. Instead, stroke upward on his back. It may help to alternate burping positions. If he hasn't burped in a few minutes, don't be concerned. Just diaper him, put him to the other breast, and then let him drift off to sleep as he finishes nursing.

The American Academy of Pediatrics no longer advises parents to lay their babies down to sleep on their stomachs or their sides. Instead, the academy recommends that the safest sleep position for most babies is on the back. If you have questions about this, discuss it with your baby's doctor, since there are some circumstances in which some babies should be placed on their stomachs.

Bowel Movements

While your baby was still cradled in your womb, her bodily organs began to function. At about the sixth month of fetal life, a mass of cast-off cells from her liver, pancreas, and gallbladder began to form in her intestines, remaining there until birth. This tarlike dark green substance called meconium is excreted in her bowel movements during the first couple of days after birth. Its elimination seems to be speeded up by the ingestion of colostrum.

Once the meconium is out of your baby's system, her stools will range in color from a golden daffodil yellow to a yellow-green to a brownish tint, and they'll have a seedy appearance. The "seeds" are all that is left undigested and unused from your milk. The bowel movements of a breastfed baby are usually looser and more frequent than those of a formula-fed baby. They smell milder, too.

When you're changing your daughter's diapers a few days after birth, you may notice some pink staining from the vagina. This "false menstruation" is due to hormones secreted by the placenta just before birth. It will stop in a day or two and is nothing to worry about.

Your Baby's First Posthospital Doctor's Visit

Make an appointment to see your baby's doctor within two to five days after you leave the hospital. At this time, the doctor will examine your baby, and you will report on the number of stools and feedings your baby is having in a 24-hour period. If you cannot see the doctor right away, call him or her with this information. Depending on your report, the doctor may want to see you and your baby immediately, or may refer you to a lactation specialist, or may ask you to come in within a week or two after delivery to weigh and examine your baby and to observe your nursing technique. If your doctor is not providing help with breastfeeding technique

or problems, ask for a referral to a private lactation consultant in your community.

During this visit, the doctor will evaluate your baby for the presence of jaundice (see discussion on page 127). She or he will also perform a complete physical examination, including weighing and measuring the baby, evaluating the status of breastfeeding, recording the information in a chart, and guiding you on correcting any problems.

Your Baby's Weight After Birth

Most newborns lose weight in the few days after birth, mainly because of their elimination of birth fluids and meconium. Breastfed babies tend to lose weight for the first two to three days, until the mother's milk becomes more plentiful. Women who have borne previous babies usually produce a full supply of milk more quickly.

A loss of 5 to 7 percent of birth weight is not uncommon, although the occasional breastfed baby may lose a bit more than that. However, a weight loss of more than 7 percent may indicate that your baby is not getting enough to eat. We used to believe that breastfed babies regained birth weight more slowly than formula-fed babies, but now this seems to be more a result of restricting nursing sessions, making them too short and too far apart. Your baby will gain weight faster if you nurse

frequently and for as long as your baby wants to stay on the breast.

If your baby is not back to birth weight by two weeks of age, seek help in determining whether he is nursing properly.

Do not weigh your baby yourself. This activity is anxiety provoking and usually not necessary. A babys' weight fluctuates greatly, and many home scales are not accurate. Lactation consultants sometimes weigh a baby before and after a feeding to find out how much milk he drank, using very accurate scales.

And don't compare your baby's weight gain with that of other babies. Different babies gain weight at different rates, and there is a considerable range among normal, healthy infants.

To check to see whether your young baby is getting enough nourishment, use the criteria that follow. To help keep track of feedings, urination, and bowel movements, many mothers find it helpful to keep a simple log. In fact, software for this has been developed (by a mom) that you can program into your laptop, cell phone, or PDA (www.babblesoft.com). Of course, the old reliable pencil-and-paper technique still works. The following information focuses primarily on the very young baby, but also is applicable to babies several months of age.

Is My Baby Getting Enough Milk?

This is the big question to which every mother wants a resounding YES! answer. Fortunately, there are some solid criteria so you may be able to answer the question yourself. The following checklist is adapted from one that Marvin S. Eiger, MD (coauthor of the earlier editions of this book) suggested that his patients follow.

Your baby is probably getting enough to eat if you can answer yes to all of the following questions. If you cannot, call your baby's doctor right away.

Your Baby's Urine and Stools

The evidence in your baby's diapers is the most important sign of adequate milk intake.

❖ Does your baby have the number, color, and size of stools at the ages indicated in the box on the facing page?

Your baby should be having regular bowel movements in a quantity of at least one tablespoon (½ ounce) or more. Some babies have a stain in the diaper after almost every feeding. After the first few days, the stools should be yellow and loose, with small curds. They may smell and look like yogurt, or like a mix of cottage cheese and mustard. They should be fairly messy to clean up. (Sorry about that!) But they don't stain as much as the stools of formula-fed infants.

If a baby over five days old is passing dark or hard stools or fewer than those listed in the table, this is a sharp warning that she is probably not getting enough nourishment. If your baby is two weeks old or younger and goes two days without having a bowel movement, call your doctor, since this may signal a problem.

However, if your baby is one month or older, is nursing well, and shows no change in appearance or behavior, there is no cause for alarm if she goes up to seven days without a bowel movement, even if she has been having them every day till now. You can wait for four or five days without a stool before calling your doctor, and the likelihood is that the doctor will reassure you that healthy

Judging Intake by Output

DAY OF BABY'S LIFE	STOOLS PER DAY*	COLOR OF STOOL	SIZE OF STOOL
1 to 2	1 to 2	blackish, tarry	from a smudge to about 1 tablespoon each
3 to 4	3 to 4	brownish-blackish	about 1 tablespoon each
4 to 6	4 to 6	brownish-yellowish	about 1 tablespoon each
6 to 30	6 to 10 (normally)	yellowish	1 to 2 tablespoons or more (after each feeding)
30 and later	may be infrequent (up to 7 days without a stool)	yellow	variable

*If mother's milk is a day or two late coming in, as is common with first-time moms, count her first day of lactation as baby's day one.

babies of this age often change their bowel habits abruptly and that there is nothing to worry about.

For a helpful chart illustrating how your breastfed baby's bowel movements may look and how you can keep track of them, go to www.lactnews.com/products/diaperdiary. You can download one copy of "Diaper Diary" or buy pads of 50.

❖ By the third or fourth day, does your baby have six or more very wet diapers per day, with colorless or very pale urine?

Today's disposable diapers are so absorbent that they rarely feel wet. To check for urination, pinch the bottom of the diaper: If the padding does not spring back to its original shape, the diaper is wet. Also, if it's wet, it will feel heavy. If you're willing to sacrifice one diaper, you can pour a couple of ounces of water on it and then heft it to see what a wet diaper feels like. Another technique is to put a tissue inside the diaper and see if that gets wet. Or you could use cloth diapers for the first few weeks. (They make good burping cloths—and, eventually, great dust cloths.)

If you see a pink or reddish "brick dust" stain on your baby's diaper after the first couple of days of breastfeeding, this may mean that she is not getting enough milk. This kind of stain is caused by the formation of uric acid crystals in concentrated urine. It's common within the first couple of days because the baby is not taking in sizable amounts of colostrum. But if you see it after the fourth day, you should call the doctor to see whether your baby is gaining enough weight.

Your Baby's Appearance and Behavior

If you can answer yes to the following questions, your baby is eating enough.

❖ Does your baby seem satisfied and content for an average of two to three hours between feedings in the first month or two?

❖ In the first month or two, does your baby nurse at least eight to ten times in every 24-hour period, for ten to twenty minutes on each breast?

❖ After three days of age, when you open your baby's mouth during a nursing session, can you see milk inside and is the inside of your baby's mouth pink and moist?

❖ Is your baby's skin soft, supple, and resilient?

❖ Does your baby have bright eyes, good color, an alert manner, and a smooth head, with no dent that might indicate a sunken fontanel (the soft spot on a baby's skull)?

❖ By the third month, is your baby nursing six to eight times (often on an irregular schedule) in a 24-hour period, and does the baby seem content for up to five or six hours at least once during the 24 hours?

Your Baby's Weight

❖ At your baby's first doctor's visit, was his initial weight loss less than 7 percent of birth weight? (Breastfed babies should normally have an office visit within two to five days after early hospital discharge, then at seven to fourteen days of age, and again at one to two months.)

❖ Did your baby return to his birth weight by two to three weeks of age?

❖ Is your baby gaining an average of 4 to 6 ounces a week (about one-half ounce a day) or a pound a month? These are averages: Different babies gain at different rates and the same baby's growth is variable from week to week. Weight gain should be measured from the baby's lowest weight since birth, not birth weight.

Your Nursing Experience

❖ Can you hear swallowing sounds when your baby is at the breast, in a ratio of one or two sucks per swallow for the first five or ten minutes of nursing?

❖ Do your breasts feel fuller before a feeding and softer afterward?

❖ When you nurse from one breast, does milk drip from the nipple of your other breast? Can you feel the tingling of a let-down reflex as you begin to nurse? The presence of either of these signs affirms that your milk is flowing, but their absence does not mean that it is not.

NOTE: Do not test for hunger by offering your baby a bottle after a nursing. Many infants have such a strong urge to suck that they'll often take milk from a bottle even when they are not hungry. (Doing this may sabotage the course of breastfeeding, since some babies enjoy the ease of getting milk from a bottle and are less motivated to work harder at the breast.) The only time you want to supplement with formula is if your baby's doctor recommends this.

Jaundice in Infants

Mild jaundice is extremely common in newborns. It is almost always harmless, and almost all jaundiced babies can continue to be breastfed. In people with jaundice, the skin, the mucous membranes, and the whites of the eyes take on a yellowish tint because of deposits of the chemical bilirubin.

Everyone's body has bilirubin. Bilirubin is an antioxidant that helps to protect the body against oxygen-containing chemicals known as free radicals, which can cause damage to cells in the body. Red blood cells break down in our bodies slowly and steadily all the time, and special cells convert the breakdown products of these red blood cells into bilirubin. Bilirubin is then transported in the blood to the liver for further metabolism and is then excreted into the small intestine, and from there into the large intestine, from which most of the bilirubin leaves the body in the stool. One reason to monitor your newborn's diapers is to be sure that she is having enough bowel movements to excrete the bilirubin.

Babies are born with a surplus of red blood cells, which was needed to transport oxygen in the womb. The excess red cells are rapidly broken down during the early weeks of life, producing a large quantity of bilirubin. Jaundice normally occurs in newborns because the quantity of bilirubin is greater than the immature liver of the newborn can process and excrete. In addition, a large amount of the bilirubin that the liver excretes into the intestine is then reabsorbed by the intestine and returned to the bloodstream. This process of increased bilirubin production, decreased excretion, and increased intestinal reabsorption assures that normal newborns have a modest level of bilirubin in the blood stream and tissues to act as an antioxidant to protect tissues from excessive oxygen injury.

Very rarely, a baby's bilirubin levels can rise so high that bilirubin is deposited in the brain and causes the grave condition known as kernicterus (also known as bilirubin encephalopathy), which can result in brain damage. Today no baby should develop brain damage from untreated jaundice, since jaundice can be recognized early and treated promptly.

How to Tell If Your Baby Has Jaundice

You can learn how to recognize signs of jaundice. In natural daylight or bright fluorescent lighting, check your baby for a yellow discoloration of the skin. Press your fingertip on the tip of your baby's nose, forehead, or thigh for a few seconds. A healthy baby's skin will look white after you take your finger away. If the baby is jaundiced, the skin will look yellow after you remove your finger. In a jaundiced baby with a very dark complexion, it's harder to see the yellow color on his skin, but it shows up in his gums when you let him bite down on your finger.

The yellow color appears first on the face, then on the chest, stomach, arms, and legs. Your doctor may want to determine the intensity of the jaundice by measuring the concentration of bilirubin in the baby's blood. She or he can do this either by drawing a small amount of blood from the baby's heel or by a new method in which a device measures the bilirubin in blood levels simply by touching the skin.

If your baby's skin looks yellowish; if the whites of his eyes or his abdomen, arms, and legs are yellow; and if he is hard to wake, fussy, or not nursing well, call your doctor right away. Chances are that it will be just normal physiologic jaundice (see below), but it's always better to err on the side of caution. The doctor will test your baby's blood to measure the bilirubin levels. These tests may be repeated, sometimes as often as several times a day, to monitor bilirubin levels. If the doctor determines that these levels are high or if the levels are rising rapidly, he or she will start quick treatment, which is essential.

Types of Infant Jaundice

Four basic kinds of jaundice appear in young babies.

Physiologic jaundice: Normal jaundice is common in both formula-fed and breastfed infants. In fact, nearly every newborn has an increased bilirubin level in the blood, and more than half of all full-term infants and four out of five premature babies become clinically jaundiced (visibly yellow). The yellow tinge of eyes and skin usually appears about the third day after birth and peaks at four to five days. Physiologic jaundice is harmless and does not need to be treated. It will go away by itself, usually by two or three weeks in a breastfed full-term baby, three or four weeks in a premature infant. (For more about preterm and nearterm infants, see Chapter 16.)

There is no reason to suspend or stop breastfeeding, nor to give supplemental formula or water to breastfed babies with physiologic jaundice.

Breast milk jaundice: This is apparently caused by the presence of a substance in most mothers' milk that increases the rate of reabsorption of bilirubin from the intestine. This type of jaundice is a normal extension of physiologic jaundice, and, again, nothing to worry about. Your doctor can make the diagnosis by ruling out known causes of pathologic jaundice (a more serious condition, discussed on the next page) with a few simple laboratory tests on the baby's blood. Breast milk jaundice shows up in about two-thirds of normal, exclusively breastfed infants. It appears 5 to 7 days after birth, peaks around days 9 to 12, and remains for several weeks or even as long as two to three months. In fact, current medical opinion is that instead of being considered a disease, this is normal and expected—and that formula-fed babies' lower bilirubin concentrations are the abnormal situation. In almost all cases, there is no need to stop breastfeeding.

If bilirubin levels are very high, your doctor may advise one of the following:

✤ Phototherapy (see "Treatment," page 131) while continuing to breastfeed

✤ Supplementing breastfeeding with formula

✤ Occasionally, in severe cases, temporary interruption of breastfeeding for 24 to 48 hours. If the bilirubin concentration in the blood drops, the baby probably has breast milk jaundice. However, current medical opinion maintains that breastfeeding should not be interrupted only for the purpose of establishing a diagnosis.

Starvation jaundice of the newborn: (previously called breastfeeding jaundice—or more correctly, breast non-feeding jaundice): This describes an abnormal type of jaundice developed by some breastfed babies as early as the first week of life or later in infancy. This is not due to breastfeeding itself but to the fact that the baby is not receiving enough breast milk. The mother may not be nursing frequently enough, the baby may not be suckling properly, or the hospital's practice of giving water or glucose water to the infant may be reducing her stimulation of the mother's breasts and, as a result, inhibiting milk production. This, then, is the equivalent of adult "starvation jaundice," which appears in most animals that fast for 24 hours or more.

The solution to this kind of jaundice is not to stop breastfeeding, but to correct the problem with more frequent and more effective breastfeeding. To prevent the onset of this kind of jaundice, neonatologist and jaundice authority Lawrence M. Gartner, MD, states, "No breastfeeding mother and baby should be discharged from the hospital until breastfeeding is proceeding optimally."

To see whether your baby is getting enough nourishment, review the criteria on page 124. Improved management of breastfeeding and increased frequency of feeding are usually all that is necessary to bring down the bilirubin level. Occasionally, supplementation of breastfeeding with formula may be needed while the mother's milk supply increases.

When to Seek Immediate Help

For You:

If you experience any of the following, do not wait to seek help. The sooner you deal with problems like these, the better your chances for solving them quickly. Call your doctor, midwife, or lactation consultant if you experience:

❖ *Painful nipples.* Breastfeeding should not hurt. There is a difference between tenderness and pain. Some temporary tenderness is not uncommon, but painful, bleeding, and cracked nipples are signals that something is wrong. In almost all cases, with help, you can heal very quickly.

❖ *Fever, aching, and/or chills.* This is an almost certain sign of an infection, possibly mastitis. If caught and treated early, you do not need to stop nursing.

❖ *A small red lump on your breast that is painful to touch.* This may signal a clogged duct, which can lead to mastitis if it is not treated.

For Your Baby:

❖ *Signs of dehydration.* Although dehydration is relatively rare in babies, if it does occur, it can be extremely dangerous. But again, if this situation is caught early, it can almost always be resolved so that you can continue to breastfeed. Immediate medical help is required if your baby:

❖ Has gone more than 24 hours in the first few weeks without the number of urinations and bowel movements described on pages 124–126. Breastfed babies are never constipated, so too few bowel movements in the early weeks

---

Pathologic Jaundice: This kind of jaundice is more serious than physiologic and breast milk jaundice, both of which are harmless and not symptomatic of any illness. Pathologic jaundice results from the too rapid breakdown of red blood cells, as in blood type incompatibility between mother and child (such as Rh or ABO disease), an enzyme deficiency or other abnormality in the red blood cells (such as G6PD deficiency), or from a disorder in the liver that reduces the ability of the liver to excrete bilirubin.

This kind of jaundice may appear on the first day of life and persist for several weeks, or it may first show up later in the newborn period. Both the condition causing the jaundice and the jaundice need to be treated. These babies need breast milk even more than healthy babies do, and they should continue to be breastfed while they are being treated.

Another type of rare pathologic jaundice results from infectious or inherited diseases of the liver and other organs. The blood test will often suggest this if a certain type of bilirubin is found.

represent a very important warning signal.

❖ Repeatedly falls asleep soon after going onto the breast.

❖ Regularly sleeps longer than four hours between feedings.

❖ Has more than two bouts of projectile vomiting in a week.

❖ Is not gaining weight as indicated on page 126, or even continues to lose weight after the first few days.

❖ Seems listless, sick, or drawn, and has a weak cry.

❖ Is less active than previously.

❖ Does not have resilient skin: When you pinch it gently, it does not spring back.

❖ Is running a fever.

❖ Has a sunken fontanel (the soft spot) on the top of the head.

❖ Has dry mouth and/or eyes and fewer tears than usual.

❖ Has a yellowish tinge on her skin or the whites of her eyes.

❖ If your intuition tells you that something is not right with your baby or with you. If you think something is wrong, trust yourself and keep checking it out. If your baby is acting strangely but doesn't do it at the doctor's office, record the behavior on a camcorder or digital camera and show the recording to the doctor. If you don't feel right but you can't put your finger on the problem, consult someone who should be able to help you.

Don't ignore a problem, hoping it will go away. It's always better to nip something serious in the bud than to look back and say, "I should have done . . ."

Treatment

Virtually all jaundiced babies can continue to breastfeed. Mildly jaundiced infants do well with the procedures outlined in Chapter 5—early, frequent, exclusive breastfeeding, with help as needed from lactation specialists. More severely jaundiced babies often become sleepy and feed less eagerly and less frequently, further increasing their jaundice.

Severely jaundiced babies can be treated in the following four ways:

1. Supplementing breastfeeding with small amounts of formula: Very small amounts of formula, as little as 1 ounce (2 tablespoons), can be given if the mother is not producing enough milk. When bilirubin levels in the baby have dropped, the formula can be discontinued. For suggestions on feeding formula to your baby without encouraging attachment to the bottle, see the box on page 134.

2. Temporary interruption of breastfeeding with substitution of formula:

This might be prescribed if your baby has very high bilirubin levels, especially when the previous bilirubin levels were not known and the rate at which the bilirubin increased in the blood is uncertain. Interrupting breastfeeding for 24 to 48 hours will generally lower bilirubin levels faster than supplementing. You will want to pump or express your milk to maintain your supply during this brief, temporary break. You can freeze this milk for later use. (See Chapter 11 for suggestions on pumping, expressing, and storing breast milk.)

3. Phototherapy: Babies are put under high-intensity fluorescent lights called bili-lights. The babies wear only a diaper, and their eyes are covered to protect them from the lights. If your doctor recommends phototherapy for your baby, find out how your hospital manages this. The baby does not need to be under the lights 24 hours a day; he may be taken from them for up to 30 minutes at a time so that you can nurse him.

You can continue to nurse on cue, except for the periods when your baby is under the lights. If you have rooming-in, you may be able to have the lights brought into your room. If this is not possible, see whether you can stay with your baby in the nursery. Increased frequency of nursing may help to lower the bilirubin level. Home phototherapy is possible, but it's better to have it done in the hospital, especially for babies with risk factors. Some parents mistakenly think that they can accomplish the same result by exposing the baby to sunlight, but this can cause a dangerous sunburn and will not necessarily lower the bilirubin levels. Placing babies behind a sunny window is also not recommended because it does not reduce bilirubin levels sufficiently and may also overheat the baby.

4. Exchange transfusion: This is most often done in extreme cases of mother-baby blood-type incompatibility; when the previous methods fail to lower the bilirubin count; or when the baby shows other symptoms, as well, like lethargy, poor feeding, and vomiting. After the transfusion, breastfeeding and phototherapy should be resumed.

If your jaundiced baby is healthy in every other respect, you should be able to take him home with you at the normal time of discharge, even though you may have to take him in to the hospital or to his doctor regularly for blood tests to monitor his bilirubin levels.

As we said earlier, because mothers and babies generally leave the hospital 24 to 48 hours after birth, it's important to take your baby to your health care provider on the third to fifth day of life. This allows a trained observer to check for jaundice—as well as for breastfeeding progress, to determine whether your baby is eating enough. The most important signs of adequate nutrition are the two P's (poop and pee): the number of bowel movements and wet diapers your baby is having.

You will be paying more attention to these two P's than you ever have in your life.

Exclusive Pumping

In certain situations, a mother cannot help her baby to accomplish good latch-on and therefore effective breastfeeding. This may be because the baby has some physical problem, is premature, or has to be separated from the mother for some other reason. In some fairly rare cases, failure of latch-on may occur for reasons no one can figure out. Some of these mothers opt for exclusive pumping (also known as EPing). Under this regimen, the mother pumps her milk very frequently and feeds it to her baby in a bottle. This is time-consuming and not as emotionally satisfying as direct breast-feeding, but it does work for some women, who succeed in feeding their babies nothing but breast milk for many months. This way the baby still gets most of the nutritional value of breast milk, as well as its immunological benefits. (One recent study indicated that the concentration of ascorbic acid, or vitamin C, declines in breast milk after being in the bottle for only 20 minutes, so while pumped breast milk is better than formula, breast is still best.)

If you're considering going the EP route, talk to your doctor or lactation consultant. You can also find many stories and suggestions on the Internet from women who have done this.

Bottle-Feeding the Breastfed Baby

Although the ideal infant feeding program is exclusive breastfeeding until six months and continued nursing until one year or as long as mother and baby desire, sometimes it's necessary to feed babies supplementary formula or pumped breast milk.

Lactation specialists have generally warned against introducing bottle-feeding too soon for fear that babies who became used to the relative ease of drinking from a bottle would not make the necessary effort to get milk directly from the breast. Mothers were advised to use alternate ways to deliver milk, such as a cup, teaspoon, or nursing supplementer (see Chapter 15 for an explanation of nursing supplementers). However, since many moms and caregivers found these other unfamiliar methods too difficult and were ready to give up nursing completely, some breastfeeding advocates experimented with methods of delivering milk from bottles in ways that would not discourage breastfeeding.

One lactation consultant, Dee Kassing, IBCLC, RLC, developed a method of bottle-feeding that does not discourage babies from breastfeeding,

How to Bottle-Feed the Breastfed Baby

Here is the technique developed by the lactation consultant Dee Kassing. For more information about this style of bottle-feeding, see the Resource Appendix for information on accessing her published article.

1. Use a straight bottle, not a bent one, and a reusable bottle with a small-mouthed opening, rather than a disposable bag system or wide-mouthed bottle.

2. Use a nipple with an old-fashioned long, round shape. The nipple should not be orthodontic, stubby, or shaped like a miniature human breast. The base of the nipple should be narrow, about 1 inch (2.54 cm) across, so the baby can get the entire nipple in her mouth. The base should preferably be tapered, not bulbous. When the tip of the nipple is far back in the baby's mouth, it's in a similar position as the breast nipple would be when baby has it drawn out correctly, and will similarly help to stimulate the baby's sucking reflex.

3. The nipple should be a slow-flow nipple, unless otherwise directed by your lactation consultant. A slow-flow nipple requires the baby to make an effort during feeding, so she won't mind putting a similar effort into breastfeeding, whereas a regular-flow nipple lets the milk flow so quickly that the baby doesn't have to do as much work. Very small or weak babies, however, may need medium-flow nipples until they become strong enough to use the slow-flow.

4. Use a soft nipple if possible. Again, this is similar to the mother's nipple and has less risk of causing damage to the baby's palate.

5. Sit the baby upright on your lap rather than cuddling her in the crook of your arm, which could make her lean back. The upright position will prevent the force of gravity from letting milk flow into her mouth and will make her work for her milk with almost as much effort as she needs to expend at the breast. If baby has to work harder for her meal, she is less likely to choose bottle-feeding over breastfeeding.

6. A baby younger than two months will usually need support for her lower back. You can do this by loosely crossing your legs and setting the baby on your lower leg with her back against your higher leg. Or you can place one foot on a footstool. If you're sitting in a chair with high arms, you can tuck a pillow against the baby's back. Meanwhile, support her head and neck by placing your thumb behind one of her ears and your fingers behind the other ear. Hold her head firmly enough to keep her chin up and off her chest (see illustration).

7. Gently brush the bottle nipple down over the center of the baby's lips. Pull the nipple away from her face and center it in front of the

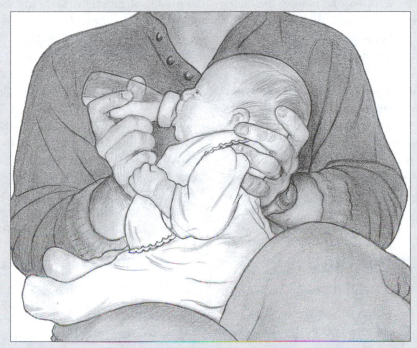

Sometimes babies who receive most of their nourishment from the breast need to get some milk from a bottle.

baby's mouth. Pause. Wait for the baby to open her mouth wide, like a yawn. If the baby does not open wide after you have paused, repeat the downward stroke of the nipple. If the baby still does not open wide, gently tap the nipple two to three times on the baby's lower lip. Then pull the nipple slightly away from her face and center the nipple in front of her mouth. When the baby opens wide, insert the nipple all the way into her mouth, so her lips touch the collar that holds the nipple onto the bottle.

8. Tip up the bottom of the bottle just enough so that milk covers the hole in the nipple. Healthy full-term babies will pause and breathe on their own. But if you're feeding a young preemie or a neurologically impaired baby, you may have to periodically tip the bottle down so that no milk remains in the nipple, and the baby can pause and breathe.

9. When there's very little milk left in the bottle, lean the baby's body back about 45 degrees. This will keep her head and neck in line, yet allow the bottle to tip for the rest of the feeding.

10. Bottle-feeding a baby this way should take about 15 to 20 minutes. If feedings consistently take 30 minutes or longer, contact your lactation consultant.

does not create nipple confusion or suck confusion, and mimics the beneficial mechanisms of nursing at the breast. For some babies, like those who are too weak to suck or those whose mothers don't have enough milk, alternate systems of feeding may still be the most appropriate, but in many cases the style of bottle-feeding described in the box on page 134 can help babies get the nutrition they need.

Meanwhile, the following suggestions may make the introduction of the bottle easier for your baby.

Buying Bottles and Nipples

❖ Avoid any polycarbonate plastic bottles that contain the chemical bisphenol A (BPA). Most new bottles do not contain this chemical, but bottles saved from an older child may have it. For more about BPA, see Chapter 11.

❖ If you buy glass bottles, get the kind made of strong, heat-resistant glass.

❖ Buy silicone nipples rather than latex, since latex can contain impurities and may cause an allergic reaction.

❖ Look for nipples with an old-fashioned long shape and a narrow base, not the flattened orthodontic ones made to look more like a human nipple "in use."

❖ Be sure *not* to buy nipples especially made for premature infants if your baby is full-term; these nipples are made of thinner rubber, and some strong suckers have been known to bite pieces off and swallow them.

❖ You can buy three different levels of nipples for babies of different ages: Stage #1 (slow-flow) for newborns up to about three months, the faster #2 (medium-flow) for babies three to six months old, and #3 (fast-flow) for older babies. All these ages are approximate, and different babies advance to the next level at different ages. When you move up to the next level, watch your baby closely to be sure the milk is not coming too fast for him.

❖ If you buy nipples that don't have holes, you can make your own hole with a sterilized straight pin, to ensure that the milk won't come too quickly.

Giving the Bottle

❖ Someone other than the nursing mom should give the bottle, right from the start. This is an ideal way for your baby's father to assume a larger role in his baby's care. The next best feeder is the person who will care for your baby when you are busy with other responsibilities, like work, school, or other activities.

❖ Introduce the bottle when your baby is not frantically hungry.

❖ To test the flow of milk, hold the bottle upside down. Milk should drip out at one drop per second. If it pours out, the nipple opening is too big; if it doesn't squirt out when you squeeze the nipple with your fingers, it's too small. In the first case, there's nothing you can do other than throw the nipple out; in the second, you can make an additional hole or two with a sterilized straight pin.

❖ If a nipple becomes cracked or torn, throw it out.

Now you'll continue to do all you can to ensure your baby's well-being—by taking good care of yourself (which we talk about in Chapters 8 and 9), by taking only those medications or drugs that will not interfere with nursing (see Chapter 10), and by enjoying breastfeeding and your relationship with your baby over the next months (discussed in Chapter 7). You're ready to continue on the great adventure of parenthood.

CHAPTER SEVEN

You Are a Nursing Family

"Some of my favorite times in the day are when I get to sit or lie down and relax
for a few minutes, cuddle my baby close to me, and let him enjoy a wholesome
and nutritious feed. Nursing is our special time together."

TRISCA New York, New York

N
o matter how much you've read, how many classes you've taken, or how many friends you've spoken to, you get a whole new understanding of what parenthood is all about when you and your baby are together at home.

Many new mothers impose unrealistically high expectations on themselves. In their eagerness to look upon childbirth as natural (which it is), they forget that recovery from it is natural, too, and that most societies around the world decree a period of rest for the new mother while she is cared for by others in the community. In a new mother's belief in her own strength and competence (which is justified), she may deny herself the means to restore that strength and enhance that competence.

You're probably more tired now than you ever thought you could be, and you wonder whether you'll ever be back to your old energetic, self-confident self. You will. And you'll get there sooner if you give yourself what we routinely grant our newly elected public officials—a settling-in time for establishing new routines and responsibilities. You need your "first 100 days," too. No one is ever fully prepared for the time and the energy needed to care for a new baby. But over the next few weeks, you'll develop your routines, enjoy your baby, and forget how hard life seemed to be such a short time before.

Consider the first couple of months after birth an orientation period. In fact, Dr. Laura Marks calls the first six weeks or so after childbirth the "survival time" (no matter how the baby is fed) as the mother gets accustomed to being on call 24/7. During this time, you'll need to let your body recover from pregnancy and birth and initiate lactation, and to let your psyche get used to the idea of being a mother. Meanwhile, your baby will use this time to get used to the world, to make the big adjustment from having everything done for her in your womb to learning how to do things for herself. The more you can smooth the transition for both of you, the sooner the fun part of mothering and breastfeeding will take over.

Your husband or partner can be enormously helpful at this time. His or her involvement can go far toward cementing the two of you as a parenting team, and the three (or more) of you as a family. Because of work commitments your partner may have, however, and because at this time another woman (especially someone who has breastfed herself) may be able to give a special kind of help, this is the time to call upon one or more people who can serve as your doula(s), as described in Chapter 4.

These first few weeks are crucial for the nursing family. You don't want to—and you don't have to—shut out the rest of your family and the rest of your life. It's especially important for your baby to bond with your partner, for the two of you to nurture your own adult relationship, and for you both to be attentive to the needs of any older children. However, your primary commitment right now is to your nursing baby and to yourself. You have to feed your baby when she is hungry; you have to get enough rest to help your flow of milk; you have to work at becoming a twosome.

Happily, allowing yourself to focus on your baby this way can free you to enjoy her more. By not feeling pressured by other demands, you can give your all to this courtship period. You can consider the worries and the anxieties of these early weeks as akin to the same kinds of tension that often accompany the period of falling in love. Because that is, after all, what parents and babies do.

Breastfeeding at Home

Probably the first thing you'll want to do after coming home from the hospital or birthing center is to climb into bed and feed your baby. This is natural and normal—and the best thing you can do for both of you. Your transitional milk may not have come in yet if you leave the hospital within 48 hours of birth. If your baby seems fussier and hungrier than he was for the past day or two, this is natural since he has used up some of the nutritional reserves he was born with and is now feeling pangs of hunger. Don't worry: Just rest and nurse whenever your baby signals that he's hungry—and that may be very frequently.

The concept of supply and demand is expressed nowhere more elegantly than in the relationship of the nursing mother and baby. Remember: The more your baby nurses, the more milk you will produce. The single best thing you can do to ensure successful breastfeeding is to be available to nurse when your baby wants you.

Still, this is easier said than done. How do you know when your baby wants to nurse, instead of wanting something else? How do you know when your breasts are supplying enough of the milk that your baby needs? How can you continue to meet your own needs as an individual and as part of an adult couple? These are just a few of the questions that arise in these early weeks. We'll talk about them in this chapter and also in later ones.

When to Nurse Your Baby

How does your baby signal that she's hungry? As the other half of the nursing duo, you'll learn how to read your baby's signals, like these common cues that she's ready to nurse:

❖ Increased alertness or activity

❖ Smacking her lips

❖ Making sucking motions

❖ Rooting (moving her head around in search of the breast)

❖ Crying, which is a late sign of hunger. It's best not to wait for this, but to feed your baby before she starts to cry. If she has to cry too much, she'll fall asleep from exhaustion, will be weak, and, as a result, will not nurse as vigorously.

You'll learn to distinguish different kinds of cries—the rhythmic pattern that often means your baby is hungry, the sudden onset of loud crying followed by breath-holding that may indicate pain, or the long, drawn-out wails that communicate frustration. You'll learn when your baby's restless stirring in the crib means that she's about to awaken and when it's just an interlude in sleep. You'll also learn when a smile means that your baby is happily enjoying solitary play, and when it means she's happy to be with you.

This learning is not instinctual; it comes through getting to know your baby and through trial and error. You'll take your cues from your baby and you'll interpret those cues. You'll recognize that your baby's healthy growth depends not only on satisfying her hunger for food and her longing to be held and cuddled, but also on her coming to realize that she has the power to influence her world. Responding to signals that your baby sends lets her appreciate this power and build on it in the future. By answering her needs as well as you can when she is small, you'll be setting your child on the road toward becoming secure and independent.

On the other hand, sometimes you'll know what your child needs better than she does. You'll recognize those times when your baby might accept your breast if you offer it, but when she might need some other kind of care, like cuddling or rocking, even more. And sometimes you'll have to take other considerations, like your own needs and those of other family members, into account. You know that caring for a baby goes far beyond offering your breast.

In general, you'll have confidence in your baby's ability to set the pace for nursing and in your ability to keep up with her. You'll nurse your baby whenever she seems to want the breast. She'll want it for the milk, of course. But she'll also appreciate the warmth of your body, the rhythms of your breathing and heartbeat, the comfort of your arms, and the feel of your skin on her face.

In the early weeks, your baby will probably want to nurse on an average of every two or three hours. She may sometimes sleep for four or five hours between feedings—and at other times want to be fed almost hourly. To stimulate your breasts as much as possible and help your baby go a little longer between feedings, after she has finished nursing from the first breast, burp her, and then offer the second breast. This way, she will get the fatty hind milk from both breasts, which will sustain her longer.

Babies vary greatly in the feeding schedules they seem to want. Some average 10 to 14 feedings during a 24-hour period for the first month; others are content with fewer. After the first month, the number of feedings needed decreases. By one month, 6 to 10 feedings in 24 hours constitute a typical range, and by three months, some babies cut back to 5 to 7 feedings in a day, sleeping through the night, while many others still want to nurse around the clock. Then, just as you seem to see a pattern in your baby's schedule, it's likely to change, possibly because of a spurt in appetite.

How to Tell When Your Baby Is Getting Enough Milk

Many nursing mothers' biggest worry is that they cannot tell how much milk their babies are drinking. Not seeing the milk level is actually one of breastfeeding's biggest advantages, since the nursing mother is not tempted to urge her baby to drain the last drop, thus taking more than he needs. If you feed your baby on cue, your supply of milk should keep up with his appetite. If you're healthy and if you take reasonably good care of yourself (see Chapter 9), you're virtually assured of having plenty of milk—especially if you don't worry too much about it.

The section beginning on page 124 lists ways to tell whether your baby is getting enough to eat. As we suggested there, it's sometimes helpful to keep a daily log of your baby's feedings, urination, and bowel movements, either on your computer or by using pencil and paper.

After you've been nursing for about six weeks, you'll notice that your breasts are no longer hard and full the way they were at first, and you're leaking less. This does not mean that you're producing less milk. The glandular changes in your breasts and the increased blood circulation caused their initial fullness. Once your milk production is fully established, your breasts may become softer and smaller, even while producing copious amounts of milk. After about a month of nursing, a woman's milk supply typically reaches a plateau of about 25 to 30 ounces a day (700 to 850 ml), or a little less than a quart a day. As long as your breasts are being emptied regularly, this level will remain relatively consistent for the next several months until your baby starts eating solid foods, at which point it will begin to diminish.

The following information focuses primarily on the very young baby, but also is applicable to babies several months of age.

Appetite Spurts

Very often babies who have been on fairly regular schedules suddenly begin to clamor for more food. This seems to occur most often at about three weeks, six weeks, three months, and six months of age. Your baby may be undergoing a growth spurt, a period of rapid growth that makes her especially hungry. Or you may be in an "activity spurt," doing so many other things that you get overtired and produce less milk. (See Chapter 8 for suggestions on taking care of yourself.) Whatever the reason, the best way to satisfy your baby's expanded appetite is to nurse more frequently for a few days to increase your milk supply.

Ways to Build Up Your Milk Production

New mothers sometimes fear that they won't have enough milk to feed their babies. They hear stories about other women who "didn't have enough milk," and they worry that they might be in this category. But when you look closely at the situations of these women, the problem can almost always be ascribed to lack of information about breastfeeding, lack of encouragement, or faulty nursing technique by either mother or baby. You need to tell yourself that millions of other women nurse their babies, and you can, too. Following one or more of the suggestions below should increase your milk supply within a few days.

❖ Nurse your baby more frequently for several days, on both breasts at each feeding. This is the single best way to enhance your milk supply.

❖ Wake your baby, if necessary, to feed him more often—about every two to three hours during the day and at four-hour intervals during the night.

❖ Pump or express milk between feedings. But don't get discouraged if your pumping yields as little as half an ounce of breast milk. Your baby is almost certainly getting more than this. Even the best pump is less effective than an actively nursing baby. (More about pumping in Chapters 11 and 12.)

❖ See a lactation specialist if your baby is not suckling well or nurses only a few minutes at a time.

❖ Cut back on your schedule. Do less. Rest more. Nap at least once a day—more often if you can manage it—or at least put your feet up. Ask someone else to help with grocery shopping, cooking simple meals (or picking up take-out food), and doing basic laundry. Most people like to help a new mother, so take advantage of this willingness now. You can always reciprocate later on.

❖ Even though everyone wants to see the new baby, ask visitors not to come for several days—or even weeks—unless they're people who won't expect you to entertain them. Let your voice mail take your phone calls—which you can return later when you're not so tired. Well-meaning family and friends can wear out the new mom.

❖ If you can, in the first few months take an occasional day or two off from work or from other obligations so that you can focus only on nursing your baby.

❖ Check your diet. Are you eating enough? Are you drinking enough? Some women find that eating or drinking more seems to produce more milk. Keeping a glass of water or juice near the spot where you nurse is a good idea. You don't need to drink any more than you need to quench your thirst, but some nursing moms find that they are thirstier than usual.

❖ Make a special effort to relax, as suggested in the box on page 145. Of course, this is hard when you're concerned that your baby isn't getting enough milk—but the more you can relax, the more milk your baby is likely to receive.

❖ Develop a few affirmations that you can repeat to yourself, such as: "I am doing the best thing I can as a mother"; "My baby is growing fit and healthy from my milk"; "My milk is my baby's perfect food."

❖ Visualize your baby at an older age, looking well-fed and happy.

❖ Virtually every culture in the world has galactagogues: certain recommended foods or substances for nursing mothers, in the belief that they help to make milk. Cheston M. Berlin Jr., MD, a pediatrician who is knowledgable about both drugs and lactation, has concluded that the effects of such potions may be largely psychological. The mother thinks that a certain substance will increase her milk supply, so she relaxes and has a good let-down reflex, thus "proving" its value.

As we have stated, though, the best way to build up your milk supply isn't what you eat. It's what, how much, and how often, your baby eats. The more often you nurse, the more milk you're likely to have.

❖ Believe in yourself and trust your body.

There is no need to offer your baby formula while you're building up your milk supply. A few ounces soon turn into a full bottle, which soon turns into several bottles, until you find that you're producing even less milk. In most cases, a breastfed baby should not be offered a bottle until nursing is well established—usually at about four to six weeks of age.

The only exception to this is if your baby's doctor (not your friends, relatives, or child care provider) feels that he absolutely needs a supplement. Your doctor may be worried if your baby is sick, dehydrated, so small that his health is endangered, or if he is not gaining enough weight. Any one of these conditions may leave him without enough energy to nurse and thereby stimulate your milk production.

If a decision is made to supplement with formula, you might try offering a couple of ounces of formula in the bottle before nursing your baby. This practice, which reverses previous guidelines for supplementation in the order of breast-followed-by-supplement, has become more widely recommended in recent years. This reversal satisfies the baby's immediate hunger and gives him the nourishment he needs, but ensures that he will get his final sense of fullness from breast milk and associate this good feeling with his mother.

Some babies do better getting their supplement like this, while others thrive more on the traditional practice of nursing first and supplementing afterward. It's not always clear which way will work best, so this is something you should discuss with your lactation consultant.

Another way of supplementing is to use a nursing supplementer, a device that lets your baby suckle at your breast (thus stimulating your milk production) while at the same time receiving formula (see page 328 for a description).

Once breastfeeding is well established, you may want to give your baby an occasional bottle of breast milk or formula. It's important to practice bottle-feeding if you will be going out without your baby at a time you would normally be breastfeeding, or if your partner or someone else (like the baby's grandmother) will be feeding the baby at times. If you'll be going back to work and your baby will be getting bottles regularly, you should start to give bottles before three months of age, since babies faced with bottles for the first time after three months often adamantly refuse to drink from them. Ideally, these bottles should contain only your breast milk until your baby is six months old.

Waking Your Baby

Babies look so angelic while they're asleep that this is a favorite time for parents to slip into the room, gaze on them with adoration—and express thanks for these precious, peaceful hours. There are some occasions, however, when you may want to gently wake a sleeping baby (for ways to do this, refer to the box on page 116):

❖ If your baby confuses night with day. Some babies regularly sleep for five or six hours during the day and cry to be fed almost every hour after you have gone to sleep. You may be able to change the inner body clock of a baby

---

Tips on Relaxing Before and/or During Feedings

Before a Feeding

❖ Lie down for a few minutes.

❖ Take an herbal bath or hot shower.

❖ Do deep breathing (like the kind you learned in your childbirth class), yoga exercises, visual imagery, meditation, or other relaxation techniques.

❖ If your nipples are tender, take an occasional ibuprofen or acetaminophen about 30 minutes before you plan to nurse. If you are in real pain, see a lactation specialist. (See Chapter 15 for suggestions on healing sore nipples.)

❖ Phone or e-mail a La Leche League leader or a reassuring friend, preferably another mother who is currently nursing or has recently breastfed her baby.

Before or During a Feeding

❖ Drink a glass of water, milk, or juice.

❖ Eat a healthful snack, such as a small sandwich, a piece of fruit, or raw vegetables.

❖ Listen, to calming music with your eyes closed.

❖ Read something light and enjoyable.

❖ Watch a favorite television show.

During a Feeding

❖ Nurse in a quiet room.

❖ Nurse lying down.

❖ Sit in a comfortable rocking chair with arms.

❖ Use a breastfeeding pillow that's just the right size for you so that your baby is well positioned to reach your nipples.

like this by waking her at two- or three-hour intervals during the day. She'll eventually realize that daytime is for nursing and nighttime is for sleep. Also, you can give her environmental cues—like keeping lights dim at night and bright during the day, even at naptime, or speaking in soft, hushed tones at night and allowing normal household noises and regular voice levels by day.

✤ If your baby is not gaining enough weight. Some premature babies and others who are unusually docile nurse obligingly when they're awake but don't wake up often enough to take in the nourishment they need. In these cases, it's sometimes advisable to wake them to increase the number of feedings. For more on the slow-gaining baby, see Chapter 15. And for more about preterm and near-term babies, see Chapter 16.

✤ If you have scheduling conflicts. If you expect other children home from preschool, if you have to go to work, or if something else is going on that would make feeding time hectic and rushed, you may be doing both yourself and your baby a favor by waking her half an hour or an hour early so that the two of you can enjoy a relaxed, quiet nursing.

How Long Should Feedings Be?

We are a clock-watching, number-counting, measuring, and quantifying society. We were this way even before watches with sweep-second hands and digital clocks came into common use, and now many of us have to fight the urge to run our lives like train time-tables. You can learn from your baby—who can't tell time—and you can use your breastfeeding experience to overthrow minute-hand monarchy and digital despotism.

There is no hard-and-fast rule for establishing the lower or upper limits of a nursing session. Some babies are goal-oriented efficiency experts who milk one breast in five minutes, go on to do the same with the other, and promptly fall asleep. Others nurse and rest ("nip and nap"), wanting to linger at the breast for an hour or more at a single feeding. If your baby seems to be nursing forever, it may be a sign that he is not nursing efficiently, and you will want to talk to his doctor or a lactation consultant to see whether he's getting enough nutrition.

Most babies seem to need at least half an hour for a feeding. Some research indicates that an actively suckling baby (past the newborn stage) will milk each breast in five or six minutes, getting only a trickle the rest of the time. Other research points to multiple let-downs at a single feeding session, with the breasts making milk as long as the baby nurses.

The best way for you to decide when it's time to put your baby down is to watch the baby, not the clock. As we pointed out in Chapter 6, you can tell when your baby is actively nursing. Listen for swallowing sounds, and look for the working of jaws and temples. If you're holding your baby properly and if your nipples are used to the suckling, you can nurse for as long as you and your baby want to stay with each other.

These feeding sessions can be wonderful opportunities to relax, put up your feet, and enjoy being with your baby. Once your nursling is latched on, you might want to watch television or read, or read to a toddler who nestles on one side of you while your baby nurses at the other. If your schedule dictates time limits for some nursings, you can provide a balance by allowing other feeding sessions to be leisurely.

What if your baby never wants to

The Popular Pacifier

Pacifiers have a long history in baby care: They're good tools for providing extra sucking time for babies who want it, for soothing a baby at times when you can't nurse her, for cheering up one twin while you're nursing the other one, and for comforting a colicky baby. But if you use them to "plug" your baby's mouth closed every time she opens it or to put her to sleep, you may be covering up other needs and creating a hard-to-break habit.

Pacifier use has been a fairly popular research topic in recent years. One study found that extensive pacifier use is associated with increased risk of acute otitis media (infection and inflammation of the middle ear). But this same study found that restricting pacifier use to the moments when a child is falling asleep effectively prevents ear infections. Other research has suggested that pacifiers may be especially helpful when babies go to sleep, for both naps and at night, and may even be helpful in preventing sudden infant death syndrome (SIDS). Some speculate that the pacifier helps clear the baby's airway and prevents the baby from sleeping too deeply and from rolling onto her stomach.

But what about pacifier use in relation to breastfeeding? Some research suggests that early use of a pacifier might lead to nipple confusion and interfere with a baby's ability to latch onto the breast. And pacifier use in the early weeks seems to lead to early weaning. On the other hand, one study of healthy nursing moms and their healthy full-term three-month-old infants found that babies who used pacifiers were not weaned any earlier than those who didn't. It seemed that babies who were having problems with breastfeeding were more likely to be given pacifiers, so the pacifier was the consequence of these problems, not the cause.

The prudent course seems to be to wait until breastfeeding is well established before going the pacifier route. But you know your baby best, and you need to trust yourself to know when a pacifier makes sense and when it doesn't. If you decide to offer your baby a pacifier, you might be unsure of which shape to buy. Different babies prefer different shapes, so see what's available, try one, and if your baby rejects it, try other kinds.

stop nursing but is over six to eight weeks old, has been evaluated by a doctor or LC, and seems to be getting enough to eat and developing normally? He may just need a lot of sucking, and you may want to offer him a pacifier after feedings. (As we said earlier, giving babies pacifiers sooner, before breastfeeding is well established, carries the risk of nipple confusion. And too frequent pacifier use can result in a baby's doing too much nonnutritive sucking and not enough at the breast.)

If You Have "Too Much" Milk

Abundance is wonderful, but plentiful milk production can cause two kinds of problems, neither of which is due to the actual amount of milk.

One can be seen when a woman's let-down is so forceful that her milk flows too quickly into her baby's mouth. The baby will gulp noisily, gasp, choke, gag, and sputter during the feeding. He may stop nursing after only a few minutes, only to burst into loud wails of hunger and frustration. A baby forced to drink too quickly in this kind of situation will swallow air, have uncomfortable air bubbles, hiccup, spit up, and be unable to satisfy sucking needs.

Oversupply can be corrected in one or more of the following ways:

❖ Express the first torrents of milk until it starts to come in a steady drip.

❖ Lie on your back or lean back in a recliner, with your baby lying on top of you. This allows the force of gravity to reduce the flow of milk from your breast and lets your baby control his intake more easily.

❖ If your baby starts to choke or spit up during a feeding, remove him from the breast, express a little milk, and after he has calmed down, bring him back to the breast.

Breast Milk Bonus

Because of breast milk's natural antibodies, which fight infections within a baby's system, this precious substance can help fight external infections, too. As we pointed out in Chapter 1, breast milk has been used for years to prevent or treat infections, and even to treat skin warts. It can also be used to treat a minor cut, diaper rash, cradle cap, dry skin, or eczema.

To use breast milk in this way, express a little onto a sterile cotton pad and dab it onto your baby's skin, air-dry the site you're putting it on, and then if it's a cut, bandage it. Be sure to change the bandage every day.

❖ Be sure your baby is latched on and properly positioned. Some babies slide down a firm full breast and clamp down on the nipple, resulting in sore nipples for the mother.

❖ Offer just one breast at a feeding. If your other breast becomes uncomfortably full, express or pump just enough to relieve your soreness and save the milk for relief bottles. This will signal your body to make less milk. Over the next few days, your milk production should decrease to a level your baby can handle more easily.

Another problem that can result from overabundance occurs when a mother has more of the high-lactose fore milk, which a baby gets when he first latches on, than is typical. A baby who drinks too much fore milk and does not get enough of the higher-calorie, more satisfying hind milk may become gassy and have frothy, loose green bowel movements. To remedy this situation, again, try offering only one breast at a feeding and let your baby suckle at that breast until he seems satisfied. At every feeding, then, your baby will drain your breast enough to take in the hind milk.

Babywearing

Babywearing is a relatively new term for an ancient practice by which a mother (or other caregiver) holds her baby against her body in a sling or baby carrier for much of the day. This way of caring for babies has many advantages: Babies cry less, spend more time in an alert state in which they learn, develop trust and emotional comfort, and gradually adapt to life outside the womb. The advantages to the adult include being able to breastfeed hands-free, doing various tasks while still being attentive to the baby, and going for walks with little fuss.

Both child-care professionals and casual observers have noticed that babies in cultures where their mothers carry them around most of the day cry less than babies in Western countries. In industrialized societies (in which babies are generally carried the least),

they tend to increase their crying bouts until six weeks of age, then gradually cry less up to four months of age, crying mostly in the evenings.

A team of Canadian researchers conducted an experiment that has helped to change baby care in the Western world. They asked some mothers to carry their babies in their arms or in baby carriers for at least three hours a day, and they asked others to carry their babies as they usually did (which was less than three hours a day) but to change their babies' environments by placing mobiles and abstract pictures of faces where the babies could see them from their cribs. The results: The babies who were carried at least three hours cried less than the ones who were not carried this much, even with the added stimuli of mobiles and pictures. Thus, the big movement to babywearing.

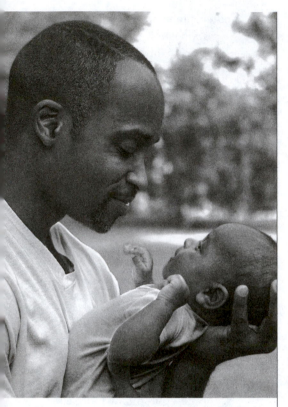

Carrying babies is a time-honored way of soothing them—and mom isn't the only one who can turn cries into smiles.

A number of books and websites give advice and suggestions about comfortable and safe babywearing, and sell a wide variety of slings and carriers to help you do this. For safety's sake, you need to be especially careful in the kitchen, going around doorways and corners, outdoors near curbs and icy spots, and within baby's reach of any dangerous or breakable objects. Bag-style slings may be dangerous for small infants, and all babies should be positioned upright and directly against the caregiver's body in any carrier. You need to be sure your baby can breathe easily, has a healthy pink color, and is not dressed too warmly in the carrier. Don't wear your baby while you cook; while leaning over a washer, dryer, or deep sink; when you're drinking or eating hot soups or beverages; or when you're in or on any moving vehicle. That still leaves plenty of opportunities for you and your baby to feel each other's rhythms—and for your baby to enjoy being held by other people, too.

When Your Baby Cries

Crying is the most powerful way—often the only way—that babies can let the outside world know they need something. It's a vital means of communication and the first way that infants establish any kind of control over their lives.

Research shows that babies whose cries are responded to seem to become more self-confident because they realize that they can affect their own lives.

By the end of the first year, babies whose cries have brought tender, soothing care cry less and communicate more in other ways, while babies of less responsive caregivers cry more. So don't be afraid of spoiling your baby by responding to her when she cries. An infant cannot be spoiled by being picked up and held; being held may be exactly what she's crying for. This teaches the baby that she can trust you to meet her needs, and this circle of trust expands as she grows to include other family members, and then others in her life.

When your baby cries two or three hours after the last feeding, you immediately know what to do—bring her to the breast. But suppose she cries an hour after a feeding? Or a few minutes after? What should you do? First, check see if she shows the earlier signs of hunger (page 140). Then you might think of other reasons why she might be crying, and try one of the suggestions in the box on page 152.

If your baby only occasionally cries soon after being nursed, offer her your breast and don't worry about the timing. But if she is regularly waking and crying oftener than every two hours, or if she often cries right after feedings, you'll want to try other ways of comforting her.

You cannot, of course, expect to keep your baby from ever crying at all. Frustration and discomfort are a part of life, and part of growing up involves learning how to deal with problems. Babies often fuss in their sleep, find a more comfortable position, and, in a few minutes, go back to sleeping peacefully. Furthermore, every baby is different. Some babies seem to need to cry lustily for a few minutes before they can let go of the waking state and fall asleep. Unnecessary handling at times like these sometimes overstimulates babies, interferes with their falling asleep, and makes them cry even more from fatigue. Constant parental management can get in the way of babies' solving their own problems. Of course, the problems they have and their ability to resolve them change as they grow.

It's often hard to tell just why a baby is crying. So much of parenthood involves learning the temperament and needs of your own child, starting in infancy. As you try different ways of soothing your baby—including sometimes leaving her alone to soothe herself—you learn how best to help her.

If your baby seems to be crying all the time; if she cries for long, unhappy periods at all different times of the day, or often after a feeding; and if nothing that you do will comfort her, call your doctor. The crying may stem from a problem serious enough to merit medical attention, such as gastroesophageal reflux (GER), which we'll talk about later in this chapter. Most likely, you'll be reassured that your baby is healthy, and you may receive some suggestions for making her—and the rest of the family—more content. (See "Ways to Comfort a Crying Baby," on page 152.)

The Colicky Baby

Some infants become fussy practically every day, often for hours, and usually in the late afternoon or early evening, and nothing you do can quiet them. The catchall term for this frustrating—and frustrated—kind of behavior is colic, and often the reason for it is a mystery.

Ways to Comfort a Crying Baby

Babies cry for many reasons, some easy to figure out, others baffling to everyone, including pediatricians. The easy ones include hunger (you can nurse him), soiled diapers (you can change him), and gas (you can burp him). If none of these solutions solves the problem, you can dig into your bag of maternal tricks, try one at a time, and see which ones your baby is most likely to respond to.

❖ Pick him up and hold him. Your baby may miss the rhythms of life in the womb, when he felt your heartbeat and breathing all day long. He may be filled with vast unnameable yearnings to be held close and cuddled.

❖ Give him kangaroo care: Hold him vertically, dressed in only a diaper, between your breasts so that you are both skin-to-skin (see page 344).

❖ Lie down and lay him on his stomach on your chest so he can feel your heartbeat and breathing.

❖ Sit with him in a comfortable rocking chair. A little rocking and cuddling can help you to relax, too.

❖ If you're nervous and upset, your baby may be responding to your mood. At times like this, it's sometimes helpful if someone else can hold your baby for a while. Meanwhile, making extra efforts to put your own cares out of your mind and to relax will help you—and may also help your baby.

❖ Take him out into the fresh air and walk with him.

❖ Hold him to your chest vertically with his head over your shoulder, and walk him around.

❖ Move him up so he's lying over your shoulder, his stomach resting on the top of your shoulder.

❖ Pat or rub his back.

❖ Burp him. A bubble of air may be causing discomfort.

❖ Change his position in the crib— try putting his head where his feet had been.

❖ Wrap him snugly in a small blanket; some infants feel more secure when firmly swaddled from neck to toes, with their arms held close to their sides.

❖ Make your baby warmer or cooler, either putting on or taking off clothing or changing the temperature in the room by thermostat, a carefully monitored space heater, or air conditioner.

❖ Give him a massage. You can learn infant massage from a certified instructor who will teach you gentle exercises, songs, games, and specific strokes to help relieve a baby's discomfort from congestion, gas, or colic. Look up "infant massage" on the Internet for help in finding a teacher.

❖ Give him a warm bath. You may even want to get into the tub with him. If you do, you will, of course, be very careful holding him, especially while getting in and out of the tub.

❖ Put him in a baby carrier next to your chest and walk around or sit with him. While you're "wearing" your baby, you can get some of your work done at the same time (like desk work, vacuuming, grocery shopping, etc.). Some of these carriers are designed so that you can nurse without taking your baby out of the carrier. (See cautions about babywearing on page 149.)

❖ Sing or talk to your baby.

❖ Provide a continuous or rhythmic sound, like music from the radio or stereo, a simulated heartbeat, or white noise from a whirring fan, vacuum cleaner, or other appliance. You can make or buy a recording of one of these sounds.

❖ Lay him tummy down across your knees and gently jiggle your legs up and down. This helps many a parent get through dinner. (Of course, you won't be drinking anything hot while doing this.)

❖ Put him in a swing seat or cradle.

❖ Turn your baby's crib into a rocker. Replace the casters (wheels) on the crib legs with an inexpensive set of springs. At first, you can gently rock your baby in the crib; when he gets bigger he'll be able to do it himself. Or get a device that will make the crib

vibrate. The Sleep Tight Infant Soother can be attached to a crib to simulate the motion and sound that a baby feels during a car ride. To find devices like these, type the words *crib rocker* or *crib vibrator* into your search engine.

❖ Take your baby out of the house for a ride in his stroller or the car. In bad weather, you can walk around in an enclosed mall. The distraction will help you as well as your baby.

❖ Lay your baby on top of a folded towel or put him in an infant seat on top of a washing machine or dryer that's been running for a few minutes. Some babies like the warmth and the motion. If you do this, be sure not to leave his side for even a moment.

❖ If someone other than you is taking care of your baby, it sometimes helps if the caregiver puts on an item of your clothing that you've recently worn (for example, a robe, T-shirt, or nightgown) so your baby can sense your familiar and beloved scent. The sense of smell is powerful in humans, as well as animals. Dog owners sometimes find that their pet is more likely to welcome a new baby into the household if the parents take home an undershirt the baby has worn and let the pet become comfortable with the infant's smell before bringing the baby home from the hospital.

❖ Dance with your baby to music from the radio or stereo (maybe with headphones—for you, not the baby).

(continued on next page)

❖ The pediatrician Harvey Karp, MD, has developed a five-step method for calming crying babies, which involves re-creating sensations they felt in the womb. He recommends swaddling (snug wrapping), holding the baby in your arms or lap and rolling him on his side or stomach (if he falls asleep, you can then lay him down in his crib on his back), making a shushing noise (which can come from a vacuum cleaner, a recording of white noise, or the like) within hearing distance of the baby, jiggling or swinging the baby, letting the baby suck on something—even a finger.

❖ If your baby is at least six to eight weeks old and breastfeeding is well established, try a pacifier. Some babies can't work up any interest in pacifiers, but others find them soothing.

❖ Remember this mantra, and repeat it over and over to yourself: "I am not a bad mother because my baby cries a lot."

❖ An important caution: If you feel that you cannot cope with your baby's crying one more minute, get help immediately. Call a relative, a friend, a neighbor, or the hotline for the Shaken Baby Alliance (1-877-636-3727). If no one is available, put your baby in a crib or other safe place, close the door, and walk out of the room for a short time until someone can come to help you or you can calm yourself. This is urgent, since some parents get so stressed by their babies' crying that they can hurt their babies. Persistent crying is the most common trigger for an adult's shaking a baby, which can cause severe brain damage or death from shaken baby syndrome.

What Is Colic?

The classic definition of colic is the rule of three: if your baby cries for more than three hours for more than three days in a week, for more than three weeks—she has colic.

No one seems to know what makes certain babies have extreme fits of crying even when they show no obvious reason for their unhappiness. When researchers compared three groups of babies in London and Copenhagen—some of whom were held for about 16 hours a day, some half that length of time, some in between—they found that all three groups had colicky crying bouts during which nothing seemed to comfort them, leading these researchers to believe that colic has a biological origin.

Most babies magically outgrow this daily crankiness sometime between six weeks and three months of age. Tincture of time seems to be the best prescription for most of these babies—that, and knowing that there's nothing that you're doing or not doing that's causing all that crying. Meanwhile, even when your baby doesn't seem to respond to your efforts to cheer her up, it's worth continuing to try, since she's at least getting a sense that the people around her care about how she feels and are there for her—and that the world is a friendly place.

What Causes Colic?

Colic does not seem to be related to personality, since many babies who cry a lot in early infancy turn out to have cheerful, sunny dispositions later on. Some people ascribe colic to the baby's getting tired late in the day, or to his responding to the fatigue of other family members, or to late-day tension in the household, or to some kind of stomach upset. Others speculate that some colicky babies are hypersensitive to stimuli that include light, noise, clothing, and even a parent's loving touch.

Sometimes this kind of regular crying seems to stem from physical discomfort, possibly due to an immature gastrointestinal tract. You can see this in the baby who draws up his legs and screams, apparently in severe pain. It's paradoxical that the typical colicky baby is an eager nurser who's gaining well, who feeds quickly, and who spits up a little bit of milk after every feeding.

If your baby seems to suffer stomach upset, you might try exploring how the baby eats and what you eat. How does he eat? Does he gulp furiously so that he swallows air? If so, this may be causing gas and fretfulness. Does your milk come too quickly? If so, your baby may be taking in too much and becoming too full, or taking in too much lactose for his system to handle. Or, despite the fact that he is taking in large amounts of milk, he may not be getting enough calories and may actually be hungry even though his stomach is full. (See "If You Have 'Too Much' Milk" on page 148.)

Many doctors believe that colic is often caused by GER (gastroesophageal reflux), a condition in which stomach contents back up into the esophagus. A more severe version of this is called GERD (gastroesophageal reflux disease or disorder). Remember what heartburn felt like when you were pregnant? GER babies seem to suffer the same feeling, but even more acutely. Symptoms of GER include pulling away from your nipple during feedings and refusing feedings, arching his back, crying loudly, and losing weight.

Treatment may include medication to reduce stomach acid, and also positioning the baby upright during feedings (so gravity helps keep nutrients in the stomach). And you may be advised to take your baby to a pediatric gastroenterologist for a diagnosis.

What are *you* eating? Research points to substances that a nursing mother ingests, especially cow's milk, as a possible cause of colic. When mothers eliminate dairy products from their own diets, their babies' symptoms sometimes go away, often within one week. However, it does take two to four weeks for the offending food to leave both the mom's and baby's systems completely. Some mothers have been pleasantly surprised to find that giving up dairy has had good effects on them, too. Other foods in the mother's diet that may cause trouble are eggs, citrus fruits, wheat products, nuts, peanuts, caffeine, and chocolate.

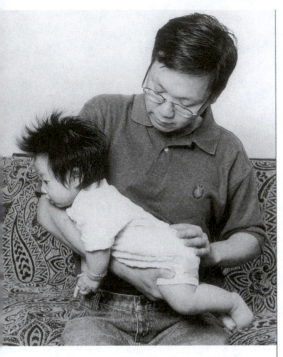

This father soothes his uncomfortable baby daughter by using the "colic hold."

None of these foods is indispensable. As you'll see in Chapter 8, you don't need to drink milk to make milk, and many different foods are good sources of essential nutrients.

If you do remove dairy or other foods from your diet, try them again a couple of weeks later. It's possible that your baby's digestive system will have matured, and you will no longer need to deprive both of you of the good nutrients in those foods. If you decide to stay away from these foods, check with a nutritionist to be sure that you are still receiving adequate nutrients from other foods or, if necessary, from supplements.

Most cases of colic, though, do not seem to be linked to anything the mother eats or anything she does. In many cases the parents are relaxed (at least until the crying jags begin) and experienced (since this isn't their first baby). Yet still their babies cry. So do what you can, don't blame yourself, and look forward to that happy day when the colic will be just a notation in your child's baby book.

What Can You Do?

Besides all the ways to soothe a crying baby listed in the box on pages 152–154, two particularly useful techniques for helping one who acts as if she has a stomachache (she draws up her legs and cries as if in pain) are:

❖ Laying her on her back and gently bicycling her legs to help her release gas; and

❖ Holding her in the "colic hold": Stretch her out horizontally on her tummy along your arm, with her head at your elbow and your hand cupped between her dangling legs, holding her by her buttocks or thigh. The heel of your hand will be applying light pressure to her abdomen. Holding a baby this way helps relieve the baby two ways: by the warm pressure of your arm against the baby's belly and by the upright or semiupright position of the baby's body. (If your arms are too short to do this comfortably, you may want to ask your partner to help out.)

And don't forget that other help is often available. Historically, mothers have turned their crying babies over to another loving caregiver for a little while so that they can get some relief. In some cultures, early evening, when many babies have their longest crying period, is known as the "grandmother's hour." This is one great benefit of having other hands to rock the cradle.

As the noted anthropologist Margaret Mead told Sally Olds, "The worst thing is just having the mother boxed up with the baby twenty-four hours a day, which nobody ever meant to have happen in the whole history of the human race."

Sleeping Arrangements

Different families handle sleeping arrangements and nighttime feedings in different ways. The following are the most common:

❖ Co-sleeping is an arrangement in which mother and infant sleep closely enough to be able to detect and respond to each other's sensory signals and cues. Room-sharing between parents and baby is a form of co-sleeping in which the baby sleeps in a crib, bassinet, or cradle next to the mother's bed, or in a side cart attached to her bed. As soon as the mother hears him begin to stir, she reaches over, brings him into bed with her, nurses him, and puts him back in his own bed. Later on the baby sleeps in a separate room.

❖ Bed-sharing represents a specific kind of co-sleeping. Here, the baby sleeps in the same bed with the adults. Typically, whenever the baby wakes up, the mother brings him to the breast, nurses, and both go back to sleep without getting out of bed. Usually, when the baby is no longer waking during the night, he no longer sleeps in the adults' bed.

❖ Separate rooms: The baby sleeps in his own room right from the start. If the parents are afraid they won't hear him cry, they might use a baby monitor or set up an intercom system between their room and the baby's. Ideally in this scenario, as soon as the baby starts to cry, the partner gets out of bed and brings the baby to the mother. After the baby has nursed, the partner takes him back to his own bed.

One of the biggest controversies in infant care today revolves around where babies sleep. There are significant health benefits in shared sleeping, which in many parts of the world is the norm, partly because it lets mothers respond to their babies most comfortably and easily during the night. One group of Mayan mothers in rural Guatemala, who keep infants and toddlers in their beds until the birth of a new baby (when the older child goes to sleep with another family member or in a bed in the mother's room), expressed shock at the idea that anyone would put a baby to sleep in a room all alone. They considered that arrangement tantamount to child abuse.

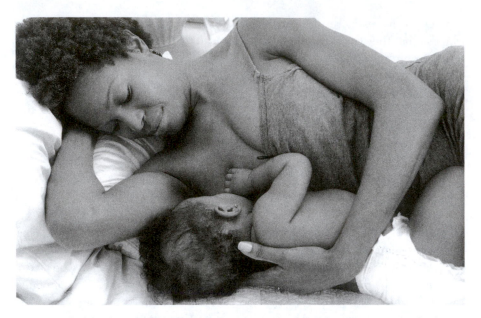

Nursing in bed can be a good way to take a rest during the day and to enjoy a cozy midnight snack. During middle-of-the-night lying-down feedings, babies get both contact and comfort, as well as food, while resting. Mom gets to rest, too.

One study found that mothers and their three-month-old infants who sleep together synchronize their sleep-wake cycles and tend to wake each other up during the night. This may prevent the baby from sleeping too long and too deeply, which may help to prevent SIDS. Infants who sleep in their mothers' beds nurse more frequently and for longer periods of time than infants who sleep separately.

The AAP recommends having infants sleep in the same room as adults, but warns against bed-sharing for fear that mothers or fathers will roll over onto their babies. Although this is rare, it can happen. The Academy of Breastfeeding Medicine, on the other hand, as well as the pediatricians who sit on the AAP's Breastfeeding Committee, maintain that there is not enough evidence to support routine recommendations against bed-sharing and that some of the studies that underlie the AAP's recommendations are flawed.

In any case, the percentage of parents who bring their babies into bed with them has doubled in recent years. According to a study of nearly 8,500 parents, almost 13 percent of infants regularly shared an adult bed in the year 2000, more than double the percentage that did in 1993; and nearly 45 percent of the parents said that they occasionally brought their infants into bed with them for all or part of the night. The numbers may be even higher, since many parents don't talk about this for fear of encountering disapproval.

Some parents sleep with their

babies because they cannot afford a crib. Such parents can get a free crib from the organization Cribs for Kids, a safe-sleep education program with many chapters around the country.

Regardless of which arrangement you choose (and usually babies experience several different sleeping environments over time), you need to make sleep safe for your baby. To do this, the following cautions are important.

Safe Sleeping for Baby Either with a Parent or Alone

By adhering to the following basic precautions, you can provide a safe sleeping environment for your baby. Keep in mind that moms and infants may combine different sleeping arrangements. For example, your baby may fall asleep in her crib, and then when she wakes up you bring her into your bed to nurse her. You both may drift off to sleep for a while, after which you may put her back into her own bed. Therefore, even if you plan to have your baby sleep in her own bed, you should be sure to follow the recommendations for safe sleeping in a shared bed also.

✤ Always put your baby to sleep on her back, not on her stomach or side. For a young baby, swaddling (wrapping the baby snugly in light blankets) may help her to stay in this position. As soon as an infant learns to fight her way out of the wrapping, give up the swaddling to prevent loose cloth in the baby's bed.

✤ Be sure that the bed or crib mattress is firm and that it fits tightly on its frame, with no more than a 1-inch space between the mattress and any side. This will prevent your baby's nose and/or mouth from getting caught in sagging or loose bedding. New cribs and crib mattresses by law must fit this standard. Check that yours have labels stating that they meet Consumer Product Safety Commission standards.

Older cribs may not meet this requirement because of wear, damage, or manufacture before current regulations. Another problem with older cribs may be the presence of lead-based paint, or splinters or cracks in the wood. New cribs may fail to meet the standard due to improper assembly. So be sure to give your crib a thorough inspection before you use it.

✤ If the crib's mattress is adjustable up and down, its highest level should be 26 inches from the top of the rail, so that when your baby starts to pull herself up she will not be able to tumble over the top rail.

✤ Bars on a crib or those attached to the side of a bed should be spaced no farther apart than 2⅜ inches to prevent a baby's head from getting caught. If you can fit a soda can between the slats, they are too far apart.

✤ Use only a fitted sheet. Never put your baby to sleep on pillows, quilts, sheepskins, or other soft surfaces.

✤ Do not use bumper pads around the sides of the crib.

❖ Put a sleeper suit on the baby instead of covering her with a blanket. Do not use quilts, comforters, or blankets in bed with baby, or anything else that could cover her face.

❖ Remove all soft items, including stuffed toys, from the baby's bed.

❖ Be sure that no objects can topple or collapse onto the bed.

❖ Be sure that the baby cannot get tangled up in her clothing, and that there is nothing in the bed that can catch the clothing and ensnare the baby.

❖ If your baby is six to eight weeks old and breastfeeding is well established, consider giving her a clean, dry pacifier when putting her down, but don't force her to take it (see discussion of pacifiers on page 147).

❖ Do not put the baby to bed with a pacifier on a cord, or with anything around her neck.

❖ Do not put the baby in a bed close enough to curtains, drapes, or Venetian blind cords that she could reach or get caught in.

❖ Do not put the baby on a plastic mattress or sheet covering.

❖ To prevent overheating, keep the baby's room in a temperature range of 68° to 75°F (20° to 24°C), keep the baby's bed away from the heat vent, and do not overdress her. If the baby is sleeping with you, dress her more lightly to allow for your own body heat.

❖ Do not let any plastic bags remain on the floor, on the bed, or nearby where the baby could roll over and fall into them.

Guidelines for Safe Bed-sharing

In the United States and other Western countries, bringing a baby into the same bed with the parents or partners is highly controversial. If you do decide to do this, you need to adhere to the guidelines specified here.

❖ Examine the structure of the adult bed closely to be sure the baby cannot get trapped between the mattress and the wall, bed frame, headboard, footboard, bed railings, other furniture, or anything else. Parents often move the bed against a wall in the belief that this will prevent their baby from falling onto the floor, but there is a danger of the baby's getting wedged between the mattress and the wall because parents may fail to notice when the mattress has come away from the wall.

Babies who learn how to rock from side to side, roll over, raise themselves up on their hands and knees, or propel themselves by pushing against a flat surface can often move to a corner of the bed, but if they become wedged between two objects they may not have the strength and coordination to free themselves. And you never know when a baby will reach this stage until he is actually doing it.

❖ Be sure the bed is low enough and the floor is covered with a firm but soft covering so that if the baby does fall out of bed, he will not be injured.

❖ If either you or your partner weighs more than 175 pounds, you need to be extra cautious about the way you bed-share. Be sure to use an extremely firm mattress.

❖ The safest bed-sharing arrangement is for the family to sleep in a large queen- or king-size bed, with the baby next to the mother instead of between the parents.

❖ Do not put the baby to sleep on a waterbed, sofa, or recliner.

❖ Do not leave an infant alone on an adult bed.

❖ Do not smoke in bed or near the sleeping baby.

❖ Do not let older children—including toddlers—sleep next to the baby.

❖ Be sure that your pet cannot climb onto the bed with your baby.

❖ Do not let your baby sleep with you if either you or your partner is usually a deep sleeper; if either of you has taken any medication that could make you sleep soundly; if either of you is overtired or is a smoker; or if either of you has had alcoholic drinks or any recreational drugs that could make you sleep heavily.

❖ When both partners sleep in the same bed with the baby, each one needs to mentally acknowledge the presence of the infant in the bed before falling asleep. Anthropologist James J. McKenna says, "This is a mental note like the car stickers that say BABY ON BOARD; but in this case the message is BABY IN BED. Most healthy, undrugged parents sleep lightly when they know that the baby is in the bed with them."

Whatever way you decide to arrange your family life is up to you. Babies grow up happy and healthy under all manner of sleeping arrangements. Basically, your choice will depend on your own views and personal preference.

Sleep and Lack of It: Night Feedings

It's the middle of the night, and everyone, including the family dog, is sleeping peacefully. Everyone, that is, except your new baby, whose lusty bawling pierces your sleep. You wonder when that happy day will come when you can once again know a night of uninterrupted sleep. Hard to say.

The age at which babies stop waking for night feedings seems to be an individual characteristic unrelated to size at birth, weight gain afterward, the amount of food eaten in a day, or whether this food comes from breast, bottle, or jar. Babies seem to be born with differing needs for sleeping and eating. While the average newborn sleeps about 16 hours a day, one healthy baby may sleep only 11 hours, while another sleeps 21. After three months, babies become more wakeful in late afternoon and early evening, and by six months more than half their sleep takes place at night.

An occasional baby gives up middle-of-the-night feedings as early as six weeks; many give it up at about three months; and many others need it for a few months longer. In the early weeks, you need those night feedings as much as your baby does, so that your breasts will continue to be well stimulated and will not become engorged and uncomfortable by morning.

Night feedings are easier if you don't bother changing the baby's diapers unless she's drenched or uncomfortable. If a diaper change is necessary, let your partner do it so you can get your rest.

Encouraging a Baby to Give Up Nighttime Nursing

If you don't really mind getting up at night, there's no age by which your baby has to sleep through, so you can just wait until he gives up night feedings himself—and try to catch up on your own sleep by scheduling a nap during the day.

But if your doctor says your baby is growing well, if he is nursing often and well during the day, if he's at least 12 weeks old, so your milk supply is well established, and if getting up with him leaves you exhausted and irritable, you may be able to encourage him to sleep for longer stretches at night. (Some anthropologists say that human beings in various cultures regularly sleep in two shifts, with an hour or two of wakefulness in the middle. Seems that young babies have read these textbooks.)

Still, if you want your family, young and old, to follow the typical Western sleep schedule, sometimes one of the following will help:

❖ Try nursing later at night, maybe at midnight, to see whether this will hold your baby till early morning.

❖ Let your baby fuss (not scream) for five or ten minutes when he wakes during the night. If he's not too hungry, he may go back to sleep.

❖ If your baby sleeps in a separate bed, let your partner comfort him, maybe by rubbing or patting his back or speaking softly to him. From very early on, your baby associates your looks and your smell with feeding. If you go to his side, he'll expect to nurse. This is why someone else is often more successful in getting him back to sleep.

It's best to take your baby off the breast as soon as she falls asleep, since letting an infant sleep on the nipple (even yours) may cause dental cavities. Saliva does not flow as well at night and cannot wash away bacteria in the mouth. This is, of course, especially important for babies whose teeth have started to erupt. There's a good argument also for taking your baby off the breast when she's sleepy but not completely asleep. If you do this with at least some feedings, day and night, you will help her learn to fall asleep without needing to nurse, so that when she's older she'll be able to go to sleep on her own.

If your baby is sleeping in your room, you'll probably hear her make many sounds throughout the night, including little snuffles and whimpers, the equivalent of an adult's talking in his or her sleep. If she is really awake and wanting food, you'll want to nurse her before she cries in earnest. But if she seems to be making these little sounds in her sleep, you can wait until she wakes before you put her to the breast.

❖ One mom we know stayed in a hotel room for three nights while the baby's father and grandmother took care of the baby. She nursed during the day and left the house after the early evening nursing. By the time she came back home to sleep, the baby wasn't waking at night anymore.

❖ If the baby cries when you leave after putting him to bed, go back every few minutes so he can be reassured by your (or your partner's) presence. If you sit with the baby in the room, stay quiet and look away so he won't think it's playtime.

❖ If your baby is on a night shift—sleeping during the day and up a lot at night—reorient him by waking him up and nursing him every two to three hours during the day, and keeping him awake by taking him out, bathing him, playing with him, or sitting him in an infant seat where he can see interesting things and people.

❖ You might also teach your baby to distinguish day from night by keeping the lights on during the day, even during naptime, and not making an effort to be quiet.

❖ Although some parents feed their babies solid foods in the belief that this will help them go longer between nursings at night, there's no evidence that this does any good. The American Academy of Pediatrics recommends breast milk alone for six months, but some pediatricians do suggest starting solid foods at about four months, depending on individual needs. (Suggestions for starting solids are given in Chapter 17.)

❖ Offer a pacifier, if your milk supply is well established and your baby is at least six to eight weeks old.

Ways to Guard Your Rest

The Telephone

To protect your privacy and rest, take precautions like the following:

✧ When you and your baby want to rest, turn off the ringer on your home and cell phones.

✧ Change the message on your voice mail to something like: "I can't answer the phone right now. Please leave your name and number and I'll call you back when I can." Or indicate when someone else will be home to answer the phone.

✧ Return phone calls while lying in bed at a time when it's convenient for you.

✧ Ask people to communicate by e-mail, and answer your messages on your timetable.

The Doorbell

To prevent being disturbed by unexpected callers or delivery people, hang a notepad and pen on your door, next to a sign that says something like this: "Please don't ring the doorbell. We can't be disturbed now. Please leave a note."

Gradually your baby will go longer between night feedings until one morning you'll wake up after sleeping for five or six hours, breasts full, wondering what's the matter, and dashing to your baby's side. Nothing is wrong; your baby has just slept through the night for the first time.

The Joys of Nighttime Feedings

It's hard for an exhausted new mother to think of night feedings as anything but a burdensome sleep-robber to be ended as soon as possible. Yet many women have found that they welcome and enjoy them more than they ever thought they would—especially if they're able to nap or at least rest during the day.

Women who like night feedings talk about the warm feeling of nursing in bed, surrounded by the people they love. They talk about the special feeling of being the only two people awake in the house. They talk about the serenity of being alone with their babies. They talk about the slightly illicit feeling of slipping out of bed in the middle of the night and sitting with the baby and a snack in front of a late TV show, or immersed in a good book. These days, some moms will sit in front of the computer in the middle of the night, where they can go to a site like www.breastfeeding.com, click on "Things to Do While Breastfeeding," and enjoy videos, info about celebrity breastfeeders, and other online features that can be accessed with one hand.

Other mothers who long for these nighttime feedings to end often find with some surprise that years later they look back upon them with nostalgia. Still, if you're in the latter group, you may find the suggestions in the box on pages 162–163 helpful.

Sleep for Mom

Weariness seems to be the lot of every new mother, and even after warnings from friends who have already been through it, this feeling of exhaustion is something that few moms are prepared for. Right after your body has undergone the aptly named labor, you have more responsibility but get less sleep. If stress and fatigue kept women from breastfeeding, none of us would be

here today. Our early forebears had no other choice but to breastfeed, and it certainly didn't stop them from having babies. However, the better you feel, the easier breastfeeding will go—and everything else in your life, too—so it makes sense to get as much rest as possible.

If you have always slept best on your stomach, you can continue to sleep in this position as long as you have a good milk supply and this position is not painful for you. Some women find that sleeping on their stomachs during the early weeks of nursing causes leaking or puts uncomfortable pressure on their breasts. But if it feels good, do it. You may be more comfortable wearing a sleep bra (see Chapter 9). You need your sleep, however you get it.

Diapers, Revisited

Remember that your breastfed baby's bowel movements and habits are quite different from those of a formula-fed baby. A grandmother or friend who is used to formula-fed babies may look at your baby's stools, become worried about her health, and alarm you. So put their minds and your own at ease.

Your baby may move her bowels quite frequently, possibly after every feeding during the first month. Then her pattern may change abruptly to infrequent movements. She may even go more than seven days without a movement, as noted in the table on page 125. Breastfed babies tend to

excrete less waste than formula-fed infants, because human milk is digested so completely.

Sometimes there's only a stain on the diaper; this is not diarrhea. Sometimes your baby strains a bit; this is not constipation. These patterns are normal and healthy. Straining reflects the fact that the soft stool of a breastfed baby may be hard for her to expel. Because babies digest breast milk so well, there's less bulk in the stool. You may be able to help your baby have a movement by "bicycling" her legs (moving them up and down as if she were riding a bike).

Constipation is rare among breastfed babies and is not defined by frequency (or infrequency) of stools or by straining at a bowel movement. A hard stool does signal constipation. If your baby seems to be in pain when she tries to move her bowels, try drinking 6 ounces of prune juice or 8 ounces of apple juice yourself once or twice a day. If this doesn't help, call your baby's doctor. She or he may suggest giving the baby 1 or 2 ounces of pear juice diluted with water or 1 teaspoon of Karo syrup in a 3- to 4-ounce bottle of breast milk.

On the other hand, your baby's stools may become looser in response to something you have eaten—large quantities of fruit juice, for example, or certain foods in the cabbage family.

Try to determine the offending food and avoid it. Don't take a strong laxative, because this can give your baby diarrhea, and don't give your baby a laxative.

Some babies go several days without moving their bowels. After the first month or two, this is common. But if your baby doesn't move her bowels for a week, check with your doctor. And be forewarned: When the baby begins to move her bowels again, a great deal of soft, unformed stool may appear in several diapers in a row.

To prevent infection in either you or your baby, wash your hands after diapering and before nursing her.

What Is Your Baby Like?

All new babies have certain characteristics in common. They all have facial configurations particularly suited for nursing—the receding chin and flat nose that let them get their faces in the right position at the breast, and the well-developed cheek muscles they need for suckling. They all cry when they want something, they all feed often, and they all need to be taken care of. They're all tiny, dependent, defenseless, and incredibly appealing.

However, we now know scientifically what parents have always known—that each baby comes into this world with a unique personality. Studies that have followed children from birth into adulthood have found that individuals differ greatly right from the beginning in such characteristics as activity level;

regularity in biological function (hunger, sleep, urination, and bowel movements); adaptability to change; acceptance of new situations; sensitivity to noise, light, and other sensory stimulation; mood (cheerfulness or crankiness); distractibility; intensity of feelings and responses; and persistence. From the time each of us draws our first breath, we have our own distinctive temperament.

Furthermore, children's temperaments influence the way we respond to them. A cheerful baby is treated differently from a fussy one, an active one from a docile one, and a predictable one from one with very irregular patterns.

Since you'll respond to your baby's personality, it's helpful to try to figure out his temperament and to accept his uniqueness as an individual. You may recognize your child immediately in the following profiles, or decide he's a combination of several, or realize that his personality is different from anything described here. Whichever way your baby is, the important thing for you to do is to accept and love him for the way he is, not for the way you would like him to be.

The Alarm Clock: She has an inner clock that wakes her regularly, about every two hours in the early weeks. She sleeps about the same time every day, tends to move her bowels at about the same time every day, is hungry at regular intervals, and in general has predictable patterns. She's easy to live with and easy to take care of.

The Nonconformist: This is the baby who tries parents' souls. He sleeps for two hours one morning, for 15 minutes the next, and not at all the third. He's ravenously hungry Monday morning and totally uninterested in eating on Tuesday. He offers few clues to his wants. If left to set his own feeding schedule, he innocently runs his mother ragged.

This child benefits from parental guidance in helping to regulate his living patterns, but as one mother said, "Trying to schedule him is like walking up the down escalator." You may have to ride with his nonschedule for a while, and end up compromising somewhere between the regularity you would like and the irregularity that comes naturally to the baby.

There is probably more of a pattern to your baby's activities than you think. Try keeping a log of the times he nurses, the times he sleeps, and the times he moves his bowels. After a few days, you may find a certain rhythm that was not apparent at first.

The Good Eater: She comes to the breast with a good appetite and an inborn knowledge of technique. She eats well, suckling so enthusiastically that she develops blisters on the middle of both upper and lower lips. These don't bother the baby; the skin falls off, another blister forms, and the cycle repeats itself till the baby's lips become used to her energetic nursing.

The Waiter: He doesn't become interested in nursing until about the fourth or fifth day. He may be sleepy from childbirth medication, or he may not feel like exerting himself until his mother's milk flows copiously. This baby needs to be seen by a lactation consultant or a doctor to be sure he isn't on the road to serious trouble.

The Dawdler: She's a slow eater who nurses for a few minutes, then rests awhile. Other times she mouths the nipple, tastes the milk, and then sets to work. She takes the milk in her own good time and cannot be hurried.

The Dozer: He likes to sleep, especially at mealtimes. You may be able to rouse him by dabbing him on the forehead with a sponge dampened with cool water; expressing a little milk into his

How to Discourage Biting

A baby who is actively nursing cannot bite, since her tongue extends over her lower gum and if she bit down, she'd bite her own tongue. Biting happens most often toward the end of a feeding, or when a baby is about to fall asleep. Babies are smart! Once they realize that every time they start to bite, they get taken off the breast, they learn that this kind of behavior isn't getting them what they really want, and they'll stop. The following suggestions work well:

❖ As soon as your baby starts to bite down on your breast, break the suction by inserting your finger in the corner of her mouth and withdraw your breast.

❖ As you take your breast away, look your baby in the eye and say "No" firmly but gently. Do this every time your baby tries to bite. Do not smile when you say this; your baby may interpret this as a game you're playing. You might even look at your baby with a sad expression. Any baby old enough to bite can read facial expressions.

❖ One mother we know began socializing her children by saying, "That hurts Mommy. We don't hurt other people," as she took her biting baby off the breast. She repeated this same litany over and over again as her four children grew into toddlers, providing a continuing way to teach them not to bite, kick, hit, or otherwise hurt others.

❖ If your baby is teething, you can massage her gums with your finger, give her a cold washcloth to bite down on just before you nurse her, and give her special teething toys and soothers. If she has begun eating solids, you can give her teething biscuits or bagels. (Watch her closely to be sure she doesn't break off a piece that she can choke on.) If the baby seems to be in pain, you can use an over-the-counter pain reliever like infant acetaminophen (Tylenol).

❖ Try putting her down, walking away for a moment, and then returning to put her back on the breast. When you return, be gentle as you tell your baby, "Be gentle." While this may seem like punishment, it's not. It's discipline (a word that comes from the Latin for "education"). By interrupting breastfeeding when your baby bites the breast, you're teaching her that biting and nursing are not compatible, and that biting is not acceptable. This is only one of the many lessons you'll be giving her in the years to come.

❖ If you can anticipate when the biting is likely to start, take your baby off your breast ahead of time. Keep your finger close to her mouth and watch her carefully; as soon as she stops nursing actively or looks playful, remove her from your breast.

❖ Quietly say your baby's name while drawing her close to you; this distracts her and gets her back to nursing.

mouth; taking off some of his clothing; leaning him forward on your lap; walking your fingers up his spine; or massaging his legs and arms. Playing with him before a feeding may encourage him to stay awake, and changing diapers after the first breast may wake him up enough to take the second. (For other ways to wake a sleepy baby, refer to the box on page 116.)

The Biter: He comes down hard on your breast, chewing it as if he had been born with a mouthful of sharp teeth. However, even an infant can learn not to bite the breast that feeds him. For ways to discourage biting, see the box on the facing page.

The Overeager Beaver: She becomes so excited at feeding time that she moves her head quickly from side to side, grasps the breast, then loses it and ends up screaming in frustration. Handle her gently, speak to her softly, keep putting her back on your breast. Try to nurse her before she gets frantically hungry, even if you have to wake her sometimes to do it. Eventually, she gets the idea and settles in.

The Spitter: Chubby and healthy, she may continue to spit up milk after nearly every feeding until she's almost a year old and you're convinced that you, the baby, and your home will always smell like cheese. (The smell is a lot milder while she's on breast milk alone.) If the spit-up milk shoots out forcibly in what is known as "projectile vomiting," call your baby's doctor. Otherwise, don't worry.

The Lopsided Nurser: She develops a preference for one of your breasts. She's not lopsided, but you may soon get that way. What to do?

❖ If one breast is producing more milk than the other, offer the less full one first at every feeding: Your baby will drain it better and encourage it to produce more; when it does, you can go back to alternating—if your baby is agreeable.

❖ Express or pump milk from the less favored breast and save it for a relief bottle.

❖ Switch nursing positions: Hold your baby more vertically or in the clutch (football) hold (see page 107), or nurse lying down.

❖ Try the slide-over technique. Using the cradle hold (see page 106), start your baby on the breast she prefers. When it is time to switch, slide her over into a clutch hold at the other breast, without changing her lying position. A pillow on your lap makes it easier to do this smoothly without disturbing her.

❖ If you can't influence your baby to give both breasts equal treatment, forget about it and pad your bra on the smaller side when you go out. When you stop nursing, you'll regain your symmetry.

The Unhappy Archer: He pulls away from your nipple during feedings, arches his back, and cries loudly. Babies who do

Cutting Down on Spitting Up

Many babies spit up milk after nearly every feeding, but as one experienced family doctor says, "In a healthy baby, spitting up is a laundry problem, not a medical problem." To minimize spitting, try the following suggestions.

✤ If your baby seems to be gulping down milk at a fast and furious rate, try feeding him more often instead of waiting until he's desperately hungry.

✤ If you're engorged, your baby may be swallowing air as he latches on. To relieve engorgement before a feeding, express a little milk and apply a warm or cold compress (whichever feels better) to your breasts. Of course, if you're feeding your baby often enough, your breasts are less likely to become engorged.

✤ If your milk is coming too quickly at the beginning, express a little or let some flow into an absorbent cloth before nursing.

✤ If your baby seems to be taking in more than he can handle, nurse on one breast only at each feeding.

✤ Prop your baby back at a 30-degree angle; if he's still awake 20 to 30 minutes after a nursing, burp him. This helps the milk settle in his stomach and discourages it from coming up with the air bubble.

✤ When you do burp your baby, do it gently.

✤ Have an ample supply of bibs and burping cloths wherever you are. Wear washable clothing for the spit-up duration, which may last several months.

---

this sometimes are diagnosed with GER (gastroesophageal reflux; see the discussion on page 155).

The Playgirl/Playboy: Practically every baby falls into this category at some time—usually at about four or five months. By this time babies are more aware of the world around them and eager to show how much they love you. He'll suddenly pull away in the middle of a feeding to flash you a bright toothless smile. Or she'll turn her head in response to a voice or footstep. He'll stroke your breast or face with his dimpled little hand. She'll play with the buttons on your blouse.

This is such a beautiful way to cement a loving relationship that you should make every effort to relax and enjoy these longer, more playful feedings. If you occasionally want the feeding to go more quickly, nurse in a dark, quiet room free from distractions.

Years from now, you may look back and see how these nursing behaviors predicted how your child's personality would develop.

What Will You Call It?

You may not be able to imagine a time when your baby will be talking and asking for "num num" or "nursy" or "titty," or some of the other words that sound so cute just between the two of you, but that might bring a blush to your cheeks if uttered, say, at your employer's family Christmas party.

So think ahead. You may be nursing long after your child has learned to talk. Use a hand signal or a word for nursing that won't embarrass you if your child says it in public. Instead of using a more explicit word for nursing, one mother always asked her baby if he wanted to drink. When he started to talk, his word for nursing, "dra," was a code word between him and his mother. This mother's second child transformed "drink" into "gingky." Her third would ask for "mee" for "milk." The daughter of another mother, who would ask, "Do you want me to feed you?" came to call nursing "feed'ly," a code word that the outside world didn't know and didn't need to know. Her second baby asked for "more," and that became her special word for nursing.

Life as Part of a Nursing Family

It takes a couple of months for you and your baby to become attuned to each other. The first few weeks you're both busy learning how to nurse and the next few, you're perfecting the art. During this time you come to know what to expect of your life together.

You learn that there are days when everything goes smoothly—and days when nothing does. You learn that there are days when your baby is cranky and days when you're cranky. You learn that you can cope with all these ups and downs because that's what life is all about. By the time these first couple of months have passed, the trial-and-error period is over. You don't have long lists of questions about breastfeeding. You know what to do—and you go about doing it. You and your baby are a nursing pair.

CHAPTER EIGHT

Diet, Exercise, and Your Health

"Since I changed my eating habits while I was pregnant,
I've been surprised at how much more energy
I have and how much better I feel. I had intended
for my baby to reap the benefits of my healthier diet,
but as it turned out, we both did."

KAREN Baton Rouge, Louisiana

A
s a nursing mother you take it for granted that you need to take care of your baby. The good news for your baby is that even if you don't eat well—even if you're anemic, in fact—you can still give your baby the best nutrition in the world, your healthy breast milk.

But what about you? At the same time that you're caring for your baby, you need to take care of yourself, as well. In this chapter, we talk about how your diet, your activity level, and the process of breastfeeding affect your well-being and your post-childbirth weight. We also discuss how to deal with baby blues and postpartum depression. In Chapter 9, we'll talk about how you look. And in Chapter 10, we'll talk about how various medicines and drugs affect both you and your baby.

Diet: What You Eat, What You Drink

Just as you "eat for two" during pregnancy, you continue to "eat for two" during the time when most or all of your baby's food intake comes from your milk. Sorry, but this doesn't mean that you eat twice as much as you normally eat. It does mean that what you eat is reflected in the milk you produce. And it also means that you'll be eating more than you did before you became pregnant—but certainly not double the amount.

Eating smart can provide what your body needs for the most part, and can also improve the way your body uses vitamins and minerals. It's a good idea to keep taking your prenatal vitamins, and take them with orange juice, not milk. (Vitamin C enhances the absorption of iron, while calcium inhibits it.) However, don't make the false assumption that the vitamins can replace a well-balanced diet. Supplements don't supply the necessary carbohydrates, proteins, fats, fiber, and other nutrients found in food.

If you were eating well before you became pregnant, you won't have to make any significant changes during the first three months of pregnancy. Then you'll only need to eat a little bit more (about an extra 200 calories a day) for the rest of your pregnancy. plus an additional 300 calories as long as you are breastfeeding exclusively— that is, feeding your child nothing besides your breast milk. If your eating habits have been catch-as-catch-can, this is a good time to improve them. You'll benefit and your baby will be off to the best possible start.

Even if your diet is not optimal, your breast milk will in almost all cases still be good. (A recent study in India found that even the babies of anemic mothers did not develop iron deficiency by six months of age.) However, you won't feel well with a poor diet, and how you feel is important for how well you'll be able to take care of your baby, regardless of how you feed her. Also, researchers caution that a diet of highly processed foods—which are often high in sugar, fat, and preservatives (otherwise known as junk food)—during pregnancy and lactation could result in overweight, diabetic children.

Over the past few years American eating habits have undergone many changes. Many of us have become more nutrition-conscious, and in line with our new awareness we've been eating more fresh vegetables and fruits; more fish, pasta, dried beans, and peas;

more whole-grain foods; more low-fat milk and yogurt; and less red meat and whole milk. All these changes are in line with current guidelines for sound nutrition during pregnancy and lactation.

Guidelines for Healthy Eating

In 1992 the U.S. Department of Agriculture (USDA) released the Food Guide Pyramid to demonstrate graphically the key aspects of a healthy diet. However, many nutritionists took issue with some of the recommendations, and in 2005 the USDA released a revised version called My Pyramid.

We prefer the pyramid developed by the Department of Nutrition at the Harvard School of Public Health (see illustration opposite). This pyramid is based on the latest nutritional science and is not affected by any commercial interests, one criticism leveled at the USDA pyramid.

Harvard's Healthy Eating Pyramid emphasizes an overall healthy eating pattern for adults. It does not give portion sizes. Its message: Eat a variety of foods, as long as the amount you eat of any particular food or type of food is in proportion to its place in a healthy diet. On this plan, a healthy diet includes more foods from the base of the pyramid than from the middle, and foods at the top should be eaten sparingly, if at all.

Basically, if you follow the pyramid, your diet will consist of:

❖ A large percentage of whole-grain foods (brown rice, whole wheat pasta, and oats, for example), fruits and vegetables, and healthy fats and oils.

❖ Somewhat smaller amounts of fish, poultry, and eggs, along with nuts, seeds, beans, and tofu.

❖ A still smaller proportion of dairy (preferably low-fat milk, cheese, and yogurt).

❖ And very small amounts of red meat, butter, potatoes, refined grains (white rice, bread, and pasta), salt, and sugary drinks and sweets.

❖ The entire pyramid rests on a broad base of daily exercise and weight control.

To figure out how much food you need, calculate your own daily calorie requirements. Figure out the amount that keeps you at a stable, normal weight, and then add 500 calories while you're nursing. For example, a woman who is 5 feet 4 inches tall and normally weighs 120 pounds probably needs about 2,200 to 2,700 calories a day while she's breastfeeding.

Eat foods that have a high proportion of nutrients for the calories it

The Healthy Eating Pyramid

USE SPARINGLY:
red meat & butter;
refined grains: white rice,
bread & pasta; potatoes;
sugary drinks & sweets; salt

DAIRY
(1–2 servings a day)
or vitamin D/calcium
supplements

DAIRY

HEALTHY FATS/OILS:
olive, canola, soy,
corn, sunflower,
peanut & other
vegetable oils;
trans-fat-free
margarine

FISH, POULTRY & EGGS

**NUTS, SEEDS,
BEANS & TOFU**

**WHOLE
GRAINS:**
Brown rice,
whole wheat
pasta, oats,
etc.

VEGETABLES & FRUITS

**HEALTHY
FATS/OILS**

WHOLE GRAINS

**DAILY EXERCISE &
WEIGHT CONTROL**

Adapted from The Healthy Eating Pyramid, copyright © 2008. For more information about The Healthy Eating Pyramid, please see The Nutrition Source, Department of Nutrition, Harvard School of Public Health, http://www.thenutritionsource.org, and *Eat, Drink, and Be Healthy,* by Walter C. Willett, M.D. and Patrick J. Skerrett (2005), Free Press/Simon & Schuster Inc.

contains. Empty calories—highly processed foods that fill you up without fulfilling your nutritional needs—deprive both you and your baby. You can eat the right kinds of foods and enjoy them, too, with flexible dietary guidelines. Read labels—your cereal choice shouldn't have sugar as its first or second ingredient. Don't top your vegetables with gobs of butter. To be sure you're eating well for you, consult your doctor (or a registered dietitian or a nutritionist with a degree in nutrition—to find one, see the Resource Appendix), and become knowledgeable about nutrition in general.

Components to Pay Special Attention To

A healthy diet includes nutrients in many different categories, each of which plays a role in keeping you healthy. In the following pages, we talk about recommended amounts of calcium, vitamin D, iron, protein, DHA, and folic acid, and foods that contain them.

Calcium: Calcium is an important mineral in the diets of all women to prevent osteoporosis, a thinning of the bones that causes widow's humps and fractures later in life. Calcium is also important for healthy teeth.

Currently, the average American adult gets only 500 to 700 milligrams (mg) of calcium per day, but the National Academy of Sciences' recommendations for adequate intake are 1,000 mg daily for 18- to 50-year-olds

of both sexes, including pregnant and nursing women. If you're eating a well-balanced diet, including foods rich in calcium, you will be getting enough of this mineral. The Healthy Eating Pyramid recommends one to two servings of dairy foods per day (or the equivalent in other foods or in supplements). It's always best to get your nutrients from the grocery store rather than the drugstore—that is, from food rather than supplements.

Women who have ever breastfed have half the risk for bone fractures as women who did not nurse babies, and the longer a woman's lifetime lactation lasts, the lower her risk of fracture. This seems to be one more proof that nature really wants women to breastfeed. While nursing mothers lose some bone mass during lactation, by one year after weaning, their bone mass is completely restored, no matter what they eat.

Milk is an excellent source of both calcium and protein. But if you don't like or can't tolerate milk, you can obtain both these nutrients from other sources. However, if you don't drink at least 1 cup of milk a day, you may want to increase your intake of protein and calcium. Other good sources of calcium include yogurt, calcium-fortified orange juice, cheddar cheese, tofu, canned salmon or sardines (with bones), dark leafy greens (like kale, mustard, collard, or turnip greens), dried beans, and broccoli.

Vitamin D: Vitamin D is just as important as calcium for both your baby and you. In fact, it helps your body to absorb the calcium in food. In recent years, vitamin D deficiency has shown up in some breastfed babies, leading to rickets, a softening of the bones. Although extreme vitamin D deficiency is rare in the United States, some research has found that up to 78 percent of breastfed babies who did not receive supplemental vitamin D were deficient. For this reason, the American Academy of Pediatrics now recommends vitamin D drops for breastfed babies within the first few days of life. (For more about vitamins for your baby, see Chapter 17.)

This vitamin is important for you, too. Vitamin D is a complex hormone that helps to regulate immune system function and helps prevent such immune disorders as multiple sclerosis, rheumatoid arthritis, type 1 diabetes, and cancer, in addition to helping to protect you from osteoporosis (a loss of bone density later in life), as well as periodontal (gum) disease.

You should be getting 1,000 IU (International Units) of vitamin D per day, either in a supplement or in food. You should take a vitamin D supplement if you don't drink at least 3 cups of vitamin D–enriched milk a day or the equivalent in other dairy foods. This is especially important if you have a dark complexion, since some dark-complexioned women excrete less vitamin D in their milk than do women with light skin. You can also get vitamin D through normal exposure to direct sunlight. If you're not a milk drinker or you get little exposure to sunlight, ask your doctor to order a blood test for vitamin D.

Iron: Lean red meats and organ meats (liver and heart) are rich sources of zinc and iron in readily absorbable forms. You can increase your iron intake by eating iron-fortified cereals, cooking acidic foods like tomato sauce in cast-iron pots (some of the iron from the pots will leach into the food during cooking), and choosing darker cuts of fish and poultry. Since acidic and vitamin C–rich foods improve iron absorption, another easy way to increase your intake is to eat foods in these nutritional combinations (for example, drinking vitamin C–rich orange juice with iron-fortified cereal, or eating meatballs with tomato sauce). If you drink a lot of tea, take it between meals, since large quantities taken with meals may interfere with the absorption of iron.

Protein: The Department of Nutrition at Harvard's School of Public Health recommends up to two 2½- to 3-ounce servings of protein-rich foods a day for the average person. This means that healthy portions of meat, poultry, and fish are much smaller than those served in most restaurants. One serving of meat or fish is only about the size of a deck of playing cards or the palm of your hand.

Next to human milk, eggs contain the most usable protein in the human diet. More than half the protein is in the white, which has no fat or cholesterol, whereas the yolk has both. While you can eat as many egg whites as you want, it's probably best not to eat more than four yolks a week, including those you use in cooking. In some recipes you can use egg substitutes or two whites to equal one whole egg. Other good sources of protein are lean cooked fish, meat, or poultry; dried beans or peas; cottage cheese; chili with meat and beans; tofu; nuts; and sunflower and pumpkin seeds.

Peanut butter is also a good source of protein, but as of this writing the medical community isn't in agreement about whether pregnant and nursing moms, especially those with a family history of allergy, should eat it (see page 181).

DHA: The long-chain fatty acid DHA (docosahexaenoic acid) is important for your baby's brain and eye development and is also thought to raise IQ scores in childhood. DHA occurs naturally in breast milk—if the mother's diet contains fish, red meats, organ meats, and eggs. Most infant formulas now have DHA (those that do cost about 15 percent more than those without it), but the jury is still out as to whether the additives in formula offer the same benefits to babies as the DHA in breast milk, or whether they might even be harmful.

DHA is also important for adults—especially for mental health, cognitive functioning, and vision. You give your DHA stores to your baby during pregnancy and lactation, and it takes more than nine months after giving birth to return to your normal DHA levels. For this reason, some physicians and nutritionists have begun to encourage pregnant and nursing women to take a DHA supplement, which is available over the counter from pharmacies and health food stores. However, such supplementation is still controversial, because so far there's no scientific evidence of how much DHA is needed and whether there are indeed actual benefits for mothers or their babies.

Folic Acid (Folate): This B vitamin is crucial in the diets of women of childbearing age, especially for women who are considering pregnancy, and also for those who are already pregnant or lactating. The vitamin is important for ensuring the health and normal development of both mother and infant; it is especially important for preventing certain birth defects. Research also suggests that it may reduce the risk of heart attack.

Current daily folic acid recommendations from the Institute of Medicine of the National Academy of Sciences are 400 micrograms (mcg) for nonpregnant, nonlactating sexually active women; 600 mcg during pregnancy; and 500 mcg during lactation. To obtain essential amounts of folate in food, a breastfeeding woman needs to consume at least 2,000 calories daily or take a multivitamin pill with 400 mcg of folic acid.

You can get a good folate intake by eating whole-grain products like bread, rice, pasta, and cereals, or those made with enriched or fortified flour. Other foods high in this nutrient include citrus fruits and juices; spinach, cauliflower, broccoli, and asparagus; dried beans and lentils; and beef, veal, chicken, or turkey liver. However, the U.S. Public Health Service still recommends a supplement for women of childbearing age.

The Vegetarian Diet

A meatless diet can provide a healthful eating pattern if you choose your foods carefully. However, maintaining a vegetarian diet that provides all the nutrition a pregnant or nursing woman needs can be somewhat of a challenge: First, you need to get enough calories from your diet, and second, you need to get enough protein. It would be a good idea to consult a dietitian or nutritionist to be sure that you're meeting your baby's nutritional needs, as well as your own. To find a professional, see the Resource Appendix.

✤ Getting enough calories. Since plant products are lower in calories than animal foods, it's sometimes hard to take in enough calories. If you eat no meat, fish, or poultry, but do eat eggs and dairy products (ovo-lacto vegetarian) or dairy products alone (lacto-vegetarian), you'll have an easier time getting all your nutrients. Be aware, though, that if you're eating large quantities of cheese as a substitute for lean meat, you may be taking in too much fat.

✤ Obtaining enough protein. Your need for protein, vitamins, and minerals is higher when you're pregnant and nursing. Therefore, vegetarians—and especially vegans, who eat no animal-based foods—have to be especially aware of food choices and the way to combine plant-food proteins to make them "complete," that is, containing all the essential amino acids. Amino acids are the building blocks of proteins and are essential for human health. Of the 20 amino acids found in proteins, our bodies can make only 10; the others must come from the foods we eat every day.

Animal-based foods like chicken, fish, eggs, dairy products, beef, and pork are rich in amino acids. Some plants, such as dried beans (black, kidney, great northern, red, and white beans), peas, soy, nuts, and seeds are sources of protein, but since they generally lack one or more of the essential amino acids, they need to be combined with whole grains.

Most cultures in which people don't regularly eat meat have developed combinations of plant foods that provide complete proteins. Some Latin Americans, for example, eat beans with either rice or corn, and in Nepal, villagers typically eat rice with lentil sauce at every meal. You don't have to eat these food combinations at the same time; eating them over the course of a day is fine.

A vegan's breast milk lacks sufficient DHA, the omega-3 fat found in fish (discussed in Chapter 1), and essential amino acids. If you ordinarily follow a vegan diet, you'll be helping your baby if you eat eggs and dairy products during pregnancy and lactation. If you're a vegan, you can get some DHA from walnuts, canola or soybean oil, grains, green vegetables, ground flaxseeds, or a flaxseed oil supplement.

If you have been a vegan for several years, you and your breastfed baby should be taking vitamin B_{12} supplements. Your breastfed baby will also need vitamin D supplements (see Chapter 17).

A Healthy Vegetarian Diet

For You: While you're eating for two, your daily needs include six or more servings of grains; two to three servings of dried beans, nuts, seeds, eggs, or meat substitutes; three or more servings of vegetables (one or more of dark leafy greens); two to four servings of fruit (at least one citrus); and two to three glasses of milk or its calcium equivalent. You may need supplements that include vitamin B_{12}, vitamin D, calcium, iron, zinc, and folic acid.

The above servings are minimums; you'll need more food than described here to get enough calories. If you maintained a healthy weight before you became pregnant, you should now be eating about 500 calories more than you were eating then, or about 200 calories more than you ate during pregnancy.

For Your Child: You need to be especially careful that your infants and young children obtain enough protein to stay healthy and grow properly—especially after weaning. They also need reliable sources of vitamin B_{12}, vitamin D, calcium, iron, and zinc.

Beginning at six months of age, your child will need more protein in his diet—regardless of whether or not you continue to breastfeed. He'll need extra protein sources until he's about five or six years old. In infancy, he can obtain protein through pureed tofu, cottage cheese, and pureed and strained legumes.

Fasting

Some religions stipulate that believers neither eat nor drink for various periods of time, which might include a 24-hour span, or a month's worth of daily abstinence from sunrise to sunset. However, most religious strictures exempt people with special medical needs, including pregnant and breastfeeding women. While you're nursing a baby under one year of age, you need energy from adequate nutrition, and your baby needs a plentiful supply of milk. Fasting is generally not recommended while nursing.

What You Drink

Liquids are important, especially while nursing, since you need fluids to make milk. A good rule of thumb is to drink to satisfy your thirst. This usually turns out to be about six to eight glasses of fluid a day, including water and other beverages like milk, juice, coffee, and tea. Remember, though, that the caffeine in the beverages you drink may wind up in your milk and make your baby more wakeful. Although we've all heard that it's important to drink eight glasses of water a day, there's no scientific evidence for this recommendation.

Pay attention to what your body tells you. No matter how busy you are, don't disregard your body's signals. You'll probably become thirstier while you're nursing, and especially when you perspire during exercise or in hot weather. Besides thirst, another sign that you're not drinking enough is the color of your urine. If your urine is dark in color, showing that it's very concentrated, you need to drink more. On the other hand, if you're feeling overfull or bloated, you may be drinking too much. Actually, too much fluid (more than 12 glasses a day) may decrease your milk production. In other words, as in "Goldilocks and the Three Bears," you need neither too little nor too much—but just the right amount.

One way to get enough fluids is to keep a pitcher of water and a glass close by your favorite nursing place throughout the day. (This is better for the environment than buying water in plastic bottles.) A cup of water, milk, soup, fruit juice, or other liquid should become part of your routine before each nursing. Although caffeinated beverages like coffee, tea, and cola are diuretics (that is, they increase the excretion of urine from the body), when taken in moderation they don't lead to dehydration.

Should You Avoid Any Foods While You're Nursing?

About 6 percent of American children under age three have a food allergy. If you have no food allergies yourself, and neither you nor your baby's father has a family history of allergy, most of the foods you eat won't cause problems for your baby. There's no overall evidence that restricting the diet of a pregnant or nursing mom *with no history of food allergy* will prevent allergic reactions in her child. Exclusive breastfeeding for six months, with no

solid foods until after that time, is the best way to prevent allergies.

However, if there is a family history of allergy or if any of your children have food allergies, check with your doctor. Standard advice has been for mothers to avoid peanuts and foods that contain them (like peanut butter), other nuts, and seafood while nursing, since elements of these foods can be passed to the baby. Many allergists have suggested not giving these foods to a child with a family history of food allergy until age three. And for children showing signs of allergy, mothers may be advised to avoid eggs, dairy, and wheat. However, recent research suggests that giving some of these foods early in life seems to prevent allergy (see Chapter 17). At this time, the jury in the medical community is still out, so be sure to talk to your pediatrician before giving your baby these foods.

Some foods eaten by a nursing mother seem to affect her baby adversely in other ways. Cow's milk is an offender for some women. Some nursing babies who have shown symptoms of colic (see Chapter 7) showed fewer symptoms when their mothers stopped drinking milk or eating dairy products for a while. Daily exercise and weight control—both key elements affecting your health—form the base of the Healthy Eating Pyramid. To maintain a well-balanced diet, eat more foods from the bottom of the pyramid and less from the top. It may take from two to four weeks for these foods to be eliminated from your and your baby's systems. In some cases, all the symptoms have disappeared when

Avoiding Harmful Environmental Substances

In Food

✤ Fish is a wonderful food for everyone, and especially for pregnant and nursing women. However, so much of our fish supply is currently contaminated that you need to be careful about which fish you eat until you wean your child. To avoid unsafe levels of mercury and other harmful chemicals, don't eat local freshwater fish unless your state health department or department of environmental conservation pronounces it safe. If there are no advisories, eat local fish no more often than once a week.

✤ Eat no more than 12 ounces of cooked fish per week, and choose from a variety of different species, fresh or canned.

✤ Eat no more than 6 ounces of white albacore canned tuna per week, and no more than 12 ounces of light tuna.

✤ Wild salmon has fewer contaminants and less mercury than farmed salmon (unfortunately, it's twice the price).

✤ Choose smaller fish like cod, whitefish, pollock, mahi-mahi, halibut, haddock, flounder, sole, catfish, crawfish, tilapia, squid, sardines, herring, anchovies, and shellfish. These species, which are lower on the food chain, are less likely to contain chemicals.

✤ Don't eat large fish like shark, swordfish, tilefish, king or Spanish mackerel, Chilean sea bass (toothfish), fresh tuna, grouper, marlin, eel, or orange roughy. Bigger fish are more contaminated because they eat the smaller fish.

✤ Don't eat raw shellfish.

✤ Peel or thoroughly wash fruits and vegetables to get rid of pesticide residues.

their breastfeeding mothers gave up dairy products. And we've received anecdotal reports from women who seemed to have more milk when they stopped eating dairy products.

It takes an estimated four to eight hours between the time you eat a food and the time it affects your milk, with liquids traveling faster than solids. If you can find any relationship between certain foods that you eat and your baby's reactions, it's easy enough to avoid these foods. No one food is essential. If you keep a food diary of what you eat and how your baby reacts, you can see if there's a correlation between the two.

If your baby is colicky, avoid all dairy for a while. If her symptoms go away, you may have nailed the cause of her distress. However, you may try to drink a little milk again a couple of weeks later, since your baby may be able to tolerate it then. But if she reacts with colic, this is a sign to eliminate it from your diet.

✥ Cut away the fatty portions of meats, poultry, and fish (dark sections and skin), since pollutants tend to be concentrated in the fat.

✥ Avoid dairy products rich in butterfat.

In Your Environment

✥ Avoid using pesticides and stay away from places where they're used, but if you must use them, use the nonspray kind.

✥ Ventilate your house well; babies absorb more pollutants through the air they breathe than through what they eat or drink.

✥ Don't use antibacterial soaps, deodorants, skin cleansers, toothpaste, and cleaning solutions. These products contain chemicals, they don't clean any better than ordinary ones, and they contribute to drug-resistant bacteria in our bodies and in the environment.

Minimize your use of antibacterial lotions, shampoos, and other personal care items.

✥ Don't give your baby breast milk or formula in polycarbonate plastic bottles (with the number 7 in the recycling triangle on the bottom), which can leach bisphenol A (BPA). (More about this in Chapter 11, including suggestions for alternatives.)

✥ Become active in organizations that pressure governmental agencies to eliminate harmful substances from the environment. (See the Website Appendix.)

✥ Remember that research consistently shows that even in a world contaminated with many chemicals, human milk is still the best food for human babies.

If your baby is showing other symptoms of milk protein allergy, like hives or bloody stool, call your pediatrician and don't start eating dairy again until the doctor says it's okay. It's still possible that once the baby's digestive system matures, and you can eventually introduce dairy back into your diet. If you do give up dairy for a long time, be sure you're still receiving enough nutrients from other foods.

Foods implicated to a lesser extent include eggs, citrus fruits, wheat, and chocolate. Some allergists have commented that the foods babies react to are often those that the mother had eaten in large amounts while she was pregnant, giving rise to the possibility that the baby may have been sensitized to them in the uterus.

Nursing babies sometimes suffer from gas after their mothers eat foods from the cabbage family, like broccoli or brussels sprouts, especially if these foods give the mother gas. Others become wakeful after their mothers drink caffeinated beverages or eat a lot of chocolate. Herbal teas can make some babies crampy, and some teas can cause serious problems. Stick to reliable brands and drink only in moderation.

Many foods that a mother eats can color her milk and also the baby's urine. For example, lots of spinach will turn milk green, shrimp or crawfish will turn it orange, and, in one case, a three-month-old baby's bright pink urine was traced to her mother's drinking a particular soda. None of this is necessarily harmful—even though it may be startling to see.

All the foods you eat flavor your milk, which is a good thing since it gets your baby used to the diet of your own culture. However, an occasional baby with a discriminating palate may not like the taste of, say, vanilla, mint, or blue cheese—just some of the flavors that come through breast milk. She may even reject your milk. As you'll find throughout your parenting career, children are unpredictable. In one study, a group of infants nursed longer, sucked more, and drank more when their mothers' milk smelled like garlic, compared to when that flavor was absent. These pint-size gourmets may have become accustomed to their mothers' garlicky diets while still in the uterus. On the other hand, one nursing mother found that her baby got sick whenever she had eaten something with garlic in it. Then she remembered that her husband suffered cramps after eating garlic, making her think that the baby might take after Dad.

You'll also want to avoid certain foods to minimize the risk of passing on environmental chemicals in your milk (as detailed in the box on pages 182–183). For the most part, however, you can eat any nourishing food you want without fear that your baby will be affected.

Protecting Your Baby and Yourself from Harmful Environmental Chemicals

Many women have been alarmed by sensational media reports about the presence of chemical residues in breast milk. Such reports rarely mention that formula, made with cow's milk and water, is also likely to contain such chemicals. The truth is that yes, there are environmental contaminants in breast milk, just as there are in air, in water, in foods, and in practically everything that human beings consume. We live in a polluted world and mother's milk reflects that, but a recent overview of studies found that not breastfeeding a baby poses more of a threat than does exposure to any agent found in breast milk. Furthermore, the disease- and infection-fighting qualities of breast milk help babies to combat the harmful effects of polluting substances. Even those ecologists and researchers who are most concerned about the contamination of our environment still maintain that breast milk is the ideal food for babies.

Since some harmful chemicals have been banned or restricted since the 1970s, their levels are declining, although they're still in the environment and probably will be for years to come. Furthermore, new substances have come on the scene, including, for example, some in widely used flame retardants. Also, various chemicals are in personal care products, and since anything we put on our bodies can be absorbed and has the potential to appear in our milk, it's a good idea to go easy on your use of scented body lotions, perfume, and the like during pregnancy and lactation.

What, then, should a nursing mother do? If you think you have had unusually high chemical exposures (as in the workplace), consult your doctor. Having your milk tested is not practical, since few labs can do the analysis, it's very expensive, and the wait for results might be so long that your child could well be in school by the time they are in. For special precautions that you can take, see the box on page 182.

The Take-Away on Eating During Lactation

✤ No matter how poor your eating habits may be, your breast milk will still be better than any formula. But you won't feel as good if you don't put the right foods into your mouth. The best reason to eat well is for your own sake.

✤ The usual diets of many Americans are low in fruits and vegetables. As a nursing mother at the 2,200-calorie level, eat a minimum of seven servings a day, including one citrus fruit (a rich source of vitamin C) and one serving of a vitamin A–rich fruit or vegetable. Some nutritionists suggest eating a variety of colors: The darker the green vegetable or the deeper the orange of the squash, the more potential vitamin A it contains. Increase your intake of leafy greens.

✤ Most American diets are too heavy in fat and sugar, and too light on complex carbohydrates (whole grains, fruits, and vegetables). You can improve yours.

✤ No one food is indispensable. Allergic to eggs? Substitute 1 ounce of meat or cheddar cheese, or a quarter cup of cottage cheese, or 2 tablespoons of peanut butter (skip the peanut butter if you have a family history of allergy).

✤ Don't like or can't drink milk? You can get equivalent nutrients from yogurt or cheese, broccoli, and bone-in canned sardines or salmon.

✤ You may want to give milk a try, even if you don't ordinarily drink it. Many women find it thirst-quenching during pregnancy and lactation. If you have problems with the lactose in milk, try starting with small amounts and gradually increasing your intake (to reasonable amounts), or drink lactase-treated milk, or both. You may end up enjoying this nutrient-packed food.

✤ Want to save money? Substitute

nonfat dry milk for liquid milk, take more of your protein in low-priced beans and grains than in meats, get cheaper cuts of meat (many of which are just as nutritious as pricier cuts), and buy fruits and vegetables in whichever form is cheapest at the time—fresh, frozen, or canned.

❖ Be guided by your own body. If you're underweight to begin with or if you're very active, you'll need more calories. If you're very overweight, you probably have enough fat stores so that you can make do with fewer calories. After you start to nurse, you shouldn't be putting on weight—if you are, you're probably eating too much. If you're losing more than half a pound a week or 2 pounds a month, you're probably not eating enough.

❖ An extra 500 calories a day in your diet, in addition to calories drawn from your body fat stores, should last you through your course of breastfeeding. If you're nursing twins or a very big baby, you may need to eat more.

Losing Weight: How Much, How Soon?

Breastfeeding does not make women gain weight. In fact, it uses up calories and therefore helps to get rid of extra weight. Nature's way of providing the extra calories needed for milk production is to store up fat during pregnancy. Then lactation helps to use up these fat stores. As a nursing mother, you're more likely to lose the fat you added (especially the lower-body fat) during your pregnancy than is the woman who does not nurse her baby. If you nurse your baby exclusively for the first four months, you'll probably lose more weight than if you combine breast milk and formula.

Expect to lose no more than 2 pounds per month while you're nursing, unless you're very overweight. In six months you'll have lost 12 pounds, and by eight months, you'll have lost 16. This, in addition to the weight you lost with your baby's birth, will probably bring you back down to or close to your prepregnancy weight. This amount of weight loss will not affect your baby's growth and will not increase the concentration of harmful environmental chemicals in your milk (see discussion on page 184). It took nine months to put on all those pounds, so it's not unrealistic to expect it to take about the same amount of time to take them off.

This gradual weight loss may happen without any special effort on your part—many nursing mothers who eat normally lose about 1 to 1½ pounds a month for the first four to six months after delivery without making any special effort to shed pounds. However, about one in five nursing mothers does not lose weight while breastfeeding. And some do lose most of the pregnancy weight but seem to retain the last few pounds until they wean their babies. The best approach seems to be to wait for two or three months after childbirth to see how your body responds.

If you're losing steadily, even if it's only 1 pound a month, you don't have to do anything special about your eating habits. If you're not losing steadily, you can start to cut back gradually. By the time your baby is nine months old and is taking less milk in proportion to other foods in his diet, you can begin your plan to lose 1 to 2 pounds per week. Losing weight slowly by changing your eating and exercise habits is better than dropping weight quickly, since you're more likely to keep the pounds off. A well-planned exercise schedule is important in your weight-loss program for a number of reasons, which we'll talk about in more detail later in this chapter.

In devising your own plan, pay attention to portion sizes. How much you eat is a crucial element in any weight-loss or weight-stabilization program. For example, as we mentioned earlier, a healthy portion size of pasta is a half cup—far less than the amount served in most family restaurants.

In addition to monitoring portion size, you can do the following:

❧ Substitute skim milk and nonfat yogurt for whole milk products.

❧ Broil, boil, roast, or bake meats and potatoes instead of frying them.

What the Labels Usually Mean*

The following descriptions give information for a single serving:

Calorie-free—no more than 5 calories

Sugar-free—less than ½ g of sugar

Salt-free—fewer than 5 mg of sodium

Low-sodium—no more than 140 mg of sodium

Fat-free—less than ½ g of fat

Low-fat—no more than 3 g of fat

Light—⅓ fewer calories than, or half the fat in, the regular version of a similar food

*This information was provided by the Center for Science in the Public Interest, Washington, D.C.

❧ Eat more fish and poultry and less red meat.

❧ Eat smaller amounts of fatty meats and fatty fish.

❧ Snack on raw vegetables and fruits instead of potato chips and cookies.

❧ Eat fresh fruits rather than sweetened canned ones.

❖ While you should consume high-calorie fruits like avocados and cherries in moderation, they are healthy foods that don't provide the kind of empty calories found in snacks like potato chips.

❖ Eliminate or eat very little of high-fat cheeses, rich sauces, fatty salad dressings, sugary soft drinks and cereals, cookies, cakes, pastries, and candy.

❖ Although a mother's intake of moderate amounts of artificial sweeteners doesn't seem to adversely affect her nursing baby, there's no good evidence that these products help people to lose weight, and you're probably better off minimizing your intake of them.

❖ Read the food labels (see the box on page 187).

Still, every woman is different, and some nursing mothers retain at least some of the weight they gained during pregnancy longer than others do. What, then, to do about it?

First of all, wait a couple of months after your baby's birth before trying to shed pounds. Then, for as long as you're breastfeeding, don't diet strenuously. Don't follow a liquid diet, take any weight-loss drugs or herbal supplements, eliminate any specific food groups, or cut your calories below the recommended amount for your height and build.

Here's why: Your body needs enough nutrients to produce milk. If you cut down too drastically on what you eat, you'll be robbing yourself. Your body will maintain the quality of your milk at your expense by cutting into your lean tissues (your muscles) and your bones. You could lose muscle tone and bone density, and become anemic.

If You're Considerably Overweight: The advice against losing a great deal of weight during lactation does not necessarily hold for women who are very overweight. If you're considerably overweight, you'll have more problems nursing, and the more overweight you are, the more difficulty you're likely to have, for several reasons. The areola of a very heavy woman is often so large that it's hard for her baby to compress it enough to get a good milk supply. Also, heavier women have more trouble finding a comfortable position for nursing—and sometimes can't see their babies at the breast well enough to see if they're nursing correctly. Although a lactation consultant may be able to help with breastfeeding, it's still a good idea—for both your and your baby's health—to work out a weight loss program with your doctor and/or your nutritionist. While you're on a major weight-loss program, taking a vitamin supplement will help ensure that you have enough vitamin B_6 in your body and in your milk.

A New Look at Your Body

Some women do lose the weight they gained during pregnancy very soon after their babies are born and remain quite slender throughout lactation and afterward. You don't have to be plump to be a good milk producer. However, other women keep their more rounded contours for a longer time.

You may need to think about your weight in a new way. Just as breastfed babies grow differently from formula-fed babies, the bodies of breastfeeding mothers tend to follow a different schedule from those of non-nursing mothers. A substantial weight gain during pregnancy helps to assure a healthy baby, and part of that weight seems to be nature's way of providing energy for milk after your baby is born.

If you're a typical contemporary Western woman, you'll probably have no more than two or three children. Recognizing that during pregnancy and lactation your nutritional status has to support two lives—yours and your baby's—and recognizing the very small proportion of time in relation to your total life span that you'll spend breastfeeding, you need to ask yourself: *Can I stand being a few pounds heavier after the birth of each baby, with the assurance that after I've stopped nursing I'll lose this extra weight?* Since you recognize the value of breastfeeding, you can probably answer this question with a ringing "Yes!" You may want to talk this issue over with your husband or partner to help him or her understand and support you.

If you want to feel beautiful now, go to your closest art museum and find paintings featuring breastfeeding mothers. Chances are that most of them will be ample in size—and you'll have a lovely standard of maternal beauty to identify with. (While you're in the museum, you might welcome one bit of news from the Vatican: A church historian has called for the end of censorship of the Madonna's breasts in paintings depicting her breastfeeding the baby Jesus.) Meanwhile, enjoy your baby, enjoy your food, and enjoy your life.

Exercise: How Much, How Soon?

You may love to exercise or you may hate it. You may have barely fitted in time between your workouts to give birth to your baby. Or you may be the kind of person who has always reacted to the thought of exercise by immediately curling up in a ball. Most likely, you're somewhere in between. Wherever on the fitness spectrum you fall, you can tailor a routine to your inclinations and your abilities, even while you're nursing.

The right kind and the right amount of exercise can bring you many benefits, not only now but throughout your life. As Robert Butler, MD, director of the International Longevity Center at Mount Sinai Hospital in New York, has said, "If doctors could prescribe exercise in pill form, it would be the single most widely prescribed drug in the world." This is particularly good news for nursing mothers, for both short-term and long-range reasons.

Following an active, well-planned exercise schedule during lactation can do wonders for you. However, before you begin a postpartum exercise program, check with your doctor. Once you have medical approval, exercise can help you by:

✤ Toning up sagging postpregnancy muscles, so you'll feel and look better.

✤ Helping you lose the weight and fat you gained in pregnancy, in combination with a measure of calorie restriction. Exercise actually tends to diminish appetite while using up calories, so it's vital in maintaining a desirable body weight.

✤ Helping to heal the backache that plagues so many new mothers, as you bend and lift more than you've probably done in your entire life. It may even help to avoid back pain in the first place.

✤ Boosting your energy level—although it's not magical enough to completely overcome the fatigue that comes from not getting enough sleep.

✤ Speeding sexual recovery by tightening muscles that were stretched during childbirth. (See Chapter 13.)

✤ Slowing bone loss during lactation, resulting in higher bone mineral density at one year postpartum, compared with women who didn't exercise.

✤ Improving cardiovascular fitness.

✤ Stimulating the release of endorphins, chemicals in the brain that reduce pain, stimulate immune response, and elevate mood.

And exercise isn't only for the postpartum period. Throughout life, it helps you build your muscles, strengthen your heart and lungs, lower your blood pressure, protect against heart attacks and cancer, improve your emotional state, and possibly lengthen your life.

Weight-bearing activities like walking, running, skating, and jogging help to control fat. They also help to increase bone density, thus helping to prevent osteoporosis. Exercise reduces stress and anxiety better and more safely than drugs and therefore contributes to your mental health. One reason exercise boosts your morale is that it releases endorphins, brain hormones that give a feeling of well-being.

Find an activity you like; exercise should actually be fun. You can share the pleasure, too, as bicycling, skating, dancing, and other vigorous activities form a good basis for lively family and other social outings. And you'll be a wonderful role model for your children, offering them one more tool for forging a healthy life.

A well-planned exercise program won't have any adverse effects regarding breastfeeding. Moderate to strenuous aerobic exercise has no negative effects on either your supply of milk or the quality of your breast milk. However, women who exercise to the point of exhaustion may find that their babies reject the breast because the taste of their milk has changed.

Postpartum Exercise

If you want to develop an exercise program, you can begin within twenty-four hours of childbirth if you are in good shape. Start easy, build up gradually, and use common sense. If you had an episiotomy, you may want to wait until you're no longer sore before you undertake vigorous exercise. Don't start exercising if you have heavy vaginal bleeding, pain, or a breast infection in the first six weeks after delivery. When you're ready, check a local gym or community center for a postpartum program or look for a book about exercise after childbirth—and check with your doctor before starting.

Begin by doing pelvic tilts, deep breathing, and Kegel (pelvic floor) exercises (see the box on page 279). Kegels will also help if you have minor incontinence after childbirth. All of these are safe to do right after delivery. In a few days, you can move on to exercises to tighten your stomach muscles and stretching and bending exercises.

Don't overdo it! Pregnancy-related changes in your body persist for about four to six weeks. Pay attention to what your body tells you. Warm up slowly, rest between exercises, and stop before you feel tired. Fatigue is an enemy of successful breastfeeding. At the beginning, it's more important to establish your milk supply than to preserve your reputation as an athlete. If you develop any unusual symptoms, like pain, increased vaginal bleeding, dizziness, faintness, or shortness of breath, stop what you're doing. Call your doctor if symptoms persist after you stop.

The amount of exercise you do will vary, depending on how active you were before you gave birth. If you were very sedentary or if you're now anemic or very overweight, do only limited exercise, and be sure to get your doctor's approval.

One way to monitor your progress is to keep a chart of the number and kinds of exercises you do each day. You'll be able to see how much more you can do as the days go by, and you'll feel proud of your efforts. If you feel good about an hour after exercise, you'll know that you haven't overdone it. However, if you feel tired, drink extra fluid, which will help you replace your body fluids and relieve fatigue. The next day, cut back your exercise level, and build up more slowly.

Developing a Regular Exercise Schedule

Shortly after breastfeeding her newborn daughter, the Olympic swimmer Dara Torres successfully swam to qualify for the Beijing Olympic Trials, and two years later, in 2008, she earned a silver medal. Another woman we know, who had been running regularly for fourteen years, ran eight miles a day before she became pregnant and continued to run during her pregnancy, cutting down her distance to two miles a day in late pregnancy. She even did one last short run as her labor was beginning. Within one to two weeks after the birth of each of her five children, she began running again. She has breastfed them all and has always produced plenty of milk. Why does she do it? Here's what she says:

"I feel better overall if I exercise regularly. I run to stay fit and have a chance to be outdoors every day. Running helps control my appetite and weight but lets me eat more! It also sets a good example for my kids; they run and participate regularly in various activities."

These women, of course, may not remind you of anyone you know, least of all yourself. While just reading about this vigorous a schedule will exhaust most of us, it's heartening to see that it can be done. It clearly shows that less ambitious exercise programs are certainly feasible.

Figure out what you like to do and what's comfortable for you to do—and then keep doing it on a regular basis. It's better to exercise three or four days a week than to do it every day, giving your muscles a chance to rest between workouts. It's also good to vary your activity rather than do the same exercise every day. And it's better to develop a routine than to exercise on a sporadic, catch-as-catch-can basis. Breaking up your routine into three ten-minute sessions is just as valuable as exercising for a straight half hour. It might be easier for you to find these ten-minute segments of time than to find an uninterrupted half hour.

The most important thing to realize is that you're doing the best thing you can for your baby by breastfeeding, and that, as one mother said, "I know that everything else I do is gravy." If you work at it, eventually you'll lose your extra weight, you'll go back to your former measurements, and you'll be able to resume your previous exercise program. For the duration of nursing, do what you feel good about doing—and feel good about yourself. For suggestions for exercising while breastfeeding, see the following section.

An Exercise Guide for the Nursing Mother

❖ Schedule your exercise around your breastfeeding. Working out immediately after nursing your baby is best for several reasons.

1. Your breasts are not full and uncomfortable, and your baby won't be hungry for a while. Some women nurse first thing in the morning (sometimes even before the baby is fully awake), put the baby back to bed, and then exercise.

2. Extremely strenuous exercise can change the taste of breast milk, making an occasional baby reject it. Flavor change may be caused by a normal, short-term rise in lactic

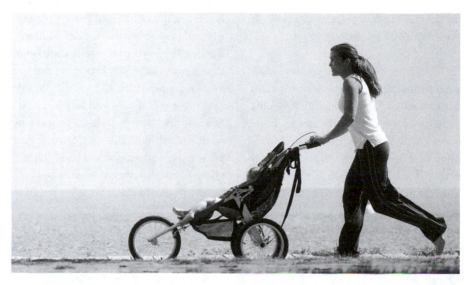

Jogging while pushing a specially designed stroller gives mom exercise and baby fresh air. It's one of several activities you can fit into your own schedule.

acid concentration after extremely vigorous exercise. Lactic acid levels are less likely to rise after moderate exercise, and in any case are not harmful to infants. Most babies are not bothered at all. However, some who don't like the taste may want to nurse again a short time later.

3. If you choose an activity for which you don't have to meet anyone's schedule but your own, you'll be more flexible in fitting exercise into your day. One working mother told us about her late-night schedule: Three nights a week, after nursing her daughter at about 10 P.M., she runs for half an hour with a friend (along a well-lit course).

✤ You may not always be able to exercise immediately after a feeding. If you find that you'll need to nurse your baby soon after a strenuous workout, take the time to cool down, drink a glass of water, shower or rinse off your breasts (if your baby doesn't like the salty taste of perspiration), and perhaps change your clothes. You may be able to postpone the feeding long enough to avoid a temporary change in the flavor of your milk.

✤ Choose an activity you enjoy, so that you'll keep on doing it. Among the wide range to choose from are walking, running, jogging, cycling, dancing, inline- or ice-skating, cross-country skiing, yoga, and jumping rope. Swimming is excellent for building muscles and body tone, but it's not as effective as weight-bearing exercise for controlling fat and building bone density. Its effectiveness depends partly on the individual person and partly on the amount of swimming you do.

❖ Strenuous arm exercises can sometimes have a negative effect on breastfeeding. If you regularly lift weights or do other demanding exercises involving repetitive arm movements, resume slowly and see how it goes. If all goes fine, keep going. However, if you notice the beginning of a clogged milk duct or any other problem, cut back immediately and try again later.

❖ Start your exercise program with very short sessions of a few minutes at a time, three times a week, and gradually increase the frequency and duration of your exercises. If you're exhausted one hour after stopping, cut back—you're doing too much.

❖ Warm up and stretch before doing aerobic exercise, and cool down and stretch afterward. The after-exercise stretch is the more important one, so if you have to skimp on time, shorten the before-exercise stretching.

❖ Drink a glass of water before beginning to exercise, and another glass afterward. A good rule of thumb is to drink 4 to 6 ounces of water for every fifteen to twenty minutes of exercise. It's important to replace fluid lost while exercising. Drink more in hot weather.

❖ Find an exercise buddy, a friend you can work out with two or three times a week. Although this compromises your flexibility, the benefits of exercising with a friend may be worth the extra planning. For one thing, you'll motivate each other to keep up with the program, and for another, your workout will do double duty as a social get-together. But don't fall into the trap of judging yourself by what your friend can do. This is your personal program, and you need to exercise according to your own rhythms.

❖ Concentrate on activities you can do without leaving your baby or at times when someone else can be with the baby. You might work out on a stationary bicycle or other at-home equipment, jump rope, or follow a DVD. One mother's at-home routine includes low-impact aerobics three mornings a week with a DVD and nightly ten-minute spot-toning exercises. She even persuaded her husband to join her in the spot-toning.

❖ Walking is excellent exercise, and if you take your baby along in a sling or carrier while you walk, the extra weight will use up more calories. This is another activity that can do double or even triple duty: As you walk with your baby, you're both getting fresh air. And if you meet a friend, you'll have adult company. Or you might run or power-walk early in the morning or at night when your partner or older children are home to watch your baby.

❖ If your favorite exercise program involves going to a gym or class, treat yourself to a sitter or barter babysitting time with a friend. Some gyms and health clubs provide child care, a service that can accustom your baby to being with other people and can help you make friends with other mothers. Again, this will do double duty as a social outing as well as a physical one.

❖ Dress comfortably. Wear underpants that don't ride up, rub, or constrict. Wicking fabrics like polypropylene absorb sweat best. Of course, shorts and a T-shirt work just fine.

❖ Wear a supportive bra. If you're full-figured, a nursing bra may not provide enough support, so invest in a sports bra in the larger size you need now, and change into it for your exercise sessions. Or wear both. Wearing a sports bra during jogging or other strenuous exercise helps to prevent the uncomfortable bouncing that can stretch the fibrous bands in the breasts and contribute to sagging.

❖ Invest in equipment that will encourage you to keep exercising— whether it's a baby jogger (shown on page 193), a treadmill, a set of steps, or whatever else you may need.

❖ Incorporate exercise into your daily life by taking the stairs rather than an elevator whenever you can, walking to errands instead of driving, and doing active chores at home.

❖ Most of all, enjoy your exercise as a time to care for yourself.

While you're taking care of your physical health, be sure to pay attention to your emotional health, as well.

How Do You Feel—and Why Do You Feel This Way?

As the mother of a new baby, you are in one of the most intense periods of your entire life. You're likely to be swept up by a dizzying array of emotions, including excitement, joy, and a deep sense of inner satisfaction—as well as worry, disappointment, and possibly even depression. (If you're experiencing these latter feelings, be assured that there are a number of things you can do to lift your mood, which we suggest on pages 198–199.)

You may look at your baby sometimes—perhaps when you have just been roused from a deep sleep, or when your nipples hurt, or when you turn down yet another invitation because you can't, or don't want to, get a babysitter—and think, *Motherhood isn't all it's been cracked up to be.* If you do, you're not alone. Practically every mother alive has at one time or another had this thought. No matter how much you longed to have a child and how much you love him, he has wrought vast changes in your life.

The birth of a baby marks a major transition point in both parents' lives, but it's usually much more marked for the mother, since your life is apt to change more than the new father's. Even in these liberated times, most of the responsibility for raising children falls to the mother in most homes. Even if you'll be working full-time outside the home, you'll probably still be the parent who finds the child care and takes your child to the caregiver, who stays home when your child is sick, who keeps track of what needs to be done. Studies show that married working mothers generally handle 70 to 80 percent of child care and household duties in addition to their paying jobs.

Some new mothers are guilt-ridden when they realize that they feel no great surge of love when they first see their babies. But maternal love may take time to develop. In one classic study, only half of a group of fifty-four new mothers said they had had positive feelings when they first saw their babies (and only 13 percent identified these feelings as love); about a third reported having had no feelings at all. It took most of the mothers about three weeks to begin to love their babies; by three months, the loving tie was usually firmly set.

As a breastfeeding mother, you're apt to be particularly conscious of your involvement in your baby's care and your primary responsibility for that care. And if you're experiencing any problems in breastfeeding, you may feel like a failure. No matter how much you love your baby, you may chafe at his complete dependence on you. As you become aware of these feelings, you may be overwhelmed by shame because

you "know" that mothers are supposed to love their babies all the time, twenty-four hours a day, seven days a week. This is one of the things we think we "know" that are not necessarily so.

Are You Feeling Blue?

You may find yourself losing your temper over little things, or crying at the slightest provocation. You may have problems eating, sleeping, or getting up in the morning. In a severe case, you might even lose interest in everything and everybody. To make matters worse, you may worry and feel guilty about the depression itself.

The first thing you need to know is that your reaction is not abnormal for either breastfeeding or formula-feeding moms. The second thing is that it's not your fault! The low feeling that many new mothers feel soon after their babies' birth is generally called the "baby blues." It was reported as long as 2,000 years ago by Hippocrates, and was sometimes called milk blues or milk fever, because it often comes a few days after birth, along with the first appearance of milk. Approximately half of all new mothers experience these baby blues, and second-time mothers are more vulnerable than the mothers of first babies. Then there is a more troubling—and fortunately, less common—reaction known as postpartum depression, which affects some 10 to 20 percent of new moms (see page 200).

What causes these low feelings? At one time, they were blamed on changes in a new mother's hormonal balance, but no compelling evidence has been found for this theory. Another, newer explanation is that stress increases a mother's risk of depression, in part by increasing inflammation in many parts of the mother's body, which affects her immune system. Both physical and psychological stressors—like pain, a difficult birth experience, lack of support, or problems with breastfeeding—can produce these changes. The good news for nursing mothers is that breastfeeding reduces stress, and thus inflammation, and therefore breastfeeding can often help to prevent postpartum mood disorders. Furthermore, most treatments for depression are compatible with breastfeeding (talk to your doctor about what would be best for you), and nursing will help you connect with your baby while you get better.

The combination of bodily changes along with life changes packs a double whammy for the new mother. You now have to transform the entire rhythm of your days to fit your new baby's needs. Both you and your husband or partner are suddenly catapulted into new feelings of responsibility, and naturally your relationship is affected. If you have older children, you need to help them adjust to the new baby, and you have to divide your time so that everyone is taken care of. Then there are new financial responsibilities, new sleeping arrangements, and new routines for the entire family. Your new baby's personality may be a factor. If your baby cries a lot, sleeps little, and is slow learning how to nurse, she will

pose special challenges. All this when chronic fatigue is likely to make all your other problems seem worse.

Before you have a baby, it's impossible to know what life with one will be like. Most women—including adoptive mothers—find that taking care of a newborn is more exhausting and time-consuming than they had ever imagined. Your sleep is constantly being interrupted, and your body is working to recover from your labor.

In our society, the typical new mother tends to lack self-confidence in her maternal ability. You know motherhood must be really hard because there are so many books telling you how to handle your children's psyches, how to raise their IQs—even how to feed them at your breast. And if the professionals disagree about the best theories of child rearing, how can you have confidence that you know what's best?

Stressful experiences during childbirth and breastfeeding may provide a fertile soil for baby blues to develop. Having idealized both, some women find that neither experience has lived up to their expectations. They're disappointed in themselves, feeling that they have not quite measured up. Women who had planned to have a completely unmedicated delivery and then needed anesthesia, women who had practiced their breathing exercises and then needed a cesarean delivery, and women who have a rocky start with breastfeeding or who have to wean their babies sooner than planned are apt to forget that the ultimate goal of childbirth and child rearing is a healthy baby and a healthy mother.

Ways to Boost Your Postpartum Morale

Many new mothers find the following measures help them to feel better:

❖ Take care of yourself. You can't meet your baby's needs if you don't meet your own.

❖ If you're employed, take as long a maternity leave as possible.

❖ Eat a healthy diet that includes foods you enjoy. Try not to rush your meals. Enjoy a healthy pick-me-up snack now and then. Foods containing omega-3 fatty acids and DHA are especially beneficial to new mothers. Take vitamin and mineral supplements as suggested by your doctor.

❖ Get as much rest as possible. If you can, nap during the day when your baby sleeps to make up for losing sleep at night. Ask your partner to bring the baby to you during the night, if the baby is not sleeping in or near your bed.

❖ Develop an exercise routine. If you haven't followed one before, this is a good time to start. You need those endorphins. A postpartum exercise class (either "Baby and Me" or one with child care available) will also help by getting you in touch with other moms.

❖ Deal with breastfeeding difficulties immediately. Don't wait to resolve problems like sore nipples,

engorgement, a clogged duct, and the like. (See Chapter 15.) And if relief doesn't come very soon, call your doctor or lactation consultant.

❖ Forget about housework for now. The board of health won't come after you if there are dustballs under the bed or full wastebaskets in every room. Do what you absolutely have to do, and let the rest wait.

❖ Ask for specific kinds of help from your husband or partner, your relatives, your friends—and don't forget how much help your older children can be.

❖ Work out an arrangement so that your partner can spend more time at home and do more in the home, at least for a while.

❖ Pay for as much help as you can afford. It's a sound investment in your comfort and peace of mind.

❖ Cut back on outside responsibilities. Let someone else collect the union dues, bake the cookies, staff the hot line, chair the meeting.

❖ Schedule—and then take—some time for yourself *every day,* even if some days it's only 15 minutes to read a magazine or listen to music. Or you could set aside a few minutes for meditation, playing the piano, writing in

Then, in an age when women are urged to have it all, many learn that having it all at the same time can be overwhelming. Combining career with motherhood is much harder than most

women expected it to be. As a result, you may feel that there's something wrong with you—rather than with the unrealistic expectations that only a supermom could fill. No mother is perfect, and you your journal, taking a bubble bath, or just taking what one mom calls her ten-minute sanity walk.

❖ Bring laughter into your life: Watch a comedy on TV or DVD, sign up for a daily joke e-mail, or read a funny book.

❖ Go to www.breastfeeding.com and click on "Things to Do While Breastfeeding."

❖ Pay at least glancing attention to your appearance; you'll feel better if you look better.

❖ After the first week, get dressed every day. At first, staying in your pjs may help you get your rest, since people won't expect too much of you. After one week, though, it can be dispiriting to find yourself still in your bathrobe at dinnertime.

❖ Get out of the house for at least a short time every day, either with or without your baby.

❖ Join a group for breastfeeding mothers (like those sponsored by La Leche League, your pediatrician's office, or a local family service agency). Other new moms have similar problems and feelings and can often help you with yours.

❖ Acknowledge your negative feelings. Cry when you feel like it, and get anger out safely by hitting a pillow.

❖ See a mental health professional who will give you short-term counseling or cognitive therapy to help you deal with stress and think more positively.

❖ If your symptoms last more than a couple of weeks, are especially troubling, or include any thoughts about harming yourself or your baby, see a psychiatrist (an MD) who can discuss options to help you get through this period, like psychotherapy and antidepressant medication. Be sure the doctor knows you are breastfeeding. If the medicine is not listed among those in Chapter 10 that are safe for your nursing baby, check with your pediatrician and/or La Leche League (see the Resource Appendix).

❖ Also check with your doctor before taking any herbal, homeopathic, or other alternative remedies. Not all substances that grow naturally are safe for breastfeeding mothers (see Chapter 10). Your local La Leche League leader can also provide resources to share with your doctor.

Making an effort to take care of yourself may well make you feel better. But if doing just one of these suggested things seems overwhelming, read "Postpartum Depression" (page 200) carefully and seek help.

don't have to be perfect, either. You just have to do the best you can.

Ideally, as a breastfeeding mother, you should feel empowered that your milk is helping your baby to bloom.

However, because of cultural pressures, your confidence may actually be undermined by the fact that you're the exclusive supplier of your baby's food. When a formula-fed baby cries, or has frequent or sparse bowel movements, or sleeps too little or too much, a mother (and the people around her) will blame the formula or the baby's personal inclinations. When the same thing happens with a breastfed baby, the first reaction may be to blame the breastfeeding. You worry that your baby's not getting enough milk, or that your milk isn't good enough, or that you're doing something wrong. Unhelpful remarks from other people often feed this anxiety. No wonder your confidence is shaky and your feelings can run away with you.

Breastfeeding itself has been shown to be protective against depression, but if you're having major problems with nursing—if your baby isn't gaining enough weight or if you have developed a medical condition that makes it difficult to continue nursing—it's not surprising that you should be upset. Almost always, with the right help, you will be able to overcome such difficulties and to move beyond them.

In most cases, the blues will leave as suddenly as they came. To help them go away, you may want to try some of the suggestions in the box on pages 198–99.

Postpartum Depression

If you're still feeling low, with troubling symptoms (like those listed under "Depression" in the box on the opposite page), more than two weeks after your baby is born, talk to your doctor. She or he may want to check your thyroid hormone levels, which may be causing your problems. If they're normal, make an appointment to see a mental health professional, such as a psychiatrist, to investigate treatment options.

The most important difference between the milder blues and clinical depression is that the blues are temporary and will pass soon, usually within a couple of weeks. Clinical depression, on the other hand, needs more attention and treatment.

You're at higher risk of depression if you have experienced it before or during pregnancy, have a family history of depression, had a difficult or complicated pregnancy and birth, have experienced many life stresses recently, or have a baby with special needs. If you have any of these risk factors, speak to your doctor sooner rather than later.

In deciding on therapy, you need to weigh the risk of treating depression against the risks of not treating it. Depression has very serious physical and emotional consequences for the sufferer and also for her baby. Although you want to take as few drugs as possible while you're nursing, if you're advised to take medication for depression, ask your baby's doctor whether it's safe for you to breastfeed. The risk to the baby of a depressed mother may be greater than the risk of the mother's taking antidepressants.

Although there's some limited evidence of problems in the first few months in children whose mothers took antidepressant medication while pregnant, these problems are generally not serious and appear to get better over time. However, the research in this area is sparse, and it's hard to

Differences Between Postpartum Blues and Postpartum Depression*

	BLUES	DEPRESSION
Time of Onset	3 to 14 days after delivery (sometimes after a helper goes home or partner goes back to work)	Any time in first year after delivery, often in first three months
Duration	A few days, up to a couple of weeks	At least two weeks, but often longer
Incidence	From 30 to 84 percent of new moms; average, 56 percent	10 to 40 percent of new mothers
Symptoms	Mood swings, crying easily, headaches, forgetfulness, restlessness, irritability, negative feelings toward baby and other family members	All those experienced with the blues, plus anxiety, despair, problems with sleeping and eating, feelings of helplessness and hopelessness, irrational fears about baby and self, sometimes including a fear of harming the baby
Treatment	Balanced diet, vitamin and mineral supplements and exercise as suggested by your doctor, help in caring for the baby, emotional support from family and friends, psychotherapy or counseling (especially cognitive therapy, which helps you to think positively); for a list of suggestions, see page 198	All those recommended for the blues, plus foods or supplements containing omega-3 fatty acids, bright light therapy, and antidepressant medication, if prescribed by doctor and not harmful to baby (see Chapter 10)
Prognosis	Good!	Good!

*This chart is adapted, with permission, from one prepared by Kathleen A. Kendall-Tackett, PhD, IBCLC, clinical associate professor of pediatrics at Texas Tech University School of Medicine.

predict what may occur down the line. Babies whose mothers took antidepressants while breastfeeding show very few effects. Still, some medications are safer to take than others. Alternatively, many women respond to nondrug treatments for depression, including foods or supplements containing omega-3 fatty acids, bright light therapy, exercise, social support, and psychotherapy.

The decision about the type of treatment you may undergo is one that you and your doctor need to make together. For more about antidepressant medication, see Chapter 10, and for additional help, consult the Website Appendix for organizations that offer help for postpartum depression.

What You Need to Tell Yourself

We can't help how we feel about things, even though we can control what we do about our feelings. You'll learn to live with the mixed feelings you may have about parenthood as you learn to live with mixed feelings about every other aspect of life—your marriage or partnership, your work, your schooling. We learn to take the bad with the good— the dirty diapers with the joyous gurgles, the waking up at three in the morning with the bright smiles that reward us when we go to our babies, the burdens of responsibility with the all-embracing love of a child. Be reassured that you are doing the best you can for your baby. Then accept your negative feelings along with your positive ones and realize that you're neither bad nor inadequate for having them.

The thought and care that you put into your health will pay off in many ways. The better you feel, the happier your breastfeeding—and parenting—experience is likely to be. And the better cared for you are, the more both you and your baby will benefit.

CHAPTER NINE

Confident, Comfortable Nursing at Home and Away

"When an actress takes off her clothes onscreen but a nursing mother is told to leave [the theater], what message do we send about the roles of women?"

ANNA QUINDLEN *The New York Times*

Y ou're not living solely for your baby even during these months when so much of your time is spent with this newest member of your family. You're still a person with your own life and your own needs. Ignoring those needs can have negative ramifications for you and for the other people in your life, both now and in the years to come. For all these reasons, you need to care for yourself physically, mentally, and emotionally, as well as care for your baby. And yes, this means looking out not only for your needs, but for your wants, too.

Care of Your Breasts

Fortunately, you don't need to treat your breasts like fragile china. In fact, while you're pregnant or nursing, you don't need to do anything special for your breasts. You don't need to bother with any special nipple-care rituals, and you don't need any special salves or ointments.

But your breasts do need to feel comfortable, which for many women involves wearing a supportive nursing bra. On the following page, we talk about finding bras that will provide support, while making it convenient for you to breastfeed. And you do need to let your body's natural moisturizers work on your breasts by not using any drying agents on them, including soap.

If you splash water over your breasts during your daily shower and change your bra at least once a day (or more often, if you're leaking a great deal of milk), your breasts and your nipples will be clean. Furthermore, disposable or washable breast pads worn inside your bra will help protect your nipples and prevent milk from leaking onto your clothing. Change them often so they don't stay wet and foster the growth of bacteria.

Although breastfeeding women were advised for years to apply a soothing cream or ointment to their nipples after feedings to prevent or treat nipple soreness, research does not show any evidence that any of these creams or salves help. In fact, some can even do harm. If a substance needs to be wiped off before a baby nurses, the friction on the mother's breasts may contribute to soreness. Also, some salves contain ingredients that some women are allergic to; the more ingredients a product contains, the greater the possibility of a reaction. If you do use anything on your nipples and they become sore, stop using it immediately. If it was a prescription item (for treating thrush, for example), ask your doctor to prescribe a substitute.

But what if your nipples do get sore? One over-the-counter balm that some women find soothing is purified lanolin. It does not have to be wiped off before you nurse, and it won't hurt you or your baby. Lansinoh HPA Lanolin is a safe, pure brand of modified lanolin. Some women swear by hydrogel pads, which are designed to temporarily prevent nipple soreness and soothe sore nipples. They're worn inside your bra, kept in the refrigerator or freezer when not in use, and some can be worn for up to six days.

If nipple soreness persists or worsens, get help immediately. Stop using the pads or balm and call your doctor or lactation consultant. More important, keep your nipples dry by changing your bra or breast pads if they get wet from leaking milk.

Your breasts should feel good during lactation. Because they're doing something they may never have done before, however, they may feel tender on the second or third day of nursing, and possibly even later. However, you should not be hurting. Painful, cracked, or bleeding nipples are not normal. If you develop soreness that's more than mildly uncomfortable and if it doesn't go away in a day or two, take care of it immediately. You may need to change your breastfeeding technique (see Chapter 6) and also treat your nipples (see Chapter 15).

Wearing the Right Bra

Your bra is the single most important item in your wardrobe these days. Even if you're small-breasted and don't ordinarily wear a bra for support, you may want to wear one now—if for no other reason than to hold breast pads in place or to prevent milk from leaking onto your clothes. You may find that a bra provides comfortable support, especially in the early weeks when your breasts are so full of fluid. While you don't need a bra specially designed for breastfeeding, it makes life easier.

You'll need at least three bras—one to wear, a clean one in the drawer, and one hanging up to dry—and maybe a couple of extras. If you're leaking a great deal of milk, you'll want to change bras or liners often to keep your nipples from getting sore and your clothes from getting stained. If you hand-wash and hang your bras to dry, they'll last longer.

Nursing bras come in a wide variety of styles and fabrics, from no-nonsense sturdy to lacy and sexy. Some are soft; some have underwires for added support. Some have a row of hooks down the front; others have a hook at the top of each cup. You may find the front-

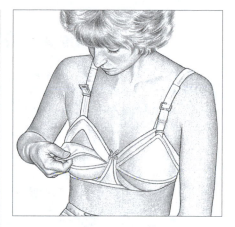

A comfortable nursing bra that lets you uncover one breast at a time, using only one hand, makes life—and nursing—easier. Some bras have a front closure rather than one in back, which can make it easier to put on and take off.

closing style easier to put on and take off, but it may make discreet nursing more difficult.

The nursing bra you bought at the end of your pregnancy may still fit during lactation if you allowed extra room. Typically, you'll need at least one size larger in the cup and one size larger in the band while you're breastfeeding. If the prenursing bra is now too tight, don't wear it. A tight bra can cause clogged milk ducts and make you miserable. Try one style at a time. And if you like one after wearing it for a couple of weeks, order more by phone or online, or ask someone else to pick them up for you. For tips on bra shopping, see the box on page 206.

During the early days of nursing when you're heavier and your breasts are larger, you may want to use a bra extender. Available in department and fabric stores, these extenders consist

Finding the Right Nursing Bra

A bra that fits right may help to maintain your breast contours, and one designed for function will simplify breastfeeding. Keep these points in mind when you go shopping:

✤ When trying on a bra, lift your breasts up into it and adjust the straps.

✤ The cup should support the entire lower half of your breast in a natural position and should completely and comfortably cover your breast. Put the bra on and hold your arms straight down at your sides. If it fits properly, your nipple line will be level with a point midway between elbow and shoulder.

✤ When you sit down, the bra should stay put.

✤ The band around your chest and back should fit snugly, neither binding nor slipping up and down. To test this, put your hands on your hips and look at yourself, front and back, in the mirror.

✤ Be sure you can uncover your breast generously enough so that the fabric of the bra doesn't put concentrated pressure on any one spot on your breast and leaves enough room for your baby to latch on well.

✤ Look for a style that lets you uncover one breast at a time, using only one hand.

✤ All—or at least 90 percent—cotton or another absorbent fabric is best. Avoid polyester cups, which don't breathe, and those that are only cotton-lined.

✤ The straps should be wide and adjustable, preferably padded or cushioned, and not elastic. This is especially important for women who wear size D cup or larger.

---

of a band of fabric or elastic that can be attached to the band of your bra to make it comfortable for your temporarily larger size.

Protect Yourself from Leaking Milk

You may feel a wonderful sense of abundance when your breasts produce so much milk that it drips even when you're not feeding your baby. You may also not want to walk around with nice round spots where your breasts meet your blouse. Although you need not feel embarrassed by public evidence of this wonderful way of nurturing your baby, you may not feel like announcing your lactational status to the world. (See the suggestions beginning on page 210 for clothing that is least likely to show telltale signs of leaking.) Of greater concern is the fact that excess

❖ Some nursing bras used to have plastic-lined cups—do not buy these! They'll trap moisture, which may lead to nipple problems.

❖ Be careful about underwires. Ideally, avoid them. Even if they don't dig into your breast tissue when new, the wires tend to shift and can dig in after the bra is washed. This can block milk ducts, depriving your baby of some of your milk and putting you at risk of a plugged duct or breast infection. So be aware of these possible problems.

❖ The band should be completely straight and rest at or below your shoulder blades. If it rides up, the bra is too big. If it feels tight, try a larger cup size.

❖ When buying a bra before your baby is born, allow for some growth afterward. You'll want a little extra room in the band and in the cups, so that you can fit nursing pads inside. Even a bra that you already wear on the loosest hooks may be too tight once your baby arrives.

❖ The bra should not be so tight that it leaves marks on your skin under your arms, under or across your breasts, or over your shoulders.

❖ Stay away from low-cut push-up bras. These tend to cut across the fullest part of your breast and put pressure on the tissue.

❖ If you're small-breasted and don't need the support of a structured bra, you may prefer to wear a simple stretch bra that can be easily pulled up for nursing rather than a bra designed specifically for breastfeeding.

❖ If you want to wear a sleep bra, look for one that doesn't have hooks in the back and is stretchy enough so you can pull it over your head. Some have a crossover front design that lets you easily slip out one breast for nursing.

moisture trapped next to your breasts can irritate your skin and cause problems.

Leaking is common in the early weeks. But even though you continue to produce ample supplies of milk, it generally stops being a problem within a couple of months. Many moms worry that their milk is drying up because they stop leaking. Leaking seems to be a pressure-release mechanism that isn't as necessary later on, when mom's supply has had a chance to adjust to baby's needs.

Meanwhile, you can protect your breasts and your clothing from leaking milk by lining the inside of your bra with disposable nursing pads. Look in your local pharmacy or big discount store for pads without gauze lining, since gauze can stick to your breasts and cause painful hairline cracks in your nipples or breast tissue. If you want to save money or if you find that *any* disposables you try stick to your skin, buy washable, reusable pads. Look for all-cotton ones, since synthetic fibers are not absorbent.

Or make your own. Insert a folded all-cotton handkerchief in each cup of your bra. Or cut out 4-inch circles from all-cotton diapers or very soft old T-shirts, and stitch three or four circles together. They're absorbent, fold to the size you need, wash and dry quickly, and don't show through. Don't use synthetic fabrics and no-iron finishes; they're not as absorbent and may be irritating. Change pads often to keep your breasts dry.

Some women like LilyPadz, breast pads made of medical-grade silicone. They reduce leaking, have a tacky surface that makes them stick to your breasts so you don't need to wear a bra over them, and can be worn overnight or even swimming. They're especially useful for brief periods when you're wearing good clothing that you want to protect from spotting. However, the fact that they're silicone means that they don't breathe, which could be an issue. (See Website Appendix for more information.)

Although some women like to use plastic breast shells (the kind used to bring out inverted nipples as described in Chapter 4) for catching leaking milk, these shells can promote continued leaking because of the constant pressure they exert upon the breasts. Occasional use should cause no problem. If you do use them, keep them dry, and empty them often. If you're still leaking through your clothes, stop the leak by pressing your breast with the heel of your hand or your forearm.

Lumps in the Breast

Your breasts will feel different, and possibly lumpier, during lactation. If you discover a lump in your breast while nursing or during your monthly breast self-examination, chances are that it's related in some way to the fact that you're breastfeeding. If the lump is red, swollen, or painful, it may signal a plugged duct or an infection, which you can treat by following the suggestions in Chapter 15.

However, if you develop any lump that remains unchanged for more than three days, call your doctor. The chances of its being a tumor are slim, but it's always best to make certain. Breastfeeding does not cause tumors, but it does not prevent them, either. Fortunately, almost all tumors in young women are benign. Whenever you experience any unusual change in your body, have it checked out to be sure there's no medical problem. Most of the time, you'll be reassured that it's nothing serious—and on the off chance that it is something that needs treatment, you'll most likely have caught it in time.

If you need to have a breast examination, you don't need to wean your baby. If your doctor recommends a mammogram, nurse just before the procedure and ask to have the picture read by someone familiar with the lactating breast. In the unlikely prospect that you have to have a lump removed surgically, you may still be able to continue nursing on the other breast and eventually to resume nursing on the affected one.

Back Basics

Lifting and carrying your baby, bending over to diaper and bathe her, picking up all kinds of items from the floor, and pushing a stroller are all new activities—which often cause backaches in new moms.

The American Physical Therapy Association has produced a free downloadable booklet with tips on doing these basic mom activities in healthy ways (see the Website Appendix). For example, when picking a child up from the floor, use a half-kneel lift; when carrying your child, hold her close to your body and as centered as possible (in other words, don't balance her on one hip or support her with only one arm). When pushing a stroller, stay close to it, keeping your back straight and your shoulders back.

How You Look

Since how you look affects how you feel, it's worth investing a little time, effort, and money in looking good. Physical changes that come with pregnancy, childbirth, and breastfeeding are perfectly normal and natural—and are not unattractive. Without spending thousands of dollars on cosmetic surgery, you can look your best—and your best is good enough. There is a grace in motherhood that can make this among the loveliest times of your life—much more beautiful than any Hollywood notion of glamour.

This is the time to make life as easy for yourself as possible. Find a few simple self-care routines you can stick to, and make them yours. On a busy day, just running a comb through your hair and washing your face can make you feel good, as well as look good.

Custom-tailor your routine to your own priorities. Since you can't do everything you did before, concentrate on those parts of your routine that make you feel the best about yourself—and then stick to them. One woman may feel messy if she doesn't wash her hair every day; another can't stand seeing unpolished toenails; a third feels unkempt with unshaven legs. Decide what care rituals are necessary for you.

Your Hair

❖ Keep it easy to style. This is not the time to make a radical change in the way you wear your hair, unless you're going from a very elaborate coif to a wash-and-wear one.

❖ If you're considering a permanent, you may want to wait. It may not take during or soon after pregnancy, probably because of the changes in your hormonal balance. However, if you do get a permanent or color your hair, both treatments appear to be safe for your nursing baby. There's no evidence of any harmful effects.

❖ If it looks like you're losing more hair after childbirth, don't worry. This may be just a game of catch-up. It's normal to lose a certain amount of hair daily when you're not pregnant, but this hair loss decreases during pregnancy, possibly because of increased blood flow. Then after the baby is born, normal growth and shedding of hair resumes.

❖ If you hate the way your hair looks, put it in a ponytail if it's long enough or find a cute cap to wear.

Your Skin

❖ Your skin may appear blotchy during and soon after pregnancy. Be patient. This, too, will return to normal.

❖ Whenever you think of it, put some unscented hand or body lotion or baby oil on your body. A loving way to ease back into intimacy with your partner is to give each other body massages. You can do this even if you don't feel ready to become sexually active.

❖ Stretch marks occur when skin loses elasticity as a result of weight gain and are often hereditary—if your mother had stretch marks, you're likely to get them, too. Think of them as the "service stripes" of motherhood.

Your Nails

❖ Keep your nails short and buffed rather than long and polished. Aside from the danger of scratching your baby, long nails are more likely to break.

❖ If you miss the polish, go wild on your toenails. For one thing, it's wonderful to know that you can reach them again, and you might enjoy the undercover glamour.

Dressing in Nursing-Friendly Clothes

You probably don't need to buy anything special to wear while you're nursing. Most likely you already have enough suitable clothing to wear as is, or with minor alterations. However, now that you can put away your maternity clothes (at least most of them), picking up a few new things may give your spirits a lift. And there are lots of choices out there. A growing number of companies specialize in making clothes for nursing women, which are generally equipped with disguised slits in strategic places.

Look in the pages of parenting magazines for ads for clothes to wear while breastfeeding, which you can usually order from catalogs by phone, mail, or online (type "breastfeeding clothing" into a search engine). Almost all mail-order houses make it easy to return items if they don't fit or don't look as good in person as they did on the page.

However, don't go overboard on shopping until after your baby is born, since there's always the possibility of an unplanned cesarean. And after a cesarean birth with a midline incision, you won't want anything elastic around your waist until the incision heals.

✤ Choose washable and wrinkle-resistant clothes that don't need ironing.

✤ Sweatpants or yoga pants are ideal for your first postpartum wardrobe. They come in a range of colors and are perfect with a T-shirt or other loose top that hides your middle and can be easily pulled up to nurse. You can keep them on while you sneak in a nap, and they're easy to throw into the washer and dryer.

✤ Another easy and comfortable choice is leggings and a long shirt or pullover.

✤ For more formal occasions, separates—blouses and other tops worn with skirts or pants—are easier to manipulate than dresses. Wraparound skirts or skirts and pants with elastic waists are especially good, since your former waistline will be only a fond memory for a few months.

✤ Button-front blouses are convenient, but so are knit pullovers, which can be easily pulled up to allow for modest nursing. When you're wearing a button-front blouse, you can nurse more discreetly if you unbutton from the bottom up rather than from the top down. When you wear a pullover, your baby's body will cover your midriff and the pullover will cover your breast.

✤ Choose prints rather than solid colors; prints are less likely to show leaking milk. Avoid white, pale colors, and clingy materials. If you're concerned about leaking, remember to wear breast pads.

✤ Ponchos, loose-fitting cardigan sweaters and jackets, and scarves and shawls are good cover-ups for discreet nursing.

✤ Don't make the mistake of trying too soon to squeeze into too-tight prepregnancy clothes. It's bad for your morale, as well as your comfort. Besides, tight tops rub against your nipples and can trigger a let-down at the most inconvenient times. More important, they have occasionally been implicated as the cause of a clogged duct or breast infection.

✤ If you sew, you can make your own clothes or adapt those you already own. For suggestions, do an Internet search for "patterns for breastfeeding clothes." You can, for example, make horizontal seams across the bustline of a blouse or dress, or open darts below it where you can insert invisible zippers or Velcro. You can put zippers under the armholes of loose sleeveless dresses, so when unzipped, your baby's head can fit comfortably inside the garment. You can attach fake pockets over each breast with Velcro. A flip of your wrist will lift a corner of the pocket to make the breast accessible to your baby but protected from public view. However, remember that Velcro makes noise when you open it and factor this into your plan.

✤ If you work outside the home, see wardrobe suggestions in Chapter 12.

Going Out with Your Baby

Once your baby is three or four weeks old, you can get out quite easily with him or her for casual visits with friends. It's advisable to wait a little longer—at least six weeks, and preferably three months—before taking your baby into a crowded restaurant or other place where there are large groups of people. Before this time, the baby's immune system is not fully developed, so he's vulnerable to germs.

Young babies are usually very agreeable to going out and bedding down for a while in carriage, stroller, sling, carrier, car seat—or your arms. Should yours want to be fed, you're right there. A risk with this is that it seems so easy that you may tend to overdo it. If you find that you're going out so often and staying out so late that you or your baby is getting tired and irritable, cut back.

If your baby starts to cry while you're both passengers in a moving car, you may be tempted to take him out of his car seat to nurse him. Don't do it. The laws in every state require small children to be buckled into approved safety seats. (State laws differ slightly regarding the age or size of the child.) The statistics paint a clear picture: Your baby's safety depends on being securely held in a car seat, in the back seat of the car. He should never be placed in the front seat. If there's an accident, he could be seriously hurt or worse, especially in front of an air bag. Again, wait to nurse until the car is not moving. Don't try to lean over and nurse him while he's in the seat; neither car seat nor baby is made to withstand your weight.

If your baby starts to cry while you're driving, remember that your first obligation is to keep both of you safe. To do this, you need to give your full attention to your driving. It won't hurt your baby to cry for a little while if you can't pull over immediately. You can, of course, talk or sing to your baby, but you need to keep your eyes on the road and the traffic. Before doing anything more for your baby, get to a safe place where you can stop the car. It may be hard to listen to your baby's cries when you can't reach him, but because of these safety concerns, it's better than risking both your lives.

If you need to take a train, bus, ferry, or airplane, try to travel in off-peak hours, which will make for a less stressful trip. Observe safety precautions in any moving vehicle by keeping your baby in an approved car seat or safety seat, and by staying belted yourself.

Nursing in Public

Although women in some of the most modest cultures in the world comfortably breastfeed their babies wherever they happen to be, many Western societies display a bizarre and contradictory set of values.

One reason for the low breastfeeding rates in the United States is that many people view breasts as purely sexual organs, not functional ones. In our society, women's uncovered breasts are displayed openly in movies and magazines and are barely covered on beaches and streets from coast to coast. Yet our culture's insistence on defining the female breast as a symbol of eroticism has generated a taboo against showing it in public for its primary purpose: nurturing babies. Nursing mothers continue to be humiliated at, and even evicted from, restaurants, hotels, stores, and swimming pool areas.

But why should a woman have to hide herself away from normal life and from other adults because she wants to do the best thing for her baby? Today, more and more women are refusing to accept this taboo. They're nursing their babies in meetings, at parties, at concerts and ball games, on beaches, on airplanes, and in houses of worship. And they're getting support from other women, and often from elected officials.

As a result, more contemporary observers are becoming familiar with a sight that was once commonplace in Western society and is once again regaining its proper place as an acceptable practice. As women themselves accept the naturalness and the respectability of breastfeeding, cultural—and legal—acceptance of public nursing will keep pace.

Many women nurse their babies wherever they happen to be, with such skill that no one else is aware of what

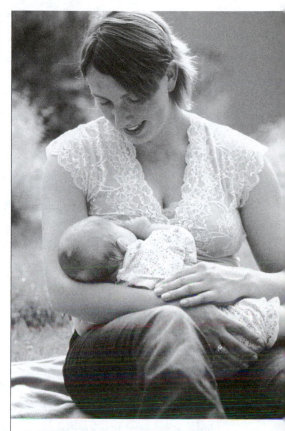

Today's women often nurse wherever their daily lives take them, confident that they are caring for their babies in the best possible way.

they're doing. Still, if you feel shy about nursing in front of other people, you don't have to do this. When feeding time comes, excuse yourself, go into another room, and feed your baby. Or begin the feeding elsewhere and then rejoin the group. Usually the time your breast is most exposed is at the start of a feeding. Once your baby has latched on, it's easier to keep your breasts covered. In a public place, you can usually find a quiet nook where you'll be relatively unobserved. Or a companion may be able to shield you from public view.

Flying with Your Nursing Baby

Babies are usually ready for their first airplane trip at about three months of age, after the fluid in the middle ear has gone away and their immune system has matured a little. You can do a lot to make your flight as comfortable and hassle-free as possible. We are indebted to two experienced mom flyers, Annie Crombie and Cullen Curtiss, for their help with this section.

❖ Know your rights. In the U.S. and Canada, your right to breastfeed anywhere you and your baby are legally entitled to be is generally understood, even in the absence of specific laws. There's no law that specifically forbids breastfeeding at any time or place.

❖ Start planning your trip as far ahead as possible. Ideally, you should have no trouble breastfeeding, but to avoid an unpleasant encounter between airline staff and nursing mothers (there have been some in the past), prepare ahead of time.

❖ Ask about the airline's breastfeeding policy. It might not have one, but if you can get something in writing (maybe via e-mail), you will have a copy of the policy with you in case anyone challenges your right to breastfeed.

❖ Choosing the time of your flight depends overall, of course, on airlines' schedules. For short flights, late morning or early afternoon may be best, so that if there's a delay, you'll have a good chance of catching the next flight out. For a long flight you may be better off with late evening, to correspond to your child's usual sleep time. Try not to fly during the busiest holiday seasons.

❖ Book a window seat, where you'll have more privacy, and near the front of the plane, where there's less turbulence. The website www.seatguru .com has seating plans for most airlines.

❖ If you can afford to, buy a separate seat for your baby, even if she's under two years old and could fly for free on your lap. The advantages of having an extra seat include safety (since you can secure her in a car seat) and comfort (more space for you and baby).

❖ If you do opt to hold her on your lap, bring her birth certificate to prove she's under two.

❖ Wear nursing-friendly clothing that can help you nurse discreetly. One comfy outfit includes stretchy pants, tank top with built-in bra, T-shirt on top of that, and zip-up sweatshirt. If you wear a nursing bra, be sure you can undo and refasten it one-handed.

✤ It's best to nurse your baby during takeoff and landing to avoid pressure in her middle ear. Such pressure may make her uncomfortable at any time during the flight, and if so, holding her upright often helps.

✤ Bring helpful accessories, like a carry-on bag with roomy compartments, nursing pillow, sling or other carrier for trips to the bathroom, and a nursing cover or clean, lightweight blanket in case you're met with a demand to cover up.

✤ If you need to express or pump and you want to do it in the privacy of the onboard restroom, you'll have more time for it if you go into the restroom while other passengers are having their meals.

✤ If another passenger complains about your nursing and you're told you can't nurse on the plane or have to move or cover up, first, calmly inform the flight attendant of your right to nurse and the airline's stated policy. Ask the attendant if she or he can settle the issue with the complaining passenger by offering to move that person. If you're still being pressured, ask for the attendant's name, and

then ask to speak with the head flight attendant.

✤ You shouldn't have to move or cover up, but if you have stated your rights and they still insist, sometimes it's easier to go along and report the incident later rather than to get embroiled in a stressful argument.

✤ If you feel you were discriminated against, follow up after you return home. Send a letter to customer relations at the airline, and if warranted, file a complaint.

✤ At this writing, Transportation Security Administration (TSA) regulations permit a mother flying with or without her child to bring breast milk aboard. Breast milk is an exception to the three-ounce rule— you may travel with a greater quantity than that; however, the TSA encourages mothers to carry only as much milk as needed to reach their destination. This may not allow for delays, though, so it's wise to take a little extra. You may keep your milk separate from the three-ounce containers of other gels and liquids in your zip-top bag. It's best to carry it in bottles that accurately show the amount in each bottle. Declare your breast milk at the security checkpoint and present it for additional inspection when you reach the X-ray.

If you feel comfortable about breastfeeding in front of others, there's no reason why you shouldn't. You need not feel apologetic or bashful about nurturing your baby in the healthiest way possible. In fact, this right is legally protected almost everywhere in the United States, as discussed in Appendix I.

Many women who never thought they could feel easy about nursing in public find that when they're out with their baby and the baby is hungry, they overcome their reluctance very quickly —often in direct proportion to how loudly the baby is crying. And the more you do it, the easier it gets. The basic ingredients for comfort are what you wear, where you go, how you act—and most of all, how confident you feel about your right to nurture your child wherever you happen to be.

You may want to practice nursing at home in front of a mirror with different kinds of clothing and cover-ups until you feel comfortable about doing it in public. It's a good idea to practice hooking and unhooking your bra cup in front of the mirror, as well.

Where You Go

If you're out shopping at a department store, you can often find a comfortable chair in a well-equipped women's lounge, in the furniture department, in or near a women's fitting room, or in the children's department. In a restaurant, try to sit in a corner seat in a booth. In a bookstore, look for a comfortable area where people can sit and read—and you can sit and nurse.

When you drive somewhere, nurse your baby in your parked car before you get out at your destination. On a bus, train, or plane, try to sit next to the window, where you'll have a little more privacy.

How You Act

You can position yourself for maximum privacy by turning your body away from the sight of passersby. Some women discourage interaction with strangers by maintaining eye contact with their babies or a companion, while others openly meet other people's eyes and smile. Either way, your body language can show your own comfort with breast-feeding and will tend to discourage disparaging remarks and complaints. Also, people will follow your line of sight. If you look away from your breast while your baby is latching on, people are less likely to notice. Nursing at the first sign of hunger is better than waiting for a crying baby to call attention to what you're doing. If you're with someone, she or he can "read" a newspaper and provide extra privacy.

Almost all cases in which women have been asked to stop nursing or to go somewhere else to nurse have ended in apologies to them. But most women would rather avoid the incident in the first place. However, should you encounter difficulty, remember that the law is on your side.

CHAPTER TEN

Drugs and the Nursing Mother

*"By taking . . . precautions in drug selection
and considering the infant's age, breastfeeding rarely
needs to be discouraged or discontinued when
a mother needs drug therapy."*

PHILIP O. ANDERSON, PHARM.D. Clinical Professor,
UC San Diego Skaggs School of Pharmacy & Pharmaceutical Sciences

From time immemorial, people have taken a variety of drugs to cure their diseases, to ease their pain, to drown their sorrows, and to achieve new levels of consciousness. During the past half-century, however, our pharmacopoeia has mushroomed incredibly: 90 percent of all the medicines available today were unknown fifty years ago. In addition, with advances in medical research we now know that any drugs that you take might affect the fetus you carry in your womb and the baby you breastfeed.

It's comforting to know that you can safely take many commonly used drugs and continue nursing your baby. It's true that most do cross into breast milk, but in most cases, they do so in such small amounts that they will not hurt your nursing baby. Still, all too often, physicians unnecessarily tell mothers not to breastfeed if they are taking any medicine, for fear that the substance will hurt the baby.

As of this writing, the FDA is about to change its labeling system to provide updated, detailed information about a medication's risks and benefits—or about the risks of failing to treat a medical condition. Up to now, drug labeling has been oversimplified, providing little guidance. Furthermore, many drug companies, fearful of being sued, stipulate that a drug is not suitable for a pregnant or nursing woman, even when there is no evidence for this statement. Of course, this overlooks the drawbacks of *not* breastfeeding.

In this chapter, we'll focus on the effects of drugs on nursing babies. We don't discuss the effect of any drugs that you take during your pregnancy. If you're pregnant while you're reading this, it is essential for you to consult your doctor before you take any prescription medication, over-the-counter (OTC) remedy or herbal preparation, or nutritional supplement, including vitamins. And you certainly shouldn't take any recreational drug. Some of these can have harmful effects on the fetus when taken by a pregnant woman.

The same holds true for breastfeeding. Drugs act differently during pregnancy than they do during lactation; just because it's safe during one stage doesn't mean it's safe during the other. Check with your doctor to be sure medications, herbs, or supplements are compatible with nursing.

If there is a medical indication that a particular drug is important for your physical and emotional well-being, in most cases you can take it. Some drugs require a temporary suspension of breastfeeding, but you can resume nursing once the compound has left your body.

The boxes in this chapter list drugs that are divided into the following categories, according to criteria that are accurate at the time of this writing:

❖ those you can usually take without fear while you are nursing (page 224);

❖ those that, if you need to take them temporarily, require a brief interruption of breastfeeding (page 226);

❖ those that, if you need to take them, will require that you wean your baby (page 225);

❖ and those that are controversial (page 226). In these cases, you'll need to weigh the risks and benefits to you and your baby, and decide whether or not to take the drug. Often there's an alternative drug that has a proven track record that is safer for breastfeeding. Sometimes you can make a trade-off, taking a drug that's slightly less effective at treating the condition but still compatible with breastfeeding.

Resources for Information about Drugs and Breastfeeding

The Drugs and Lactation Database (LactMed) is the major source of information on medications and their effect, if any, on breastfeeding. It is a peer-reviewed, fully referenced, and constantly updated database of drugs that breastfeeding mothers may be considering taking. Among the data included are the possible effects of specific drugs on breastfed infants and on lactation, and alternate drugs to consider. It is maintained by the U.S. National Library of Medicine, part of the National Institutes of Health. You can access it at http://toxnet.nlm.nih.gov.

Breastfeeding Pharmacology is a comprehensive Texas Tech University site maintained by Thomas W. Hale, RPh, PhD, about medications and lactation. He takes questions only from professionals, but anyone can search the database of answers. Access at http://neonatal.ama.ttuhsc.edu/lact. Dr. Hale's book, *Medications and*

Mothers' Milk: A Manual of Lactational Pharmacology, updated in 2010 for its fourteenth edition, also has helpful information.

You can ask your doctor to consult the American Academy of Pediatrics's book *Breastfeeding Handbook for Physicians;* chapter 12 discusses specific drugs and drug classes.

You can also contact La Leche League International (see the Resource Appendix), which has access to lactation-knowledgeable physicians on the league's Health Advisory Council, who can help to guide you and your doctor.

One other good resource, for medical professionals only, is the Breastfeeding and Human Lactation Study Center of the University of Rochester School of Medicine and Dentistry. Your doctor or lactation consultant can contact the center at 585-275-0088 (phone) or 585-461-3614 (fax).

However, these lists are only guides at best, since new drugs come on the market every day and new findings emerge about many established ones. For specific, up-to-date information about various medications and their effects on nursing babies, you can go to the resources listed in the box above. Before you take any medication—even one on a safe list—discuss it with your doctor. Factors such as the age and health of your baby and your overall health might affect how safe that drug really is.

Before we discuss medications taken while you are breastfeeding, let's look at the effects on nursing of drugs taken during labor and delivery.

Drugs During Childbirth

Biblical scholars still debate whether God's injunction to Eve, "In travail shalt thou bring forth children," implied labor or sorrow. In any case, most societies have evolved ways to speed delivery, make the mother's work easier, and lessen her discomfort. General anesthesia, which renders the woman completely unconscious, is rarely used today. If any anesthesia is used during labor and delivery, more commonly it is regional (local) anesthesia, which blocks the nerve pathways that carry the sensation of pain to the brain.

If you receive medication during labor and delivery, some of it will pass through the placenta and enter your baby's blood supply and tissues. The effect of the anesthesia in your body will wear off in a few hours, but it may take several weeks for all the drugs to be eliminated from your baby's immature system.

Babies whose mothers received a great deal of anesthesia during childbirth are likely to be quite sleepy during the first few days of life. While this does not seem to have a permanent effect on full-size, full-term babies, it does affect their early activities, including their interest in nursing. The vigorous suckling of a hungry baby is vital for establishing an ample supply of milk in the mother, so if your baby is sleepy and not interested in nursing, both you and he are at a disadvantage in building up your production of milk: You'll have to work harder at helping your baby become a good nurser.

What About Epidurals?

The most commonly administered regional anesthesia today is the epidural block, in which an anesthetic agent or a narcotic, or a combination of both, is injected into the space between the spinal cord and its outer covering to deaden sensation in the lower half of the body during delivery. Different anesthesiologists use different combinations of drugs.

The use of epidural anesthesia has increased dramatically over the past thirty years. It's easy to administer, is relatively safe since it requires only a small amount of medication, and lets the mother stay awake during delivery. Also, it can be stopped temporarily to let the mother have full control over pushing, and then restarted after delivery. However, problems with epidurals may include a longer labor.

As of this writing the use of epidural blocks, especially for mothers who plan to breastfeed, is controversial. Some research reports ineffective early suckling and shorter durations of nursing by infants whose mothers received epidural anesthesia, while other research shows no effects on such babies.

What Should You Do During Childbirth?

There is no simple answer to this question. If you can avoid anesthesia during childbirth, this is best. However, you're the only person who can gauge your pain, and you're also the person who's most concerned about your child's well-being. Therefore, you, in consultation with your birth attendant, should be the one who decides which, if any, obstetric medication should be used. If you do need anesthesia, there is no reason for you to feel guilty. Most mothers who have received obstetric anesthesia have had healthy children and have gone on to breastfeed normally and happily.

You have to weigh the relative risks and benefits of pain relief. If you're in so much pain during childbirth that you're worn out and overstressed, your ability to nurse will be affected. The best thing, then, is to educate yourself ahead of time about your options, including nonchemical means of alleviating discomfort, such as breathing and relaxation techniques, massage, and visualization, either alone or in combination with lower doses of anesthesia. Many of the negative effects of a drug are dramatically dose-related, so minimizing the amount you take minimizes the risk.

It's extremely important to discuss with the birth attendant what kind of medication might be ordered while you're in labor. You have to be very clear about what you want. You might say something like: "I want to have the least amount of medication possible. I want to avoid general anesthesia. But what if my prepared childbirth techniques are not enough and I'm in a lot of pain? How can I feel more comfortable while posing the least amount of harm to my baby?"

The two of you can discuss your situation, in light of your medical history and physical condition, and arrive at a possible course of action. You should feel confident that both your needs and those of your baby are carefully considered and that you are getting the best care possible for your own individual situation.

After you and your birth attendant have agreed upon the probable procedures to be used in your situation, ask him or her to make a note of the plan on your chart, so that if he or she is not available when you go into labor, whoever is there will be guided by your wishes.

Medicines

A number of medicines taken by the pregnant woman that can cause serious birth defects in the developing fetus may cause no harm to the infant when ingested in the mother's milk. On the other hand, some drugs that may be safe for a fetus because they are detoxified by the mother's kidneys and liver may not be safe for a newborn baby, whose own system is too immature to do this important task. We cannot, therefore, apply what we know about one situation to the other.

The problem is that there's so much we don't know. In most cases, we don't know about the long-term effects of a baby's receiving drugs through her mother's milk. We don't know whether receiving drugs in infancy might cause a hypersensitivity to certain components later on. Nor do we know whether a buildup of the drug in the baby's system could cause problems now or later.

What Should You Do Postpartum?

As the most important guideline (even for people who are not nursing an infant), it's best to take the least amount of medicine possible. If you don't need it, don't take it. If you do need it, ask your doctor what the minimum effective dosage would be and what means of taking it will minimize its effects on your baby.

You should not be taking significant amounts of any medicine, even the most seemingly innocuous OTC or herbal preparation, without your doctor's knowledge. (You can take an occasional ibuprofen, which would be better than aspirin; acetaminophen; antihistamine; or other OTC preparation, such as the ones listed in the box on page 224.) Nor should you take anything for more than three or four days without checking with your doctor. This is important for your own health, as well as your baby's; you might be masking symptoms of a serious nature. Remember, not all OTC remedies are safe. There have been cases of babies who became sick after their mothers had taken OTC cough and cold remedies. Acetaminophen (Tylenol), for ex-

ample, should not be taken for more than a few days or in large doses.

In some rare cases, your medical situation might require a course of treatment that could have an adverse effect on your baby. Should this occur, you will have to make the best of a less-than-ideal situation and wean your baby, either temporarily or permanently. If this becomes necessary, you need to remember that for whatever lengh of time you have breastfed, you have given your child a good start in life. You can still provide warmth and comfort and nurturance in many other ways, and the most important gift you can give your child is a healthy mother.

If your doctor and your pediatrician give you the go-ahead, however, it's better to continue breastfeeding than to wean your baby prematurely because you're taking medicine. This is especially true if weaning would be abrupt. Sudden weaning is painful for the mother and upsetting for both mother and baby. Early weaning also deprives the baby of the benefits of breastfeeding. Therefore, it makes sense for mother and doctor to work together to solve medical problems within the context of breastfeeding, whenever this is possible. The drugs that would require early weaning are those listed in the box on page 225.

If you have to take a medicine that is thought to be harmful to your nursing baby, and if you need to take it for only a short period of time (say, a week or two), you can pump or express your milk during that time and discard it, while feeding your baby formula or previously expressed milk. This way, you'll be keeping up your milk supply, and you'll be able to resume nursing as soon as the medicine is no longer in your system. If breastfeeding has been well established, your baby will probably be eager to go back to the breast.

Ask the Doctors

Before taking any new drug, ask your doctor and your baby's doctor the following questions:

1. Will this drug pass through my breast milk?

Most drugs do, but the baby is generally exposed to less than 1 to 2 percent of the mother's dosage. In some cases, the baby's absorption may be even lower. In any case, this small amount is usually not harmful.

2. Is this drug potentially dangerous to my baby?

A mother on continuous or long-term medication for some medical condition needs to pose this question to her doctor and her baby's doctor, since the possible cumulative exposure to the drug must be considered in evaluating its effect on the baby.

3. Will this drug decrease my milk production or my let-down?

Ask your doctor whether there is any published research about the effect of a particular drug on a nursing mom's output.

4. What complications or discomfort will I experience if I do *not* take this medicine? Will they be acceptable from both medical and comfort standpoints?

Will it be safe for me to forgo treatment?

You could probably put up with a few aches and pains, but if your health is at stake, being a martyr will benefit neither you nor your child.

5. Can I safely postpone treatment until my child is older and bigger, and his more mature body systems are better able to detoxify chemicals in my milk?

Sometimes a compound that would be dangerous for a one-week-old or one-month-old poses no problem for an older baby. Also, a baby receiving only breast milk is more vulnerable than an older one who is eating other foods, as well. Sometimes it's possible to wait to be treated until your baby gets a little bigger.

6. Can I monitor my baby for possible effects and stop taking the medicine in time to avoid harming him? If so, what symptoms should I look for?

7. Is there a drug I can take instead that is less likely to affect my baby?

8. What is the half-life of this drug?

A drug's half-life is the time that it takes for the drug's peak concentration in the plasma part of the bloodstream to decline by half. (The plasma is the liquid component of blood in which blood cells are suspended.) This is one factor that determines how frequently a drug has to be taken. It generally takes from four to seven half-lives for a drug to disappear from the body altogether. For example, the half-life of penicillin is two hours; eight hours after taking penicillin, more than 95 percent of it is gone from the body. The

(continued on page 228)

Medicines That Can Usually Be Taken Safely by Nursing Mothers*

The following medicines are generally safe for breastfeeding mothers to take in the usual doses while they continue to nurse their babies. However, it's always safest to discuss the medication and length of time to take it with your doctor and your baby's doctor:

❖ acetaminophen/paracetamol (Tylenol); in recommended doses

❖ acyclovir and vidarabine, for herpes

❖ most antibiotics, including penicillin, amoxicillin, azithromycin, erythromycin, gentamicin, cephalosporins (occasionally may cause temporary loose stool in the baby; also watch your baby for signs of thrush, since antibiotics can increase the risk for this fungal infection)

❖ antiepileptic drugs, including lamotrigine, carbamazepine, phenytoin, and valproate

❖ antihistamines, in small, occasional doses

❖ antihypertensives, except for some drugs in the beta blocker category

❖ cimetidine (Tagamet)

❖ dental anesthetics, including novacaine and nitrous oxide

❖ fluconazole (Diflucan), for thrush in milk duct and on breast, or for vaginal yeast infection

❖ ibuprofen (Advil, Motrin), for mild to moderate pain and inflammation; 1–2 tablets a day for occasional short-term use

❖ insulin, for diabetes

❖ levothyroxine (Synthroid), to treat underactive thyroid functioning

❖ loperamide (Imodium), for diarrhea; 1–2 a day for up to one week

❖ metronidazole (Flagyl); the AAP recommends discarding breast milk for 24 hours afterward, since a large percentage ends up in the milk

❖ naproxen (Aleve)

❖ nystatin, for thrush

❖ phenobarbital, in small amounts; doses large enough to put the mother to sleep can make the baby sleepy, too

❖ probiotics, including *Lactobacillus acidophilus* and bifidobacteria

❖ tetracycline; short-term use—two to three weeks—is safe because the calcium in breast milk inhibits absorption by the baby

❖ tretinoin (Retin-A); safe as long as baby does not come in contact with area of skin being treated

❖ tolbutamide (Orinase), for diabetes

❖ vaccines

*Sources for this box and the boxes on pages 225, 226, and 227: American Academy of Pediatrics Committee on Drugs, 2001; Cheston M. Berlin Jr., MD, 2010; Ruth Lawrence, MD, 2009; K. Meador, MD, et al., 2008; The Drugs and Lactation Database (LactMed).

Medicines That Should Not Be Taken by Nursing Mothers

MEDICINE	REASON
bromocriptine (Parlodel)	Inhibits prolactin secretion, decreases milk supply.
chemotherapeutic agents used to treat cancer	These drugs are given precisely because they kill cells in the body. There is a danger, therefore, that even a tiny dose may have harmful effects on cells in the baby's system. They may suppress a baby's immune system, and their effect on growth is unknown.
ergotamine (Ergomar, Ergostat, Gynergen)	Doses used in medicines for migraine headache can cause vomiting, diarrhea, and convulsions in baby. May decrease milk supply.
lithium	Can cause irritability and poor feeding. Significant levels of lithium have been found in the plasma of nursing infants, and the consequence of this is unknown. The very young premature infant is perhaps at more risk than older infants.
all tricyclic agents and paroxetine (Paxil)	These antidepressants can cause drowsiness, changes in sleep or feeding, vomiting, breathing problems, irritability in infant, and possible cardiac effects. Unknown long-term effects on child's central nervous system.
atenolol, given to prevent migraine headache and also to lower blood pressure	This drug may cause slowing of a baby's heart rate, especially in preterm infants or those with impaired kidney function.
pseudoephedrine	This compound, which has been removed from most OTC products, is still found in some OTC decongestants. It may decrease a mother's milk supply because it may depress the secretion of prolactin. It is not recommended for children under 12, and therefore would not be advisable for a nursing mother.
tetracycline (long-term use)	Long-term or repeated use during lactation can discolor the baby's teeth. May also cause rash and/or thrush.
codeine	Codeine is present in many prescription cough, cold, and pain-relief medications. Although many nursing mothers have been using codeine safely for years, a small percentage of people have a genetic trait that makes them ultra-rapid codeine metabolizers. Since the body transforms codeine into morphine, the baby of a nursing mother with this trait can experience a morphine overdose, which can be fatal. The only way a person can find out if she is in this group is by a genetic test. Even babies of mothers who do not have this gene may be affected by codeine, so a mother should always consult her doctor before taking any medicine containing it. Ideally, she should take an alternate pain reliever. If the doctor believes the mother needs the codeine-containing drug, she should take the minimum dose possible and for the shortest period of time. To be safe, she should stop nursing as long as she is taking any codeine.

Medicines That Require a Temporary Cessation of Breastfeeding

When a mother needs to undergo a diagnostic procedure requiring her to take a radioactive compound (like gallium-67, iodine-123, -125, or -131, or technetium-99m), she'll need to stop breastfeeding for a little while. As long as the drug is in her system, radioactivity is present in her milk and will reach her baby. Iodine has a long half-life and enters pumped milk.

Should you need this type of procedure, you can protect your baby by doing the following:

✢ Ask your doctor to consult a nuclear medicine physician who can prescribe the agent with the shortest half-life.

✢ Discontinue breastfeeding for twelve hours to two weeks, depending on the compound and your doctor's orders. Most often, two or three days is the longest one needs to suspend breastfeeding, since the long-lasting types of these medicines are hardly ever given anymore.

✢ Before the procedure, pump your breasts and freeze enough milk to feed your baby for the period of time you expect not to be breastfeeding. Or you can use formula during this short-term interruption of breastfeeding if your baby is not at risk for allergy (see Chapter 8).

✢ Continue to pump your breasts (to maintain milk production) during the time the radioactive agent is present in your body. In fact, you can pump and freeze your milk, and use it later, since the radioactivity decays within hours or days, depending upon the medication and the dosage. Ask your doctor when the milk will be safe to feed your baby. Label it with the date so you will know when it's safe to use.

✢ Modern radiology departments can measure milk for the presence of radioactivity. You can resume nursing when the radioactivity has disappeared. This is the safest step of all.

Medicines of Concern

The effect of the following drugs on mothers or nursing babies is either unknown or variable.

Antidepressants

As discussed in Chapter 8, postpartum depression is a serious problem for both new mothers and their infants, in part because babies of depressed mothers often have difficulty getting attached to their mothers and developing interpersonal relationships. That's one reason why it's so important to treat depression in a mother. Also, breastfeeding is so important for mothers and babies that it should be encouraged whenever possible, and it may itself be an important aspect of treating postpartum depression.

The dilemma is how to treat the mother's depression with minimal risk to the baby. Very often, doctors treating depression prescribe medications belonging to a class known as selective serotonin reuptake inhibitors (SSRIs). These include drugs sold under the trade names Zoloft, Celexa, Lexapro, Paxil, and Prozac. Many physicians favor Zoloft because very little of the drug appears in breast milk. Other prescribed antidepressants, known as tricyclics, are not recommended for nursing mothers.

All antidepressants studied do appear in breast milk and in the plasma of some of the nursing infants exposed to the drugs. There have been few case reports of adverse reactions in the nursing infant. Most of these have been in very young infants (several weeks old). Reports tell of irritability, feeding difficulties, and drowsiness in nursing babies. These drugs do change neurotransmitter chemicals in the brain of the mother; their eventual effect on the neurological development of the baby is unknown at the present time. So far there is no proof of neurodevelopmental changes in later childhood and beyond in children whose nursing mothers took these drugs, but no long-term studies are available. One of the problems in studying the long-term effect of these drugs is that many of the mothers also took them during pregnancy, and separating out the prepartum from the postpartum exposure is not possible. Ultimately, this is a decision that a mother and her doctor need to make together, recognizing the importance of treating postpartum depression.

Over-the-counter cough and cold remedies

The use of these preparations is not recommended for young children, and the FDA does not even have dosing guidelines for children under two years of age. Such medications have been reported to cause breathing difficulties in very young infants, and some researchers suspect that infants may receive such medicines through breastfeeding. The FDA has published an advisory warning against the use of these medicines in children under two years of age.

Domperidone

This agent is sometimes prescribed in other countries to increase a woman's milk production, but not in the United States, where the FDA does not approve it for sale. Its effectiveness for this purpose is questionable, and the safety of the substance is of concern, especially in someone with a preexisting heart problem.

Sleeping pills

Small studies of nursing mothers who took zolpidem (Ambien), eszopiclone (Lunesta), or zaleplon (Sonata) found low levels in breast milk and concluded that these sleep aids in the usual small doses would not be harmful to nursing babies. However, some adults who have taken these pills have fallen into a deep, unrousable sleep or behaved in unusual ways that they didn't remember afterward, so a mother alone with a baby or toddler would be well advised not to take any of these.

shorter the half-life, the sooner it will disappear from your bloodstream (and therefore your milk) and the sooner it will leave your baby's body.

9. Is this a new medicine about which little is known; if so, can a more established medication be substituted?

10. Is this drug ever given to treat babies? What would you suggest if it were my baby who had this condition and not me?

If a medicine is sometimes prescribed for babies, it is generally safe when the mother takes it.

11. Is this the smallest possible dose that can be effective?

Although relatively low doses of certain drugs may not pose problems, even slightly higher doses taken for longer periods of time can be harmful to a baby.

For any medication, the starting dose should be as low as possible and the length of treatment should be as short as possible.

12. Why am I being advised to stop nursing? Is it because the maker of the medicine does not know what the effects would be? Or because there are known ill effects?

If You Must Take a Prescribed Medicine

Even if the medicine you're taking is considered safe for your baby, you still want to minimize its effects as much as possible.

One way to do this is to take it immediately after a feeding and to delay the next feeding as long as you can so that the medicine will have as much time as possible to work its way through your system before the baby's next nursing. It often helps to take a medicine just before your baby's longest period of sleep and to take a short-acting drug rather than a timed-release formulation.

Meanwhile, watch your baby closely for any unusual symptoms. These may include the following: fever, sleepiness, much longer periods of time between feedings, breathing difficulties, vomiting, unusual crying, loss of appetite, diarrhea, rash, irritability, low muscle tone, and so forth. Call your baby's doctor right away if you notice these or other possible signs of drug effects.

If you need to take an antibiotic, it's advisable to take a probiotic along with it. Antibiotics kill harmful bacteria, but they also often kill good bacteria—the ones that help to prevent the growth of harmful organisms. When these good bacteria are killed, you become vulnerable to a vaginal yeast infection. The yeast infection may then travel to your breast, which may cause thrush in your baby's mouth (see Chapter 15 for more about thrush).

Probiotics are dietary supplements or foods that contain these "good" bacteria. The most common probiotic is *Lactobacillus acidophilus*. You can buy probiotics in health food stores and pharmacies. Certain yogurts, juices, and other foods also contain active probiotics. Ask your doctor what kinds of probiotics he or she recommends.

Birth Control

Contraceptives that contain hormones include the minipill with progestin (a synthetic form of progesterone used in many medications), skin patches, long-acting injections, and under-the-skin implants. These all contain estrogen or progesterone or a combination of both. Neither estrogens nor progesterones have been associated with any change in the *quality* of breast milk. However, hormonal contraceptives may reduce the *quantity* of breast milk you produce, especially if you take them early in lactation. But they do not appear to be associated with a decrease in milk production if taken after six weeks, when the mother's milk supply is established.

Neither estrogens nor progestins transfer into milk, and long-term studies have failed to find any effect on growth in children up to eight years old whose mothers took estrogen-based birth control pills while nursing. And no effect on growth or the onset of puberty has been found in children up to seventeen years of age whose mothers took progesterone compounds.

Progestin-only pills do have some disadvantages. They are somewhat less effective in preventing pregnancy than the combined estrogen-and-progesterone pills (but since breastfeeding itself tends to protect against pregnancy, this is usually not a problem for nursing mothers), and they sometimes cause bleeding irregularities. Women with diabetes are advised not to take the progestin-only pill.

Once your baby is six weeks old it is probably safe for you to take either the low-dose-estrogen or progestin-only birth control pills or to use a hormonal patch. Before this time, however, you are better off using a barrier method or another form of non-hormonal birth control. For a full discussion of contraception during lactation, see Chapter 13, which also explains the Lactational Amenorrhea Method (LAM), a means of birth control that relies on exclusive breastfeeding during the first six months of a baby's life. In any case, it's safest to discuss your choice of contraception with your gynecologist.

Herbs and Other Natural Remedies

Many people turn to herbal, homeopathic, or other alternative remedies because they believe they're safer than artificial chemicals. However, not all substances that grow naturally are safe for pregnant or breastfeeding mothers. In fact, quite a few are not safe for anyone.

Large quantities of sage, for example, can reduce the supply of breast milk, and strong infusions of licorice can increase blood pressure. The sale of other once commonly used herbal preparations has been outlawed because illnesses have been traced to them.

Aside from the fact that very little hard scientific research has been conducted on herbal products, they are not prepared according to a single accepted formula, and as a result their effects are not predictable. There is no oversight by the FDA or any other governmental body. The active ingredients are unknown, since plant substances may have dozens of potentially active compounds. Purity is not guaranteed. Labels are not always accurate, and the substances can be contaminated anywhere in the process. The herbal tea or preparation you buy in one health food store may have a very different strength from one that you make yourself, or that you obtain from another store or source.

Many herbs are very powerful and can produce serious side effects. Some interact in harmful ways with other drugs you may be taking. Therefore, do not use them casually. Treat herbs as potent substances and use them only under the direction of someone who is extremely knowledgeable about the herb in question and its effect on a breastfeeding mother and baby, and who also knows what other medicines or substances you are taking. Avoid unfamiliar brands of herbal tea or home-brewed potions. Poisonous alkaloids may make them toxic.

The only herbal preparations that are generally considered quite safe are major brands of herbal tea, which list the contents of herbs in the tea. However, even with these, you need to use good sense. Moderation is the key. If you drink two or three cups of herbal tea a day, and if you steep them for a fairly brief time to keep the infusion mild, you probably won't run into trouble. Just avoid drinking too much or drinking a very strong mixture.

Recreational and Hard Drugs

Caffeinated beverages, cigarettes, and alcohol can affect breast milk and breastfed babies. And so can popular recreational and hard drugs.

Caffeine

You know that caffeine is present in coffee and tea, but it may surprise you to know that caffeine is also found in soft drinks, chocolate, and some OTC cold medications. Too much caffeine taken by the mother can sometimes make a baby overstimulated, jittery, and fussy. Infants do not metabolize caffeine well, and it accumulates in their system. You can still enjoy your morning cup of coffee, but ideally you should drink it after a feeding instead of before, and avoid consuming more

Minimizing the Effect of Nicotine on Your Nursing Baby

If you feel that you can't stop smoking even for the duration of pregnancy and lactation, it's still better to breastfeed rather than formula-feed. You can decrease the risk to your baby by taking these steps:

❖ Don't smoke, and don't let anyone else smoke, in the home or in any indoor space where your children are.

❖ Don't smoke while nursing. Aside from the danger of the tobacco smoke, there's the very real risk of dropping hot ashes on your baby.

❖ Cut down, smoking as little as possible, especially around your baby. The less you smoke, the less risk there is to your baby.

❖ Do your smoking immediately after a feeding rather than just before one.

❖ If you must smoke, wait two hours afterward before you breastfeed.

than three cups a day, or the caffeine equivalent in other foods and drinks. Try substituting decaffeinated coffee, or at least make your coffee half with caffeine, half-decaffeinated. And still no more than three cups a day, since even decaf contains a little caffeine.

Tobacco

If you smoke, is breastfeeding still best for your baby? Yes. Would it be better for your baby if you did not smoke, or at least cut down while you're nursing? The answer here is a more emphatic yes. It would also be better for you and everyone else in your household.

Nicotine, the main substance released when you smoke a cigarette, passes through your milk to your baby. This causes few, if any, severe toxic reactions. However, nicotine does interfere with milk production, so babies of smoking mothers gain weight more slowly than do babies of nonsmokers. Nicotine also seems to make babies sleep less. Babies of smoking mothers spend less time sleeping during the hours immediately after their mothers smoked, compared to times when their mothers did not smoke. Some research also suggests that a mother's smoking may have negative effects on her baby's tooth development. And it's possible that nicotine absorbed through breast milk can make babies fretful. The main reason given by mothers who smoke for discontinuing breastfeeding is that they "don't have enough milk," or that their babies "don't seem satisfied." It may be possible to avoid both these problems by not smoking.

Also, we know about the adverse effects of passive smoking, or second-hand smoke, that is, inhaling the smoke from other people's cigarettes.

Babies are susceptible to upper respiratory infections when the person closest to them is the one breathing smoke on them. This is true whether a baby is being fed by breast or bottle. One study found that babies with parents who smoke have higher rates of upper respiratory tract infections, but that breastfeeding protected them to some degree. These researchers concluded, "Smoking should not be permitted in households with infants." One reason for this is thirdhand smoke, the tobacco toxins that remain in household dust, swirling in the air, and are deposited on surfaces after a cigarette is extinguished. Young children are especially vulnerable to thirdhand smoke exposure because they breathe near, play on, touch, and put their mouths on contaminated surfaces.

If you're pregnant now, you probably already know that smoking causes a variety of prenatal complications. The best documented finding related to smoking is the tendency of pregnant smokers to bear smaller babies. And it's harder to establish breastfeeding with a premature or low-birthweight baby. Women who stop smoking by the time they are four months pregnant do not experience these complications.

Alcohol

Alcohol in moderation is a relaxant; in excess, it acts as a depressant. In recent years, many health-care professionals have advised women not to drink any alcohol for the entire duration of pregnancy. What about during lactation?

For a long time, nursing women were advised to drink alcohol, especially beer, to produce more milk. However, research has contradicted this bit of folklore. So don't feel you have to drink to make milk. But if you want to have an occasional glass of beer or wine, or a cocktail, it will probably not have any ill effects on your nursing baby.

Heavy drinking, however, is another story altogether. It can affect your ability to care for your baby, and it can make your nursing baby drowsy by depressing the nervous system. If you have had so much to drink that you can't drive, you should not breastfeed.

One way to tell whether you have too much alcohol in your milk to nurse is by using a test called Milkscreen that's sold online and in some drugstores. You saturate a special pad with breast milk; if the color changes after two minutes, that means that alcohol is present in your milk and you should wait before breastfeeding.

A 120-pound woman will need about two and a half hours to metabolize the amount of alcohol in one drink. One drink consists of 1.5 ounces of 86-proof alcohol, 5 ounces of wine, or 12 ounces of beer.

If you do indulge in light social drinking, you can minimize the effect on your baby by following these suggestions.

✤ Limit your intake to one drink.

✤ Wait two to three hours after drinking before you nurse your baby.

✤ If your baby is under three months old, avoid alcohol altogether, since infant livers have a hard time metabolizing alcohol.

❖ Choose drinks low in alcohol (like a champagne punch or small glass of wine or beer) or diluted with water or juice.

❖ Drink slowly. Sip from one drink all evening.

❖ Eat before and while you drink.

❖ Be sure your drink is measured when poured.

❖ Order juice or a soft drink instead of taking an alcoholic drink you don't want. You can always tell friends, "My baby is under the legal drinking age."

❖ Before drinking, express or pump and store your alcohol-free breast milk to feed to your baby in case insufficient time elapses between your last drink and the baby's feeding. Express or pump your postdrinking milk and discard it. Wait to breastfeed until enough time has elapsed since you drank any alcohol.

Marijuana

We know less about marijuana than about any other intoxicant. We do know that its most active ingredient is fat-soluble and does appear in breast milk. It's also capable of being stored in the body for one month or longer, even after a single exposure. Since studies of nursing animals have shown structural changes in brain cells and drowsiness in nursing babies after their mothers were given this drug, pregnant and nursing women should abstain from using marijuana.

Cocaine

Pregnant and nursing women should not use cocaine at all in any form. For their baby's sake, women who cannot abstain should not breastfeed—and for their own sake, they should enroll in a treatment program.

Many reports have described serious behavioral and health problems in babies born to women who used cocaine during pregnancy, which underscores the dangers inherent in this drug. Many people underestimate the risk of cocaine, feeling that occasional use at a party will do little harm. Aside from the fact that we don't know that such a pattern is indeed safe, we also don't know which people who begin as social users will become addicted. Anyone using cocaine is playing with fire, and a pregnant or nursing woman risks injuring her baby in the flames.

Amphetamines

These powerful stimulants can cause irritability and poor sleeping patterns in a breastfed baby. Therefore, pregnant and nursing women should not use them.

Barbiturates

While these drugs can apparently be taken safely by nursing mothers in the usual small medical doses, overuse of them can be dangerous to both mother and baby. For the user, they can be addictive or even fatal. They're particularly dangerous when taken with alcohol, and nearly one-third of accidental drug-related deaths are caused by barbiturate overdose. If a mother takes enough barbiturates to put her to sleep or to make her drunk, her baby will almost always be adversely affected. Again, this is a class of drugs to stay away from, especially when you're nursing.

Heroin

Women addicted to heroin are prone to bearing premature babies who have become addicted to the drug within the womb. If a mother is in a detoxification program, she will probably be taking methadone. She should consult a physician who is familiar with the effects of methadone, can control her dosage, and can advise her as to the safety of breastfeeding. If she does breastfeed, the methadone that passes through her milk will act to wean her baby from the heroin or methadone that her baby received during pregnancy. A doctor needs to watch the baby very closely for symptoms of heroin withdrawal or reaction to the methadone. Symptoms include sweating, fevers, diarrhea, vomiting, poor eating, or inconsolable crankiness. If the baby shows any of these symptoms, the doctor may prescribe medication.

A mother who continues to use heroin should not breastfeed. Heroin passes through milk and may affect the baby even more than it does the mother, causing tremors, restlessness, vomiting, poor feeding—and possible addiction.

Other Drugs

Phencyclidine (PCP) is a potent hallucinogen that is dangerous to both mother and baby. Methamphetamine seems to be transmitted through breast milk. For these, as for other "recreational" drugs, the approach is simple—don't.

As a nursing mother, you have many choices to make. Your decision about the substances to which you will expose yourself and your baby is one of the most important ones you will make for the well-being of both of you.

CHAPTER ELEVEN

Pumping, Expressing, and Storing Breast Milk

"At first, the idea of pumping my milk to feed to my baby seemed like a huge ordeal. I was bewildered by all the different kinds of pumps and didn't know how to pick one. But when I finally found one that worked for me, it made both of our lives a lot easier."

LUCY Port Washington, New York

In this chapter, we'll talk about situations in which you might want to express or pump your breast milk to give to your baby. You'll find practical, how-to suggestions that have worked for other nursing mothers, which you can adapt for yourself if you need to express milk.

What Kind of Pump Do You Need?

The following guidelines may help you choose the type of pump to rent or buy. However, every woman is different, and some women who fit into the electric-pump category may do just fine with a manual type. Others, who fit into the manual category, may prefer a battery-operated or electric pump. Only you—and your lactation professional—can decide which type of pump is right for you and your situation.

You probably want to rent or buy a hospital-grade double electric pump if:

✛ Your baby will be in the hospital, either because of prematurity or illness and you want to establish your milk supply for the future when you'll be able to nurse. If your baby is older when hospitalized and you are already experienced at pumping, you can continue to use the pump you have been using.

✛ Your baby has a physical or neurological impairment that interferes with her ability to nurse.

✛ You're trying to increase your milk supply, so you're pumping every three hours or at every time your baby would ordinarily be nursing.

✛ You're trying to relactate or to nurse an adopted baby.

Nursing mothers who work outside their homes will find more suggestions specific to their situation in Chapter 12; mothers of premature or sick babies will find help in Chapter 16.

There are several ways of collecting breast milk—by electric or battery-operated pump, by manual (handheld) pump, and by hand-expression (using your hands to get your milk flowing and into a container). The method you decide on will depend on your own individual needs and preferences, based on your own unique situation, as well as on your comfort, convenience, time constraints, and finances.

In recent years, manufacturers have responded to the double trend of increased breastfeeding rates and rising numbers of working mothers by producing a wide variety of pumps. We provide a general overview of the most popular types of pumps; it's impossible for any book to remain up-to-date on all available products.

Although some women still prefer to express their milk by hand (and this is a valuable skill to learn as a backup), pumps are usually quicker and more efficient. First we'll talk about the different kinds of pumps; then we'll offer guidelines for hand-expression.

To help you decide which pump to use, see the box above and the information in the next section.

You probably want to buy a high-quality electric pump if:

✢ You're working or going to school full-time.

✢ You want to increase your milk supply but are pumping only a couple of times a day, not at every feeding.

You probably want to buy a small (less expensive) electric pump if breastfeeding is well established and:

✢ You're working or going to school part-time.

✢ You're preparing for a brief separation from your baby.

✢ Your husband, partner, or babysitter is occasionally feeding the baby.

You may be able to get by with hand-expression or using a hand-operated or foot-operated pump if:

✢ You're caring for your healthy baby at home and you want to pump milk only for an occasional missed feeding.

✢ You want to relieve engorgement or pain from sore nipples.

✢ You're pumping less than twice a week.

✢ You're using the pump to draw out flat or inverted nipples.

Choosing a Pump

One good way to decide which pump to use is to find out which ones women seem to be happiest with. Ask a lactation consultant, other nursing mothers, or your local La Leche League leader.

You can also contact the companies listed in the Resource Appendix (some have lactation consultants on staff) and ask them to send you information about their products. Most pump manufacturers' websites have clear illustrations or photos of the different pumps they make. You can also access several websites that offer comparisons of different pumps. Start your research a few weeks before you plan to pump, if possible.

As of this writing, the following websites offer helpful information:

✢ www.breastpumpsdirect.com: This company sells pumps but is unaffiliated with any particular brand. It has good general information and offers excellent comparisons of different pumps.

✢ www.fda.gov/cdrh/breastpumps: The FDA regulates breast pumps and offers up-to-date information.

❖ www.babylovesyourmilk.com: A mother who nursed seven children researched breast pumps and gives her opinions as well as recommendations from others. She is not affiliated with any particular brand.

❖ www.amazon.com: Type "breast pumps" into the search box. You'll see descriptions of pumps with user ratings.

❖ www.epinions.com: Type "breast pumps" into the search box. You'll find descriptions of pumps, as well as user ratings.

❖ Although the information given in this book is accurate at the time of writing, new products are constantly being introduced, old ones discontinued, and prices changed. To find the most up-to-date information, type "breast pumps" into your Internet search engine.

Whichever pump you choose, you need to look at the instructions and see whether the pump is easy to assemble, use, clean, and take apart. In a store, ask to practice assembling and taking apart several different display pumps. For health reasons, you usually can't return a pump once you have opened the packaging. And if a pump is defective, you'll probably have to send it back to the manufacturer, not the store.

Important features to look for in any pump include:

❖ Gentleness: It should not hurt your breasts or nipples. The pump's breast shield, or flange, should fit comfortably, so that your nipple does not rub against it. (The flange is the plastic or rubber part that fits over the nipple and areola.) Some pumps offer different flange sizes that make all the difference in the world when it comes to comfort and efficiency.

❖ Fit: The flange needs to fit properly so that as the nipple is pulled into the nipple tunnel, it is not rubbed or squeezed and has a little wiggle room. Depending on the size of your nipples you may need the standard size (24 mm), the large (27 mm), or the extra large (30 mm). Nipple size can increase from the pressure of pumping, so check your size after you pump. If pumping hurts even at low suction, you may need a larger flange. Ask your lactation consultant or pump manufacturer for help in gauging size (see the Resource Appendix).

❖ Comfort: The pumping motions of a hand-operated pump should not put stress on your elbow or forearm muscles.

❖ Effectiveness: The pump should drain your breast almost as well as your baby does and stimulate further production of milk, and it should do this fairly quickly.

❖ Safety: It should be easy to clean so that bacteria do not accumulate to spoil your milk.

❖ Portability: If you plan to carry the pump to and from work, it should be lightweight and easy to carry.

✤ Convenience: The fewer separate parts, the better. Additional parts should be available without having to buy a new pump or kit.

✤ Sound level: Some pumps are so noisy that it could be awkward if you plan to pump at work or elsewhere. Listen before you buy.

✤ Open or closed system: In an open-system pump, milk particles can enter parts of the pump that can't be cleaned, mold may grow in the tubing, and milk is exposed to the outside air, all of which may result in contamination of expressed milk. In a closed-system pump, there's a barrier between the pump tubing and the breast shield, so that no outside air can reach your milk. This protects your pumped milk from any airborne contaminants at your workplace, such as smoke, chemical residues, or other toxins. Although open-system pumps can be kept quite clean by thorough washing (and sometimes sterilization), closed-system pumps are easier to clean.

Used Breast Pumps

This is one piece of baby equipment that can pose health risks if you borrow or inherit one from someone else—unless it's a pump designed with special barriers to prevent contamination from one user to another. If the previous user had a fungal infection like thrush, if her breast milk contained any viruses, or if she had cracked or bleeding nipples and her pump was contaminated with blood, you and your baby may be at risk. Home sterilization methods cannot eliminate all pathogens that may be present in the pump.

Types of Pumps

Let's look at the three basic types of pumps: electric, battery-operated, and manual or hand-operated. The kind you'll choose depends on how much pumping you'll be doing and your reasons for pumping. If you'll be pumping your milk daily to be given to your baby while you're at school or work, see the suggestions in Chapter 12 about the equipment you'll need and the pumping schedule you may want to follow.

Choosing an Electric Pump

With any electric pump, you should have some kind of backup method to use in case of an emergency, like a power failure or a situation where you're not near a source of electricity. Some electric pumps can be converted to manual ones; if yours can't, you may be able to run it on batteries or get an adapter to run on your car's cigarette lighter. Or you may buy a handheld pump or learn hand-expression for backup.

How do you know which pump to choose? Two criteria are the number of times it cycles in a minute and the strength of the suction. The best pumps mimic a baby's suckling very closely. You can do this to some degree with a manual pump by beginning your pumping with a rhythm of fast, short bursts. Once you feel your milk flowing, you can slow your pace.

Hospital-Grade Fully Automatic Electric Pumps: These allow women to collect milk from both breasts simultaneously and are the easiest, fastest, most comfortable, and most efficient way to collect breast milk. While your pump is doing the work, you can read, talk on the phone, watch television, or do paperwork. You can control the degree of suction and the cycle speed to imitate your own baby's suckling pattern. The most efficient electric pumps, the fully automatic ones that hospitals use and you can rent, cycle about 50 times a minute, which is comparable to a baby's rhythm. These pumps also mimic a baby's nursing pattern: suck, release, and relax. These high-grade pumps apply strong suction to the breast, comparable to the suction a baby applies.

If you're collecting your milk for a premature or sick baby who cannot yet nurse, if you plan to collect milk to be fed to your baby while you're at work or school, or if you plan for some other reason to collect your milk for longer than a couple of weeks, this is by far the best way to do it.

The biggest drawback is expense. The most popular hospital-grade electric pumps currently cost about $1,200. However, they can be rented on a weekly or monthly basis from pharmacies, medical supply houses, hospitals, and childbirth education groups and La Leche League chapters. Most of the kits for these pumps have a closed system, and thus they can be sterilized and used by more than one woman. Be sure that the pump you plan to rent has a closed system.

It may be well worth the expense to rent a hospital-grade electric pump for a while, and it's sometimes possible to get a lower price if you contract to rent over a period of several months. The price of renting is still less than the cost of formula for an equivalent time period—and the happier you are with your pump, the more likely you are to transition to breastfeeding and to breastfeed for a long time.

There are ways to soften the blow to your bank account. If your doctor says that breastfeeding is essential for some medical reason (such as your baby's prematurity or allergy to cow's milk) and if pumping is necessary, check to see whether your medical insurance will cover the cost of buying or renting a pump. Or you may be able to join with other nursing mothers to ask your employer to buy a top-of-the-line pump to keep at your place of work. In a case like this, each user would have her own personal kit. And many retail outlets, in stores and online, offer discounts.

If your income level is low enough, you may qualify for a program that lends pumps to low-income moms. Some WIC programs (see page 19) lend electric pumps, and their records indicate that women who use the pumps end up breastfeeding longer than women who don't.

High-Quality Portable Electric Pumps: High-quality portable electric pumps, which work by a small motor powered by electricity or batteries, cycle less often, but you can adjust the suction settings and cycle speeds. Most women find them quite satisfactory for frequent pumping. They run about $200 to $400 and are the most popular choice of working mothers who will be pumping for several months and need to take the pump to work with them. These models come in stylish options and provide for pumping of both breasts at once. Some are hands-free, and usually have backpacks or briefcase-type carriers that hold the pump itself, its accessories, and a cooler bag and ice pack for temporary milk storage. Some have a rechargeable battery and cable adapter for use in a car. They make great shower or baby gifts (you can drop hints).

Smaller, Economy Electric Pumps: These hand-held electric pumps are smaller still and cost anywhere from about $70 to $150. The motor is not as strong, but these pumps may fit the bill if you're pumping only once a day or less. They come in double and single models. Hand-held pumps vary in weight; some weigh less than a pound.

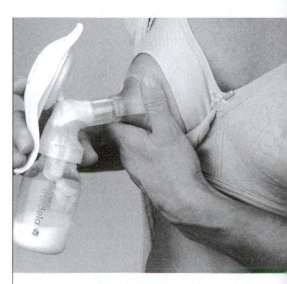

Women who pump once a day or less often find that a simple hand-held pump suits their needs.

Hand- or Foot-Operated Pumps

These simpler pumps (which typically run $35 to $50) are usually small enough to fit inside a purse, tote bag, or briefcase, and work by a handle that you squeeze or move up and down. Some women who usually use an electric pump will use a manual pump at times when electricity is not available. They are designed to pump from one breast at a time. For double-pumping, some women use two separate pumps.

To Use with Most Pumps: Easy Expression Hands-Free Pumping Bra

This aid to pumping comes in two styles, a strapless zip-front and a less expensive pull-on halter type. It's not meant to be used as a bra and should not be worn all day. The bra holds breast pump flanges in place so you don't have to. You simply attach the flanges to your breasts via openings in the bra's cups. It fits most electric pumps and allows the wearer to pump milk from both breasts while being able to write, use the computer, or do other simple tasks. It comes in a range of sizes from small (32–34, AA–B) to extra-extra large (46–48, G–H). You can have the bra fitted to your size in a retail store, but if that's impossible for you, you can find it online, along with reviews, under "pumping bra."

Hand-Expression

Manual expression is a valuable skill to have, since you can do it at any time, without any equipment other than your own body and something to collect the milk. Some mothers prefer it over other methods because it's more natural, it doesn't cost anything, and it's ready when you are. However, it requires practice to become proficient, and some women never get milk from this method. Others get so good at it that they wouldn't express any other way. Here's how to do it:

❖ Wash your hands and be sure your fingernails are clean.

❖ Before proceeding, massage, stroke, and shake your breasts (see the instructions on page 246).

❖ Position a clean cup, a thermos, or a wide-mouthed jar below your breast.

❖ Hold your breast with your thumb above and your first two fingers below, about 1 inch or 1½ inches behind the nipple. For most women, this is the

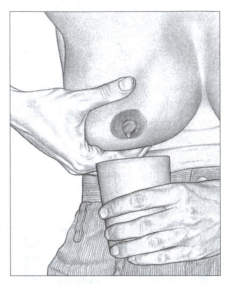

It takes practice to become efficient at hand-expression, but many women who become skillful at it prefer it to any other method.

edge of the areola, but if your areola is narrower or wider, it's the distance from the nipple that counts.

❖ Push your thumb and fingers together and gently back toward the chest wall.

❖ Very gently roll the thumb and fingers forward.

❖ Repeat the push-roll sequence a few times until no more drops come out.

❖ Repeat this at several different locations around your nipple. Some places may be better for you than others. If you think of your areola as a clock face, start at the 12 and 6 position, then go to the 9 and 3, 11 and 5, and 1 and 7.

❖ Do not squeeze or cup the breast, slide your fingers, or pull the skin on the breast.

❖ Be sure the milk doesn't run over your fingers as it flows from your breast.

❖ If you don't get any milk the first few times, keep trying.

Breast Shells (Milk Cups)

The same kind of breast shells that are sometimes used to bring out inverted nipples (as described in Chapter 4) are marketed as a way to collect milk from one breast while you're nursing or pumping on the other. This is not a good method for collecting milk, since the milk is too easily contaminated.

Principles That Apply to All Methods of Collecting Milk

1. Cleanliness. Before you express or pump by any method, wash your hands with soap and water and clean your fingernails with a good nailbrush. Germs on your hands can contaminate the milk you're preparing for your baby.

Follow the manufacturer's instructions for keeping your pump clean, and before using the pump for the first time, sterilize the parts as the manufacturer directs. Be sure your containers are clean as well (see page 249). After you pump, wash your hands and equipment with warm, soapy water. If you're pumping for a premature or sick baby, ask hospital personnel for instructions on keeping your milk clean.

2. Time and practice. If you can plan ahead (for example, for going back to work), practice at home for a while before you need to express regularly. Consider the first few times practice sessions, just like an infant's first few feedings. Practice once or twice a day, five minutes on each breast. If you initially don't get the amount of milk you'd like, keep it up. The more you do it, the more efficient you'll become.

At first, it may take you up to 30 minutes each session to get most of the milk from both breasts. Eventually, you may be able to get it down to 8 minutes each time, but some women continue to need 15 to 20 minutes. And the amount of time needed may vary from time to time. The more you practice, the better you'll do.

3. Effect of timing. It's normal for the amount of milk you collect to vary from time to time. Quantity will depend on many factors, including how much time has elapsed since your last nursing or pumping session, what time of day it is, how established your milk supply is, and how proficient you have become. You'll most likely produce more milk early in the day and early in the week. Most women's milk supply tends to drop at about six P.M. Between seven A.M. and one P.M. is usually the best time for the first sessions; late afternoon and early evening are the worst. If you're currently nursing your baby, pump soon after the first morning feeding.

Working women often find that their milk supply diminishes during the week, so that by Friday they're giving less than they did on Monday when they had the weekend to take things a little easier. Knowing this may help you plan your schedule and accept your body's ability to yield milk. Nursing more often on the weekend helps to keep your milk supply up.

4. Take advantage of your let-down reflex. Even if you don't pump during your baby's feeding, your let-down reflex will help you produce more milk. Some of the suggestions on page 246 will help stimulate let-down. Give it a chance to get going; don't pump harder or increase the suction in the pump if you don't see any milk coming out. This will just make you uncomfortable and will not produce more milk. Time and practice will improve your efficiency.

5. Take advantage of your baby's feeding schedule. Once you've learned the basics of expressing or pumping, try to schedule these sessions at about the times your baby would ordinarily nurse. This will help keep up your supply of milk.

6. Amount of milk collected. At first, you may not get even one ounce at a time, but as you increase the frequency of pumping, you'll increase your milk yield. The amount of milk expressed does not reflect how much milk your baby gets from your breasts, since your nursing baby is much more efficient than the best pump. See the suggestions on page 246 for increasing the amount of milk you collect.

7. Experiment with breast inserts. If your pump comes with inserts that fit into the breast shield (flange) portion, see which size feels best. Try pumping with the smaller size first, and then switch to the larger one if you need to.

Pumping While Nursing

One valuable technique is pumping from one breast while you're nursing your baby on the other breast. This method enlists your baby as your partner, since you'll be getting the benefit of the let-down triggered by your baby's suckling, and your work will be easier. Also, this system tends to increase your milk supply. Double-duty nursing can fool your body into thinking that you're nursing twins; operating by the law of supply and demand, you'll produce more milk.

First, get your baby started at your breast. Use a pillow to support your baby under the nursing breast. For the first few times, when you're ready to pump, ask a helper to hold the pump in position. Then use both your hands to hold your baby while the helper is working the pump. After you do this several times, you'll get the hang of it and will be able to do it by yourself.

Alternatively, you can express or pump from the unnursed breast immediately after nursing from the other one. Or you can pump or express soon after a nursing while your baby is otherwise engaged. The amount you produce doesn't matter in these early sessions. The point is to learn the technique.

The first time you express or pump, try to choose a quiet time when you're not likely to be distracted or interrupted. Enlist as much help as you can. Ask someone to be with you—if possible, someone who's done this herself. It's wonderful to have someone to answer the telephone or doorbell, take care of an older child, or provide another pair of hands in any way you need them. This person can help you maneuver both the pump and your baby (if your initial pumping is done on the nonbaby side while you're nursing on the other side). Then get yourself comfortable—in a chair or couch, with pillows for support. And do whatever you can to relax.

To begin, use your pump's lowest setting to provide the smallest amount

---

A Note of Caution about Bisphenol A (BPA)

In 2008, the National Toxicology Program of the National Institutes of Health issued a report indicating that bisphenol A (BPA), a chemical found in some plastic products, including baby bottles, sippy cups, water bottles, and breast pumps, as well as in the linings of some cans of foods and formula, could pose health risks, including having an effect on children's development.

Products that do not contain BPA usually come with a statement that their products are BPA-free. If you're not sure, you can usually tell if a product contains BPA by the recycling code (the number inside a triangle) on the bottom of the product. Items with codes 1 to 6 do not contain BPA. Those with code 7 (or "PC" for polycarbonate) may contain the chemical, so before using it, check with the product's manufacturer. If you're using formula, use the powdered form in a can with as little metal as possible. Avoid ready-to-eat liquid formulas in metal cans, since the linings of some cans contain BPA.

Most manufacturers have eliminated BPA from their products, and some laws have been passed prohibiting its use in products containing food or drinks. Therefore, you're unlikely to find BPA in any new items that you buy, but if you're using bottles, a pump, or other items that you've saved from an older child, check to be sure none of these contains the chemical.

of suction; you'll be able to gradually increase this. And start slowly, with about ten minutes on a side; again, you'll be able to increase this. If you feel any discomfort at all, decrease the level of suction or the amount of time. Just as breastfeeding should not hurt, neither should pumping. If you're not sure you're using the pump correctly, call your lactation consultant or your pump manufacturer's toll-free number. Some women who have had problems with one kind of pump do better by switching to a different model or a different brand.

Enhancing Milk Production When Expressing or Pumping

You may want to try one or more of the following methods to increase the amount of milk you can collect for your baby. Different ones work well for different women. If you're pumping at work, for example, some of these suggestions will not apply. As with the rest of this book, take the suggestions that make sense to you, see which ones work, and stick with them.

❖ First, take care of yourself: Get as much rest as possible, and be sure you're drinking enough water throughout the day.

❖ For two to five minutes before you begin, do deep breathing or some other relaxation exercise.

❖ Drink a cup of hot decaf or major brand of herbal tea before beginning, to help you relax and stay hydrated (see page 180). If your baby is not sensitive to cow's milk products that you eat or drink, try warm milk.

❖ Make yourself as comfortable as possible. If you can, sit with your feet up.

❖ Massage your breasts. If possible, just before you begin to pump, lay a warm towel on your breasts for a minute or two—the towel is helpful, but not essential. Then massage your breasts gently, one at a time, starting from the top and moving around the sides and the bottom, moving your fingers in a circular motion. With your fingertips, stroke yourself lightly from the armpit, from above and below the breast, and from the middle of the chest toward the nipple. You don't need to massage or stroke the nipples themselves. (If necessary, you can massage your breasts even while you're dressed.)

❖ Pump both breasts at the same time, using a good electric pump.

❖ If you're expressing from one breast at a time, switch breasts at least once during each session—and preferably twice—to ensure maximum draining. Usually, you'll collect less milk from the second expression than from the first.

❖ Prop a photo of your baby in front of you, smell your baby's sleeper, or play a recording of her sounds.

❖ Visualize your baby in your mind. Imagine what she looks like, sounds like, feels like, and smells like when she nurses.

❖ Pump frequently. It's better to schedule three pumping sessions of no more than ten minutes each than to schedule two sessions for fifteen minutes each. It yields more milk, it's more efficient, and it's also more comfortable, since it will cut down the likelihood of breast injury from too much pressure exerted for too long. When they first start using a pump, some women get sore nipples from pumping more than seven or eight minutes on a breast.

❖ Make the time go faster while you're expressing or pumping by talking with a friend, listening to music, reading, or watching television.

❖ If you don't need two hands to express, hold your baby while you're pumping.

❖ Wear comfortable clothes that cover your shoulders, so you don't get chilled.

❖ Listen to music that you associate with nursing. This works best if you play the album initially during actual breastfeeding sessions; then when you're expressing, hearing the same music may help evoke the memory and the sensations you felt then. (Handel's "Water Music" gets high marks from women who enjoy classical music.)

How to Handle Expressed and Pumped Breast Milk

If the temperature in the area where you're pumping is higher than 72°F (22°C) and you cannot refrigerate the milk, store it in a clean, tightly closed container. Put the container in a cooler or insulated bag with ice or ice packs. Keep the cooler out of the sun and away from heating units, and refrigerate it as soon as possible.

Refrigerated milk will keep well for three to seven days. If you have more milk than you'll use within this time, freeze it immediately. Pour your expressed milk into clean four-ounce plastic or glass bottles or ice cube trays so that you can defrost small amounts. Be sure the bottles are not made of polycarbonate plastic, which could leach the chemical BPA (see the box on page 245). You may want to freeze milk in one- and two-ounce quantities in the bottles or in clean ice cube trays so you can thaw only as much milk as your baby will drink.

Remember that, once thawed, milk should not be refrozen. It's better to give your caregiver two separate bottles with just a small amount of milk in each one. Keep an extra stock in the freezer so you won't get nervous about running out.

Bottles don't need to be sterilized if the milk has been kept cold, but they do need to be washed thoroughly after each use to be sure that no milk particles are left. See the facing page for specifics about bottle washing.

One of the qualities of human milk is its ability to slow the growth of bacteria. In the first six to ten hours after expression, human milk kept in a capped clean container does not grow bacteria, even at room temperature (66° to 72°F/19° to 22°C). Ideally, you'll cool or refrigerate your milk as soon as possible, but if for some reason you can't, you can still collect it.

If you have a refrigerator with a freezer compartment, breast milk will keep in that compartment for two weeks. It will keep for three to four months in a separate-door freezer that you open fairly often. If you have a frost-free freezer, protect your milk from the warming cycle by making an igloo: Surround the milk on the top, bottom, and all sides with ice packs or bags of frozen veggies. In a deep-freeze unit that is not opened often and that maintains a consistent temperature of 0°F (−18°C), your milk will keep for six months. For more detailed instructions on storage times for breast milk, see page 250.

Be prepared for the unexpected, which will always happen. One working mom dropped and broke her thermos of that day's expressed milk—and saved the next day by expressing while she nursed that evening and the next morning. Her baby was already sleeping through the night, so the mother set her alarm to wake herself up every three hours all night long to express enough milk for the following day. Thanks to the law of supply and demand, her breasts responded to the frequent stimulation.

Storing Collected Breast Milk

When storing breast milk, you need to be careful about the containers you use, how you clean them, and how long you store the milk.

Containers

Four-ounce plastic BPA-free nursing bottles that you can use for both storage and feeding are standard with most pumps. They're solid and sturdy, and a safer way to store breast milk than plastic milk storage bags, which can leak or become contaminated with bacteria if they're pierced by anything.

However, some women like disposable milk storage bags. These bags lie flat in a freezer, are easy to stack, and thaw quickly. They need very careful handling to avoid spillage and puncture, they sometimes split when frozen, and they absorb odors from nearby foods (although babies don't seem to mind milk that smells like the garlicky sausages in the next container). Double-bagging or putting the bags in a freezer-quality zip-top bag may overcome some of these difficulties.

Cleaning and Sterilizing

If you're collecting milk to be given to your baby, sterilize all your equipment before using it the first time—bottles, nipples, pumping equipment, and ice cube trays if you'll be using them to freeze your milk. After this initial sterilization, you don't need to keep sterilizing. You just need to wash everything thoroughly after each use.

A dishwasher that heats water to 180°F (100°C) will sterilize everything well enough. Check to be sure all the pump parts can be safely washed in the dishwasher. Wash nipples and plastic items on the top rack. First, use a bottle brush and nipple brush to remove any milk scum, and then wash thoroughly in the dishwasher or a basin of hot soapy water. Rinse well to remove all the soap.

In order to sterilize just a few things (bottle, cup, bottle caps, nipples, funnel, etc.), pad the inside of a large soup pot with a clean towel and fill it with enough water to completely cover the items you're sterilizing. Bring the water to a boil over high heat; then turn down the heat just enough so that the water continues to boil gently. After five minutes of boiling, remove the nipples with sterile tongs. Place the nipples on a clean, dry towel. Allow the other items to boil 15 minutes longer. Do not touch the rims of the bottles or the insides of the caps. Place all the other items on the clean towel.

If you're going to take milk to the hospital for a sick or premature baby or for donation to a milk bank, the hospital or milk bank will probably give you instructions. If not, or if you want to freeze the milk for your own future use, sterilize your containers and equipment as above.

Helpful Suggestions

❖ Use a nontoxic marker to label each container of frozen milk with the date so you'll use the oldest milk first. If you're taking it to a babysitter, child-care center, or hospital, put your baby's name on it.

❖ Don't fill bottles or storage bags to the top. Milk expands as it freezes, so no more than 3.5 ounces should go into a 4-ounce bottle.

❖ You can collect milk a little at a time, chill it in the refrigerator, and add the cold milk to milk that's already frozen. It will have a layered or striped look that won't affect its quality and will disappear after it's thawed and swirled around to combine. Be sure to chill new milk before adding it to frozen milk, since adding warm milk can defrost the top layer of the frozen milk.

❖ You can also freeze milk in a plastic ice cube tray covered by plastic wrap. The frozen cubes (about half an ounce to an ounce each, depending on the size of the compartments) can then be transferred to an airtight plastic or glass container or a sturdy plastic bag. When you or your sitter is ready to feed your baby, put the number of cubes you need into a feeding bottle and defrost as described on page 252. This way you have more flexibility, since you can defrost only what your baby needs at one time. Since the cubes defrost quickly, it's easy to add another one if your baby still seems hungry.

Storing Your Milk

Basically, your collected breast milk will keep for several hours at room temperature if it's covered; it will keep in the refrigerator for three to seven days; and if you want to keep it longer than that, freeze it.

Use your milk as soon as possible. For one thing, milk collected when your baby is two months old won't meet his needs as effectively when he's six months old—although it's still better than formula. When you can, feed your baby refrigerated milk rather than frozen milk, since freezing may destroy some of breast milk's anti-infective properties. If you're expressing and storing milk for a preterm infant or a hospitalized baby, follow the recommendations of the institution where your baby is being cared for or has recently left.

❖ To be given to baby within 24 hours: Immediately put milk in a clean container and cap tightly, and as soon as possible put it in the refrigerator or a cooler with frozen ice packs.

❖ To be given to baby within one week: Pour into a clean container; cap tightly. Refrigerate at 40°F (4°C) or below. Although it should keep well for a week, it's best to freeze it if you want to keep it longer than three days.

❖ To be given to baby within three months: Pour into a clean container; cap tightly. Quick-cool in the refrigerator for 30 minutes. Then freeze in refrigerator-freezer unit.

❖ To be given to baby within six months: Pour into a clean container; cap tightly. Quick-cool in the refrigerator for 30 minutes. Then freeze at 0°F (−18°C) or below in the freezer of a two-door refrigerator or a deep freeze that is not opened often. Not all freezers stay cold enough for long-term storage. Check the temperature with a freezer thermometer at different places in the unit. The freezer should maintain a constant temperature of 0°F (−18°C). If it keeps ice cream very solid, it's probably cold enough.

If your freezer does not get this cold but does keep other frozen foods hard, keep the milk in the center of the freezer and use within three to four months. Frost-free refrigerators, which have a warming element, generally do not maintain 0°F (−18°C)—see the igloo suggestion on page 248.

To find out whether your milk thaws and then refreezes in your freezer, put an ice cube in a little jar and check it over the next several days. If you find that it is shrinking and the corners are becoming rounded, you'll know that it melted and refroze. This has probably happened to your milk, too. Smell the milk to see if it's still good. If you're in doubt, discard it.

✤ Keeping breast milk longer than six months: This is not a good idea. While instructions are sometimes given for keeping frozen milk for up to two years, long-term freezing alters the chemical composition of the milk: Some of the fats break down, and the milk loses some of its ability to fight harmful organisms. Furthermore, you run the risk of spoilage if you lose electrical power during that time and the milk thaws and refreezes.

✤ Do not refreeze milk that has defrosted. Thaw milk in the refrigerator, not at room temperature. Do not store in a cooler. If frozen milk has started to thaw, refrigerate it immediately and use it within 24 hours.

✤ Throw away any milk that has been warmed and left in the bottle after feeding because organisms from the baby's mouth can contaminate the rest of the milk. This is why it's best to store expressed milk in small quantities.

Transporting Expressed Milk

You can transport your milk whatever way is most convenient for you—in a thermos, an ice chest, or an insulated bag or bottle bag—as long as you keep it cold. When you arrive at your destination, make sure the milk is still plenty cold. If it isn't, don't use it.

Offering Expressed Milk to Your Baby

Both you and anyone else who feeds your baby your collected breast milk need to know the following information, so you may want to photocopy these pages to have them handy.

Don't be alarmed by the appearance of stored breast milk. It often separates, looks striped, or turns yellow, any of which is perfectly normal. If you're not sure about the quality of the milk, smell it and taste it. If it tastes sweet and good, it's fine. If it has a soapy smell due to the enzyme lipase, which breaks down milk fats, it's still safe. Babies usually don't mind this taste, but if yours does, the next time you express milk you can scald it by heating it almost to boiling (bubbles around the edges), and then quickly cooling and freezing it. Sometimes milk may smell because it has picked up an odor from other strong foods in your refrigerator or freezer. Trust your senses and your own good sense: If you smell anything like sour cow's milk, the milk has gone bad, and you don't want to give it to your baby.

Defrosting Your Milk and Feeding Your Baby

❖ About half an hour before feeding time, take the container from the freezer and hold it under tepid running water. Gradually increase the temperature of the water to hot. Swirl the bag or bottle gently as you warm it; this remixes the cream that has separated. (Since your milk is not homogenized, the fat rises to the top on standing.) It should take about four minutes to thaw 4 ounces of frozen breast milk. This method can also be used to heat refrigerated breast milk.

❖ Do not leave frozen breast milk out at room temperature to defrost.

❖ Do not heat either breast milk or formula in a microwave oven. Vitamins and other components in the milk may be destroyed, glass bottles may crack or explode, and hot spots may occur, which could cause severe burns to your baby's mouth or esophagus.

❖ Do not heat breast milk on the stove. First, there's a danger of over-heating and destroying antibodies and nutrients. Second, there's the chance that frozen milk will curdle. And then there's the all-too-common scenario of the mother or babysitter warming milk in a pan of water on the stove, running to answer the phone or the door—and coming back to find the milk boiled into the bottom of the pan.

If you don't have running warm water, heat water in a pan, and when it's warm turn off the heat and put the bottle in the pan. Test the milk on the inside of your elbow; you should barely be able to feel it. If it feels too warm, let it cool down to body temperature before feeding your baby.

❖ Gently roll or swirl the bottle again before feeding.

❖ Use breast milk that has been defrosted but not refrigerated and not heated within 12 hours. If it has been heated, use it within 30 minutes.

❖ Discard any milk in the bottle that your baby does not finish at one feeding.

❖ If you have both fresh and frozen breast milk, give your baby the fresh milk and save the frozen for supplements and emergencies, since freezing causes some loss of antibodies.

The above measures sound complicated, but most women who express milk for their babies find that once they establish a routine, they're able to carry it off. If all the steps involved with expressing or pumping your milk do become too burdensome in terms of the other claims on your time and energy, it's always possible, of course, to switch to formula. If you do make this switch, don't be hard on yourself for the change. Instead, congratulate yourself for the efforts you have made and for your contributions to your baby's health and well-being.

CHAPTER TWELVE

The Working Nursing Mother

"When I was a pediatric resident, I felt I had to make a stand for myself (and my baby). I worked hard, but made it a point to take time out every few hours to pump. It was difficult, but I showed people in the hospital that breastfeeding and working full-time is doable— and that it's well worth the extra effort. To my delight, I found that my colleagues were quite supportive of my commitment to my baby."

LAURA MARKS, MD Westport, Connecticut

Of course, all mothers are working mothers. We change diapers, we launder onesies, we scramble eggs, we clean up kitchens and bathrooms. We stay up all night with a sick baby or wrench ourselves out of a warm bed in the middle of the night to comfort a toddler scared by a nightmare. We play endless games of Candy Land when we would rather curl up with a good book. In short, as parents we do all kinds of things that are better described as work than as play.

But besides this often gratifying, often difficult family work, most parents take on other work, too. Across the world and throughout history, most parents of both sexes have always worked. Until relatively recent times, much of this work could be done without both parents having to leave their children in the care of others. Now, though, this is less often an option.

Today, almost half of all mothers of infants under six months of age are working for pay, full- or part-time, in or out of the home—the highest proportion in the history of the United States. When we use the term *working mother,* these are the mothers we refer to. And in recent years, more and more women who are working outside the home are also nursing their babies.

Yes, it can be done. Many women are doing it, and what's more, many women are enjoying combining these two activities. Working mothers often express a special appreciation of the joys of breastfeeding. Away from their babies for much of the day, they savor the special warmth and intimacy of the nursing relationship when they are home. They find that the intensity of the nursing experience helps to make up for the hours they are away from their families. Furthermore, many working mothers find that the ability to sit and nurse actually has a calming, relaxing effect on them, while reminding the baby who the real mother is!

Not that it's easy. Anyone who combines working for pay and caring for a family is bound to experience one conflict after another: You have only so much time and energy. Adding breastfeeding to your daily schedule imposes still another set of activities and concerns. Yet more and more women are so convinced of the value of breastfeeding and are so committed to their work (for reasons of economic necessity, personal fulfillment, or both) that they are determined to carry out both activities. A few years back, women were saying, "I'm going back to work. Can you help me wean my baby?" Now they say, "I'm going back to work. Can you help me keep on nursing?"

How do so many women manage to combine these areas of their lives so well? They line up the support they need—and they organize their lives for success.

Finding Support

This is one time in your life when you need as much help as you can get. Your time to assist others will come, but for now you have to reach out for any aid that others can give you. Help is where you find it.

If your husband or partner takes over some of the household chores, cares for your baby in many important ways, and provides that all-important dollop of moral support that lets you know you're doing a good job, you're lucky. Of course, this is only fair. If you're doing your part to win the bread, he should be doing his part to help make the home. If your partner provides verbal support for your efforts but not much more, you may be able to enlist cooperation by emphasizing how important his help is to your success at breastfeeding. (Ask him, for example, to read Chapter 14 in this book.)

You may be able to call upon your babysitter for help above and beyond the work she was hired for. Or you may be able to go to family members. (One mother told us of a time when she had to visit her husband in the hospital. She met her brother during a work break, he took her expressed milk, picked up the baby at the caregiver's home, and gave the baby the bottle.) Don't forget friends, neighbors, coworkers, employers, or local support groups like La Leche League, the International Child-birth Education Association, or Lamaze. It's especially important for single mothers to find people to help them through this demanding period of their lives.

If your income permits extras or if anyone wants to give you a generous baby gift, there's no better use for money at this time than buying you some help. Hiring someone to do the cleaning, the cooking, the grocery shopping, and the laundry is an investment that can pay off not only in your physical and psychological comfort, but ultimately in your entire family's well-being.

The special helper we talked about in Chapter 4 can be a lifesaver for the working mother. She or he can step in during times of emergency and lighten your load in many ways on a day-to-day basis.

Planning Ahead: While You're Pregnant and Still on the Job

The time to arrange for your maternity leave and to enlist your employer as your ally is during your pregnancy. If you have performed your work well and made yourself valuable to your employers, they will be eager to do whatever is necessary to bring you back and keep you happy. Highly valued employees can often negotiate for concessions that company policy ordinarily doesn't permit, such as longer maternity leaves, temporary part-time schedules, and the opportunity to do some of your work at home.

If your position with your company is strong, ask for what you want. You may be pleasantly surprised at what you can get. You might suggest that your personnel director contact one of the organizations listed in the Resource Appendix under "Help in the Workplace." These organizations look at employee health and support programs from the employer's point of view, emphasizing how such services can increase productivity and profits by reducing employee absenteeism and turnover and cutting child health-care costs. By meeting your needs now, your employer is likely to have a happier and more productive worker in the future.

Your Maternity Leave

It's your responsibility to tell your employer about your pregnancy before you show up in a well-filled-out maternity outfit, and before you tell your coworkers. Fairly early in your pregnancy, ask for an appointment with your supervisor to discuss your plans and your future with the company. Tell her or him how long you expect to continue working and how much maternity leave you plan to take. Before your meeting, familiarize yourself with company maternity provisions and with the law in your state, so you'll get, at the very least, what you're entitled to.

When you talk to your employer about your maternity leave, try to get four to six months. The more leave you can negotiate for (either paid or unpaid), the easier it will be for you and your baby to establish breastfeeding. Furthermore, a 2009 report showed that women who took leave in their ninth month of pregnancy (at or before 36 weeks' gestation) were less likely to have cesarean deliveries than women who worked right up to the delivery.

The federal Family and Medical Leave Act mandates 12 weeks of unpaid leave for companies that employ at least 50 workers within a 75-mile radius of one another in the United States. If you have worked for the company for at least a year (and at least 1,250 hours in this time), you are entitled to up to 12 weeks of unpaid leave during pregnancy and for a family member's illness for each year that you're employed. With this amount of time, you'll be fairly well rested by the time you go back to work, your milk supply should be well established, and your baby may even be sleeping through the night and on a fairly predictable schedule. If your company doesn't meet the criteria set forth in the act, negotiate for a minimum of four weeks' leave.

Breastfeeding and employment are compatible—and a 2009 study of 770 full-time working mothers found that those who had at least a 12-week maternity leave were more likely to establish breastfeeding and to nurse longer than were women who took shorter leaves. But even if you have to go back to work earlier than you would like, you can still have a successful breastfeeding experience.

Your Breastfeeding Plans and Why Your Employer Should Encourage You

It's not necessary to discuss your breastfeeding plans when you first tell your employer you're pregnant. After all, that is a long time away. Besides, your employer may not be interested in discussing them with you. In fact, depending on the atmosphere at your workplace, you may decide never to discuss your nursing with anyone there, but instead to privately work out your arrangements.

Many women have found, however, that talking with their employers ahead of time was helpful in enlisting support and in reassuring their bosses that their jobs were still important to them.

Good times to talk about these plans are just before you go on leave or just before you plan to return. If you do raise the issue of nursing, ask what kinds of arrangements your employer makes to help breastfeeding employees. In some companies, support is there, but workers don't know about it. During your conversation, you'll want to make the following points:

❖ Breastfeeding is not unduly time-consuming. You know other working women who have found it compatible with their work schedules, and you're organizing your life so that you'll be able to handle it, too.

❖ Mothers need not be restricted by breastfeeding. With good organization, nursing women can be away from their babies for the entire workday, if necessary (and sometimes even longer, although this is certainly a situation you don't want to encourage).

❖ In terms of your lifetime career, the period of time you'll be breastfeeding is really very short. You have shown your commitment to your work up to now, and that commitment will continue throughout and long after this important time.

❖ You may or may not want to talk about your milk-pumping needs. If you do, make the point that you'll be able to do this on your coffee and lunch breaks, so you won't need to take time from your work. If the need to take more time arises, you can make up for it by coming in early, staying late, or taking lunch at your desk. Once you have a sympathetic ear, you can ask for access to a private, comfortable place where you can pump your milk.

❖ If your employer's workforce includes a large number of young women, you might want to suggest that management consider adopting a lactation support program like the one described in the box on page 258. Such a program is inexpensive and easy to put in place. It can go far toward attracting new workers, shortening maternity leaves of the ones already there, increasing productivity by raising morale, and saving money.

❖ Despite some employers' concerns that accommodating nursing mothers will have negative effects on other workers, research has found that, in reality, other employees generally have a positive attitude toward workplace breastfeeding or milk expression.

Rona Cohen is the president of MCH Services, Inc., which helps employers set up lactation programs. She says, "There are still many challenges ahead: It is having the courage to meet these challenges that will shape our babies' breastfeeding futures."

Employer-Supported Lactation Programs

In its most recent policy statement on breastfeeding, the American Academy of Pediatrics urged employers to "provide appropriate facilities and adequate time in the workplace for breastfeeding and/or milk expression [pumping]." (For information about setting up corporate lactation programs, see the Resource Appendix.)

Employers who do have programs to support nursing mothers are doing this not out of charity, but because it makes sense for the bottom line.

The employer benefits economically from encouraging breastfeeding. Since breastfed babies are usually healthier than bottle-fed babies, their mothers are less likely to miss work than they might otherwise. Studies have borne this out: Women who continue to nurse after returning to work miss fewer days of work because of baby-related illnesses, and when they do miss work, their absences are shorter. The employer's health insurer also benefits: An internal study by the Kaiser Permanente insurance company found that breastfeeding for only six months can decrease a family's health-care claims by hundreds of dollars in their baby's first year of life.

So, not surprisingly, the employers that have provided lactation support include insurance companies: CIGNA saved $240,000 a year in health-care costs and $62,000 in prescription costs and had a 77 percent reduction in lost work time because of infant illness, resulting in an $880 savings

per participating employee. Mutual of Omaha had a $2,146 savings per participant; Aetna, $1,435.

An employer-supported lactation program may involve:

✧ A policy, agreed upon by department heads, senior administrators, and employees, that recognizes parents' responsibilities to both job and family and that is made known to employees. Many employers who don't have formal policies still provide support to working moms and dads.

✧ A policy of granting maternity leave that's long enough to let mothers establish a breastfeeding routine and milk supply before returning to work.

✧ Provision of breaks, flexible work hours, or part-time work so that women can pump their milk or nurse their babies during the workday, at a nearby child-care site or another place where their babies are brought to them.

✧ A clean, safe, and comfortable private area (not a stall in the ladies' room) where mothers can go to pump their milk. This place should be easily accessible, have lockable doors, have electrical outlets (for an efficient electric pump), and be in a place where it won't disrupt work schedules. (The Vermont ice cream company Ben & Jerry's calls its room The Milky Way. Ford Motor Company and JPMorgan Chase are among the many other companies with policies for nursing employees.)

❖ Milk storage options. Although some lactation rooms have refrigerators where moms can keep their pumped milk, Rona Cohen points to several reasons why it may be better for a mother to keep her milk with her in an insulated cold pack. "If your milk is with you," she says, "no one can take it by mistake, you don't have to worry about a power outage, and it can't pick up smells from other foods in the fridge."

❖ Providing breast pumps. An electric one with a double pumping system to be kept at the worksite, available to workers on any shift, and portable pumps for travel and off-site use. Although the worksite pump can be shared, each woman needs her own attachable kit and tubing so that her milk will not come into contact with any surface touched by another mother's milk.

❖ A water source for washing equipment in or near the pumping room.

❖ A lactation professional who is available for consultation prenatally, during maternity leave, and after the return to work to counsel and support both female and male workers on combining parenthood and employment.

❖ Developing or coordinating with existing on-site or near-site child-care programs so that mothers can go to their babies during the day.

❖ Educating other personnel about the advantages to the company—and to them—of providing understanding and support for breastfeeding and other parenting needs.

❖ Helping male employees who are new fathers understand the importance of a father's influence on the course of breastfeeding. The program instituted by Ms. Cohen for the Los Angeles Department of Water and Power included providing information about the importance of breastfeeding for the baby, and the importance of the father's support. As part of this program, the department paid for breast pump rentals for employees.

A society like ours, which prides itself on being pro-family, should provide services that help parents give their children the best care possible. Although federal, state, and local governments are more supportive now than in years past, we are still behind many other countries. The International Labour Organization, a United Nations agency, urges protection from work that might harm a new mother or her child, as well as at least one paid nursing break per day.

Of 180 countries surveyed in 2007, 107 had laws protecting working women's right to breastfeed, and in 73 countries women received paid break time. The United States is among neither the 107 nor the 73. As a result, the authors who reported this survey note, "The United States does not guarantee the right to breastfeed." Our government could do much more to encourage employers to institute family-oriented policies. Providing tax incentives to businesses that institute lactation support programs, offer day-care assistance, and help families in other ways is one goal worth working for.

Planning Ahead: While You're on Your Maternity Leave

While most of your efforts during this brief time will probably involve resting after the labor of childbirth, getting used to caring for your new baby, and establishing breast-feeding, you'll want to use these weeks at home to handle some important business.

Finding Child Care

As a working mother, the most important person in your life after your husband or partner and child is likely to be the person who takes care of your child. You need to find a caregiver who is both caring and capable. You also need to find someone who will support your breastfeeding plans.

When you interview a potential caregiver, let her (or him) know that you plan to breastfeed your baby. Be alert to her responses: Is she supportive or does she feel that it's a mistake for a working mother to nurse? If you get any negative feelings, you'll know that this person is not for you.

If she responds positively, however, you need to open up the discussion to include the following:

❖ If she has never cared for a breast-fed baby, you need to tell her about the differences in feeding schedules (breastfed babies eat more frequently),

in bowel movements (looser), and in ways of soothing the baby (for example, avoiding bottles of water and pacifiers for at least the first few weeks).

❖ Tell her the kind of schedule you have in mind, and how many feedings a day you want her to give your baby. Let her know how to thaw your expressed breast milk and how to store it if you'll be providing frozen breast milk. It's a good idea to leave a supply of frozen breast milk with her even if you provide freshly pumped milk every day. That way, you'll have a backup if your child is especially hungry one day or if your fresh milk spills.

❖ If you'll be taking your baby from your home for care, check the caregiver's home or child-care center for safety, hygiene, a pleasant atmosphere, and all the other basic criteria of a good child-care environment.

❖ If you take your baby to the caregiver, take some familiar toys to carry the smells and thoughts of home and Mommy.

❖ If your caregiver lives closer to your workplace than to your home, you may want to nurse your baby after you take him there in the morning and as soon as you pick him up at night. Be sure that this is acceptable.

❖ You may want to give or lend your caregiver a copy of this book, marking the pages she's most likely to refer to. Or you can photocopy the information she needs and give it to her.

❖ If you will be taking your baby to a day-care center, find out its policy about feeding bottled breast milk. One mother was shocked to learn that the center she had chosen would not store breast milk on site, so she would have to take in a bottle every time her daughter got hungry. The center finally agreed to accept bottled milk, but only if the mom paid extra. Ideally, the center should have a freezer as well as a refrigerator, to be able to keep a backup bottle on hand. Check your state's legislation: Some states prohibit discrimination against breastfed babies in day care.

❖ Take the time to show your caregiver how you want her to do things and encourage her to ask you about any problems or questions she may have.

❖ Be sure she knows how to reach you and your husband or partner at work.

❖ Whether you nurse at the caregiver's house or at your home, be sure that she won't give your baby a full feeding for a couple of hours before you come to pick him up so that he'll be hungry enough to nurse vigorously. It may take a few days to work out this scheduling, but the effort is worth it, since it's important for your baby's satisfaction at the breast, for your milk supply, for your comfort, and for the success of your breastfeeding relationship. If your baby seems hungry, ask your caregiver to give him a small feeding to tide him over so he won't be miserable until you can nurse him.

Making the Transition from Home to Work

Going back to work requires an adjustment for both you and your baby. You can make it easier for both of you with some planning for this transition period.

If your caregiver will be coming to your home, ask her to start work a week or two before you go back to work so that she can get to know your baby, as well as you and your routines. If you'll be taking your baby to her home, plan to take him for a few increasingly longer visits before you go back to work. First, plan on you and your baby spending an hour or so with the caregiver just to get acquainted. Then leave your baby alone with the caregiver at a time when he won't need to be fed. Then leave him for a few longer sessions that include feeding times. Finally, hold a dress rehearsal, a day when you'll be away from your baby for about the same length of time as on a typical workday. This will let you iron out any kinks in your scheduling—and will reassure you that you can handle both home and work.

If you expect to nurse in the care-giver's presence, do so during one of these trial runs. You'll be able to see how she reacts.

Introducing Milk in a Bottle or Cup

Since the key to your success in com-bining working and breastfeeding will probably lie in your baby's having feedings while you're at work, it's vital that you take special pains to help her like the bottle or cup, even if she doesn't love it. (She'll be saving her love for you.)

In our society, we have generally assumed that babies who are not breastfed need to get their milk in a bottle. But in many countries around the world, babies who cannot be nursed receive all their liquid nourish-ment in a cup, sometimes right from birth. United Nations agencies do not distribute baby bottles at all, even to babies who cannot be breastfed.

Cup feeding has some advantages: There's no danger of nipple confusion; an open cup is easier to keep clean than either a bottle or a sippy cup; you can't prop a baby alone with a cup the way you can with a bottle; and even premature babies can drink from a cup, since the swallowing reflex devel-ops earlier than the sucking reflex. However, cup feeding is more time-consuming and usually messier (even if you won't cry over spilled milk!), and, perhaps more significantly, it's an unfamiliar idea to most people—which may include the person who cares for your baby while you're at work.

If you do want to feed by cup, get your baby used to it from an early age, and ask your caregiver to feed her this way. For suggestions on cup feeding, see the box on the facing page. Some older babies and toddlers who refuse a traditional sippy cup will drink from one with a pop-up straw. If this won't work for you, you can, of course, use bottles. By and large, the earlier a baby is given milk in a bottle or cup, the more readily she'll take it. Babies con-fronted with their first bottle after three months of age often refuse it absolutely and will sooner go hungry rather than drink from this strange, hard, unwelcome container so differ-ent from their mother's soft, warm breast. This usually happens only for a few feedings, however. See the discus-sion on page 134 for bottle-feeding breastfed babies.

Neither do you want to introduce the bottle too *soon*. Ideally, you'll wait until six weeks of age to introduce it. By this age, most babies are compe-tent nursers and yet they're still flexible enough to try something new. Furthermore, the mother's milk supply is well established by now and flows easily enough to keep her baby happy. So if at all possible, try to hold off your return to work until at least two months postpartum, for both your sake and your baby's (so you both have a little time to get used to the new delivery system).

However, it isn't always possible to wait this long. If you must go to work before this time, you'll have to

Tips for Feeding a Baby from a Cup

❖ Start the feeding when your baby is calm, not desperately hungry.

❖ Pour a small amount of milk (1 or 2 ounces) into a little cup. You don't need a special cup. Any will do, although the infant sippy cups with two handles and a lid are the least messy.

❖ Seat the baby on your lap and support him in a half-upright position, and gently restrain his arms (maybe by wrapping him in a light blanket) so that he can't bump the cup.

❖ Tuck a washcloth or a bib under his chin to catch spills.

❖ Place the edge of the cup at the outer corners of your baby's upper lip, and rest the cup gently on his lower lip. This lets him smell the milk.

❖ Don't pour the milk into his mouth; tip the cup so the milk is barely touching his lips and let him lap or sip it.

❖ Don't rush the baby; allow time for him to swallow.

❖ Stop from time to time to burp him.

❖ Limit the feeding time to 30 minutes so neither you nor the baby gets too tired.

---

introduce the bottle earlier, at least a week or two before you will be going back.

You may decide to introduce the bottle gradually, so that by the time you do go back, your baby is taking one bottle-feeding every day, at the same time every day. This time should coincide with at least one of the feedings when you'll be away, so that you and your baby set a routine. Your baby may drink less than 2 ounces of milk at a time from the bottle. This is not a problem.

Since some babies accept a bottle more readily from someone other than their mother, a babysitter can often manage this transition. This is one reason why you'll want to hire the sitter before you go back to work. Meanwhile,

your baby will associate only you with breastfeeding. Waiting to introduce the bottle until your first working day may be very stressful for your baby, who will have to make two big adjustments at the same time—to your absence during the day and to the switch from breast to bottle.

When you or someone else first introduces milk in a bottle, give it to your baby when she's not terribly hungry—maybe 45 minutes after a feeding. This way, she'll be more receptive to something new and may be pleasantly surprised to find something good trickling out of it. If you usually sit in a particular chair to nurse, have someone else—your partner, for instance—offer a bottle in another chair or another room.

What If Your Baby Refuses the Bottle?

Your baby may absolutely refuse to take any nourishment from a bottle. Some go on hunger strikes if they can't have the breast; no matter how ravenous they get or how piteously they cry, they won't give in. There are a number of different ways to cope with this. One of them may work for you:

❖ If you'll be away from your baby for only one or two feedings, nurse as much as possible while you're home. Even if your baby won't take a bottle while you're gone, he'll still be getting a good supply of milk.

❖ Brush your baby's mouth with the bottle's nipple and let him grasp it himself instead of pushing it forcefully into his mouth.

❖ Warm the bottle's nipple and the milk to body temperature by running warm water over the nipple and bottle. Never warm milk in a microwave—it can get hot spots, which can burn your baby's mouth.

❖ Ask someone else to pick up your baby while he's sleeping, but almost ready to wake, and feed him milk in a bottle. Typically, he will suck instinctively and will be more likely to accept the bottle next time it's offered. Do this for a while, and then try it when he's awake.

❖ If your baby absolutely will not take a bottle, try offering milk from a cup. (For a discussion of feeding from a cup, see page 262.)

❖ Or you can start by feeding milk through a large medicine dropper or in a spoon—rubber-coated or plastic. Sometimes, once the baby has received a couple of ounces of milk this way and is not so desperately hungry, he'll be willing to tolerate the bottle for the rest of the feeding.

❖ Experiment with different kinds of milk. One mother discovered that her baby preferred fresh, refrigerated breast milk over thawed frozen breast milk. If you're feeding formula, try another brand, after consulting with your baby's doctor. Or try different proportions of a breast milk–formula mixture to get your baby used to the taste of formula. You can start with three-quarters breast milk, one-quarter formula and gradually increase the amount of formula.

❖ Experiment with different feeding positions. Have your caregiver try propping your baby against her raised legs, or holding him facing out, so he can't see her. (We don't know why this works, but some babies feed better this way.) Doing this in front of the television sometimes helps. We've also heard of a dad putting on his wife's bathrobe and tucking the bottle under his armpit, with good results.

Learning How to Pump or Express Milk

If you plan to leave your own milk with your babysitter for the feedings you'll miss, the need for pumping or expressing milk is obvious. This means you'll be pumping while you're at work.

Even if you plan to use formula for missed feedings, pumping and expressing are important skills to have. They can help you relieve the pressure of overfull breasts so that you feel more comfortable, will diminish leaking, and will keep up your milk supply. Pumping or expressing will also help to prevent the breast infections that often result from engorgement.

Learning these techniques is a perfect activity for "What I Did on My Maternity Leave." You can't expect to do your learning when you're back on the job, pressured by time, dressed for success, and in an environment that probably provides less than ideal levels of comfort and privacy. If you start doing it at least three weeks before you go back to work, you'll have time to practice and you should

be fairly proficient by the time you need to be. For instructions for hand-expressing, pumping, storing, and feeding expressed milk, see Chapter 11.

To have breast milk for your baby's first bottle-feeding, when you're still at home, make some of your feeding sessions combos: Nurse from one breast, pump from the other, and save whatever you get. Or you can pump from the other breast right after a feeding. If you haven't pumped enough for a full feeding, refrigerate or freeze what you have, and add breast milk from subsequent pumping sessions. Be sure to cool the new milk before adding it to frozen milk so the new warm milk won't thaw any of the frozen milk. If you still don't have enough, follow the bottle-feeding of breast milk with enough formula to make up a full feeding. If milk is frozen in batches, it may have a striped appearance since the cream rises to the top as each bit freezes.

Your Baby's Feedings While You're at Work

Remember that it's better to give some breast milk than none, that worrying about the possibility of your baby's going hungry may decrease your milk output. The value of the nursing experience does not depend on the volume of milk you produce—it goes far beyond that. And if you don't produce enough, you can add formula.

If you're anxious about the amount of milk you're producing, however, leave some formula with your caregiver. It's better to do this and to be able to enjoy the emotional closeness when you do nurse than to be so worried about the quantity of milk you're providing that neither you nor your baby enjoys the nursing experience.

Equipment You'll Need for Pumping Your Breast Milk

❧ A pump that's easy to carry and store, since you'll be either taking it to work with you every day or storing it at work. If you keep it at work, you'll need another pump at home. You'll also want one that's easy to clean, especially since the washing facilities at work may not be up to the standards you have at home. And you may want a battery option for times when you don't have access to an electrical outlet. The most efficient pump is electric, with a double-pumping kit. Although this is the most expensive kind of pump, many women feel it's well worth the investment in the time and energy it saves.

One model comes in a shoulder bag or backpack that stores the double pumping kit, the pump itself, collection bottles, and cooling elements. You can also buy a unit to run it from the cigarette lighter in your car, or a rechargeable battery to use when electricity is not available. For information on finding the pump that's right for you, see Chapter 11 and the Resource Appendix.

❧ Either a thermos or a cooler to use with the bottles or milk storage bags. If you use a thermos, get the kind used for fluids, not solid foods, of the best quality you can find. Before you leave home in the morning, fill it with ice cubes to keep it cold. When you express, dump out the ice, dry the inside of the thermos, and fill the thermos with your milk. If you are going to store your expressed milk in bottles or milk storage bags instead of a thermos, put frozen ice packs and the empty bottles or bags in a small cooler before you leave home. After you pump, put the bottle or bag of your expressed milk back in the cooler. When you get home, refrigerate your milk for use within a few days, or freeze it if you won't be using it within a week. To freeze the milk in small portions, you can pour it into ice cube trays and then transfer the frozen cubes of milk into zip-top plastic bags. These procedures are described in Chapter 11.

❧ Sensory cues to stimulate your let-down reflex. Involve as many senses as possible while you pump: a recording of your baby's sounds, a photo to prop in front of you, the baby's sleeper to inhale her sweet smell, and whatever you normally drink when you're nursing.

❧ A brush for cleaning the pump after each use. Besides following the manufacturer's instructions for cleaning your pumping equipment, wash your hands and equipment with warm, soapy water after each pumping to keep any bacterial contamination low.

❧ Cleaning wipes for sink and countertop—again to keep your environment as germ-free as possible.

❧ Cloth or paper towels for wiping the rim of the thermos and the pump.

❖ A washcloth for patting your breasts dry after pumping. Do not wipe. Wiping removes natural oil secretions and can cause chapping and soreness.

❖ An extra set of breast pads.

❖ A bag or briefcase, in which you can carry your equipment between work and home.

❖ Zip-top plastic bags for storing and transporting the pump parts as well as the accessories.

❖ Labels and permanent markers to mark the date of pumped milk.

Where to Express

Find a clean, quiet, private place. Ideally, your workplace provides a room set aside specifically for nursing mothers. If not, a quiet office with a door you can lock, either your own office or another that you can arrange to use, is best. A vacant meeting or conference room may be available. Some women go out and sit in their cars, using a pump that can be plugged into the cigarette lighter. Others use a women's lounge. Although there's a concern with bathroom sanitation, sometimes this is a woman's only option. One mom confessed to a special fondness for the stall designated for women with disabilities, since it's roomier and has a convenient shelf for placing her paraphernalia. If you're using an office with windows or glass walls, check for shades so that you can maintain your privacy.

When to Express

If you are hand-expressing or using a manual pump, at first it may take you up to 30 minutes each session to drain both breasts. Eventually, you may be able to get it down to 8 to 10 minutes; some women continue to need 15 to 20 minutes. Electric pumps are much faster and take no more than about 10 or 15 minutes total right from the start. The more you practice at home, the better you'll do.

Your daily lunch hour and coffee breaks should give you enough pumping time. You may be able to take a shorter lunch break and use the rest of your allotted time for longer pumping breaks throughout the day. In your eagerness to make the most of your time, however, don't neglect your diet. You need to keep up your strength. If you can't get enough pumping time during your breaks, you may be able to make arrangements to take longer breaks and come into work earlier, stay later, or take work home. Or you may be so efficient that you can do your job in less time.

How Much to Express

At first, you may not get more than an ounce of milk at a time, but eventually you can probably count on expressing three to five ounces of milk at each session. However, different women produce different amounts. You'll most likely produce more milk early in the day and early in the week, when your energy levels are highest. If you can't get enough for your baby's next-day feedings, try some of the hints given in Chapter 11. It's still worth pumping even if you get just one ounce from each side, since you can mix your milk with formula.

When you're at home, nurse your baby on cue, or even more frequently than he "requests." This will help you increase your milk supply. Don't give any bottles or cups at all when you're home.

Remember, accidents happen, but they can be dealt with. Remember the mom we met in Chapter 11? She made up for spilling her expressed milk by waking up at three-hour intervals to pump throughout the night.

Formula

If you plan to offer formula to your baby at one or more feedings, you need to make the change gradually, to avoid engorgement and the risk of breast infection. Allow between four and seven days for each feeding to be phased out. On weekends and holidays, you can maintain your weekday schedule except for one additional breastfeeding. This keeps your milk supply at a fairly constant, comfortable level. Again, you may want someone else to give those bottle feedings, since your baby may not accept them from you.

If you plan to switch to formula exclusively, the weaning process should take at least a couple of weeks. Remember that pumping alone provides some nipple stimulation and therefore some milk. (For more on weaning, see Chapter 17.) As you begin to substitute formula for your own milk, you may need to pump or express to relieve your discomfort. If so, save your milk. You can use it for your baby, occasionally substituting breast milk for formula.

Negotiating with Your Employer

If your employer is not supportive of your pumping or breastfeeding on your breaks, find out what the concerns are, and then see how you and your supervisor can work out a solution. For example, if your employer worries that you are, or will be, taking too much time from your work, reassure him or her that you'll be taking less time within a couple of weeks, once you get your routine under way, and that you'll make up any lost hours. Or you may find that you can do your pumping or nursing in a shorter time right away. If coworkers object, ask for the basis of their complaints and see how you can meet their concerns. Also, explain, calmly and reasonably, why the health benefits of nursing are so important to you and your baby.

Illinois social worker Brandi Campbell interviewed for a new job when her son was five months old. She told the interviewer that she planned to pump: "If there was going to be a problem, I wanted to know right away. There was no way I was not going to continue nursing and pumping." There was no problem, she took the job, and more than a year later, she was still nursing but had cut the number of pumping sessions.

Another woman asked the lactation consultant at her local hospital to write to her employer, explaining the benefits of breastfeeding for mother, child, and employer. Another called her coworkers together to describe these benefits. And yet another went out of her way to have her company's nursing-friendly atmosphere recognized during World Breastfeeding Week (WBW). (For more information about the World Alliance for Breastfeeding Action and WBW, see the Resource Appendix.)

As of this writing, 24 U.S. states, the District of Columbia, and Puerto Rico have laws related to breastfeeding in the workplace. These laws generally require an employer to provide unpaid break time and a private place, other than a toilet stall, for an employee to express milk. (To check the law in your state, go to www.ncsl.org/IssuesResearch/Health/BreastfeedingLaws/tabid/14389/Default.aspx and Appendix I for suggestions on finding legal help.)

Working moms will benefit from the health care bill that President Barack Obama signed into law in 2010. The bill requires employers with more than 50 workers to provide "a place, other than a bathroom, that is shielded from view and free from intrusion from co-workers and the public, which may be used by an employee to express breast milk."

Back at Work

The day you go back to your job and leave your baby in someone else's care can be emotionally difficult after having been together so constantly since the baby's birth. Your return to work can also pose practical challenges. You can make life easier on both fronts by planning your return to make it as stress-free as possible.

Your Work Schedule

Try to make your first day back at work a Thursday or Friday. This will give you the weekend to rest up, to analyze the way your workday went, and to see how you can help it go more smoothly. Try to take off the first few Wednesdays, as well: A midweek break will also make the transition easier.

If you can go back to work part-time for a while, this will be ideal. Survey after survey shows that mothers who work part-time seem the happiest with their lives, compared to full-time workers and full-time homemakers. This is especially helpful, of course, for the breastfeeding mother, especially if you go back to work before your baby is four months old. Research has also shown that mothers who work no more than 20 hours a week are likely to continue to nurse as long as mothers who don't work outside the home.

If you have the option of working part-time and can plan your schedule,

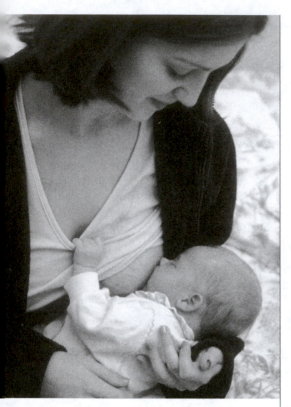

Working mothers often treasure that last nursing in the morning before they leave the baby and the first one after they return home at the end of the day. The babies love them, too.

fewer hours per day works out better for breastfeeding than fewer days per week. In other words, if you plan to work 24 to 25 hours per week, you'll do better putting in 5 hours a day for five days instead of 8 hours for three days. You'll have to weigh this advantage for breastfeeding against such disadvantages as spending more on child care or long commutes to work, and then make the decision that's best for you.

The possibilities for alternative scheduling are limitless. With some jobs, you can take some of your work home. With others, you can take advantage of flexible scheduling or of sharing your job with another worker. Some workplaces will allow you to bring your baby to work with you. Or you may be able to combine two coffee breaks into a single longer break, which you can then attach to your lunch hour, giving you enough time to go to your baby. (One mother we know meets her caregiver, her older son, and her nursing baby in a park on sunny days and in a coffee shop on cold or rainy days.) Explore the possibility of these options with your employer. Even if they never thought of such arrangements in the past, they may be willing to give one of them a try.

If your employer already provides a private place to pump, make the most use out of it. If this isn't possible, get creative. Brandi Campbell, for example, finds pumping in her car the easiest. But she also has pumped in schools, hospitals, and courtrooms. "I have pumped everywhere," she says. "I just go in wherever my job takes me and tell them I'm a breastfeeding mom and I need a private space to pump breast milk. My most unusual place was in a jail, where the men were really helpful in clearing out an office for me."

You may decide, after adding up the costs of child care, commuting, clothes, lunches out, and so forth, that the only way for you to come out ahead is to find work that you can do at home. Or you may be in a position to postpone your return to paid employment until your child is older.

Years ago, a mother who worked outside the home was criticized for leaving her children. Today, the pendulum has swung in the other direction with criticism often directed at women who are financially able to stay at home for a few years. It would be a shame if women came to accept the judgment that a person is only as interesting and valuable as her job and her income. Raising children is important work, and our society needs to recognize that every mother is a working mother. You're the only one who can decide whether this is the sole work you want to do during these years and whether it's financially feasible for you.

Whatever your decision, if you're happy with it, your children are likely to thrive. The more satisfied a woman is with her life, the more effective she is as a parent, and the better adjusted her children will be.

Your Nursing Schedule

While there are many different ways to arrange your breastfeeding schedule, a fairly typical one for a full-time working mother of a small baby with fairly regular habits may go something like this:

1. Wake up in the morning one hour before you need to begin to get ready for work. Take your baby back to bed with you for a quiet, leisurely feeding.

2. Nurse your baby again just before you leave her at the caregiver's home or the day-care center. This feeding is optional, depending on how much time has elapsed since the first one of the morning, and on your preferences and your baby's. If you do have time, it's a nice way to say "Good-bye, I'll see you soon."

3. If you're leaving your own milk for your baby's feedings, express or pump two to three times during the workday.

4. If it is feasible, nurse your baby at lunchtime, either by going to her or by having her brought to you.

5. Nurse your baby right after work, at the child-care site if you have a long ride home, or at home.

6. Nurse just before you go to sleep.

7. Nurse one or more times during the night. (This is optional, depending on your baby's schedule and the age of your baby. Many women find that getting up once during the night is not exhausting, especially if they and the baby go right back to sleep afterward, which is easier if they're sleeping in the same room.)

No one is typical, and every woman has to learn what works for her. One flight attendant, for example, went back to work after three months, making three trips a week. She chose night flights so that she would miss only one or two feedings, used a breast pump every three or four hours, put her breast milk in bottles that she packed in ice till she got home, and then froze the milk for use during her next flight.

Wardrobe Tips for
the Working Breastfeeding Mother

You may feel comfortable telling coworkers you're breastfeeding, but you certainly don't want your wardrobe to do the telling. Here are some suggestions to help you look and feel comfortable:

❖ Breast pads in your bra will prevent leaking milk from coming through and staining your clothes. Be sure to change the pads when they get wet.

❖ Pants or skirts with tops that can be pulled up or unbuttoned allow for more ease in pumping and breastfeeding than do dresses.

❖ Bright or dark print blouses or tops won't show leaking as readily as solid colors do, and they won't show the outlines of your nipples or your breast pads. Stay away from whites and pale colors; they reveal to everyone what you may want just your baby and your partner to see.

❖ Cottons and synthetic fabrics stand up best in case of leaking. Silks and linens may become stained. Clinging materials will show the outlines of nipples and breast pads.

❖ Everything you wear should be washable. Nothing should need more than touch-up ironing.

❖ If you're self-conscious about your fuller breasts, wear a lightweight blazer or loose jacket during your workday.

❖ Don't try to squeeze into too-tight prepregnancy clothes. Chances are that you're a few pounds heavier than you were then, and clothes that strain are unbecoming to even the slimmest women. Try wearing what you wore to work early in your pregnancy before you switched to maternity clothes.

❖ Tight blouses and shirts are especially treacherous: They rub against your nipples and might trigger a let-down at inconvenient times, like on the bus or in an important meeting. More important, they can cause a clogged duct or breast infection.

❖ Don't wear cotton sweaters; they tend to lose their shape after being pulled up two or three times.

❖ Wear a nursing bra to work even if you don't wear one at home. It's more convenient to be able to undo one side at a time instead of having to take off your entire bra when you pump. You'll also welcome its good support.

❖ Keep a spare blouse or sweater at work (one that can be worn with most outfits) in case you leak or spill milk on the one you're wearing.

Another mother nursed full[ ] her baby's first six weeks, the[ ] tuted formula for two daytime[ ] a day for the next two weeks,[ ] back to work after two months[ ] tinued to nurse only three[ ] day—morning, evening, and [ ]

Some working nursing[ ] schedule reverse cycle fe[ ] which they feed their babies[ ] during the evenings and at [ ] babies won't be very hungr[ ] day. Some babies seem t[ ] "up" time for these nighttir[ ] which are easier when mothers bring the baby into bed with them to nurse. If you can concentrate on the bonus of together time instead of the lost sleep, these snuggled-together sessions can be highlights of the nursing experience. (This schedule was described by Marilyn Grams, MD, who used it while nursing her babies, in her very personal book, *Breastfeeding Success for Working Mothers*.)

Travel

A job that requires travel poses special challenges. Ideally, you'll be able to postpone any trips until your baby is weaned. The next best thing is to keep trips brief, no more than overnight. If you can't do either, you still don't necessarily have to wean. The ingenuity of mothers and the adaptability of babies can be astonishing. You may be able to take your baby and caregiver with you. If so, you may be able to maintain the same basic schedule as at home. If not, you can arrange for feedings in your absence.

well as ever. One stock analyst (kn[ ] in her firm as the "Dairy Queen"[ ] with the hostility she sometim[ ] from women in her offic[ ] standing where it came [ ] "I realize," she s[ ] these women's re[ ] their own pai[ ] didn't do th[ ] they're [ ] dren [ ] did[ ]

tions on making travel easier, see Chapter 9.

Your Coworkers

Some nursing mothers find that their fellow workers, male and female alike, help them in ways both large and small. One woman, for example, pumped her milk in an office nook while a male colleague stood guard to protect her privacy. Others report that their coworkers answer their phones for them while they're on their pump breaks. Unfortunately, some mothers are targets of resentment from colleagues, who may complain about a woman's expressing milk in an employees' lounge or restroom or about her "getting away with" something that other workers are not.

Women handle their on-the-job relationships in various ways. Some don't tell their fellow workers what they're doing. Others go out of their way to let people know—and to show them that they are indeed doing their jobs as

own
dealt
s sensed
by under-
rom.

ys, "that some of
sentment came from
or regrets that they
s for their babies, or that
ot able to be with their chil-
s much as they would like, and I
n't let their remarks bother me. I
knew I breastfed because it was important for my baby, and I couldn't be
ruled by other people's derogatory attitudes and comments."

Dealing with Leaking

❖ Leaking is most common in the
first month or two of nursing, when
your breasts are full or it's nearly time
to nurse or pump, and when you're
thinking about your baby. If you can
hold off going back to work for two
months, leaking is less likely to occur.

❖ You can often prevent leaking by
anticipating when it's likely to occur

and expressing milk to reduce breast
fullness.

❖ If you do feel tingling, cross your
arms over your chest for about ten seconds. As one mother told us, "I like the
elbow pressure against my breast as I
'fiddle with an earring.' Only another
nursing mother will know what I'm
really doing."

Working mothers, like other new mothers, cite fatigue as their biggest
problem. Since it's so hard for you to
get the rest you need, you have to be
firm about cutting out everything in
your life that is not essential or enjoyable. Doing your work, taking care of
your family, and taking some time to
care for yourself should be the only
things you have to juggle during the
time you're nursing.

This is the time to cut back on the
extraneous and enjoy this precious
time of your life, so that you can look
back in later years to many happy
memories of this special shared experience. As one breastfeeding working
mother says, "It lasts for such a tiny
part of the children's lives that it needs
to be cherished."

CHAPTER THIRTEEN

Breastfeeding: A Sexual Passage

"Of course I didn't always feel sexy when I was nursing the baby. But sometimes the combination of nursing her and seeing my husband in bed next to me made me want to rush through the feeding so that Bob and I could make love."

KATE Bradford, New Hampshire

"I'm sure that nursing had something to do with my lack of interest in sex. My body was in use all day long, and by the time night came around I just wanted to draw an invisible circle around my body and say, 'No trespassing.'"

LILY Sarasota, Florida

Nursing mothers seem to fall equally into two distinct camps. Some, like Kate, experience increased sexual appetites and enjoy a much less sexually inhibited relationship with their partner. Other women, like Lily, find that they are not nearly as interested in sex for the first six months after childbirth as they had been before and will be later on.

Kate and Lily exemplify the complicated relationship between breastfeeding and sexuality. As the editor of the journal *Canadian Family Physician* has stated, "There is conflicting evidence regarding the effect of breastfeeding on sexuality postpartum. Studies show more interest, less interest, and no change in patterns of intercourse."

There's been very little research about the relationship between breastfeeding and sexuality, and the data we do have are contradictory. In one study of 567 first-time mothers who were breastfeeding, the women's responses varied widely: About half reported less sexual interest or activity and half reported no change. Overall, they tended to feel that breastfeeding had little or no effect on their sexual relationships with their partners. In another study, among more than 1,000 nursing moms, 30 percent of the women reported that their sexual relationships had improved after nursing, while only 2.5 percent reported worsened relationships. Most of the women who said they now had a better sex life had considered their sexual relationship excellent before nursing, while all the women in the other category said they had had poor sexual adjustment to begin with. What researchers do agree upon is that very few medical professionals discuss sexuality with their breastfeeding patients.

Nursing is a sensual experience. But this sensuality most often translates into a sense of satisfaction similar to the euphoria that follows orgasm rather than the intensity and excitement of orgasm. Nursing mothers most often talk about a calm feeling of completion that combines physical and emotional fulfillment. In her book *Free and Female,* Barbara Seaman describes breastfeeding as "a sensual and sensuous experience unlike any other, somewhat related to and yet different from good sex."

Sexy? Or Not So Sexy?

Some women feel sexier when they're nursing. This is perfectly normal. On the other hand, many factors can diminish a nursing woman's interest in sex. You may yearn for the intimacy that you and your partner enjoyed before your baby was born. And you may want very much to resume your sexual relationship, but be distressed to find problems that you hadn't expected suddenly getting in the way. Both you and your partner may be puzzled and concerned about what is happening—or has, in fact, already happened—to your sex life. What you need to remember is that you can—and almost certainly will—overcome any obstacles. But it may take a little time.

One condition that affects almost all new mothers and their sex lives, whether they nurse or not, is fatigue. Taking care of an infant is hard work. Furthermore, you never get a good night's sleep. Add to this the first-time mother's concern about her ability to care for her new baby and her feeling that lack of both sleep and time has made her less attractive, and it's easy to understand many new mothers' temporarily lower interest in lovemaking.

The "touched-out" feeling that Lily expressed is also common. Many nursing mothers immerse themselves so deeply in their babies' care and derive so much pleasure from the physical as well as the emotional closeness they experience from breastfeeding that they don't need this kind of closeness with their partners. In fact, they sometimes need the exact opposite—a time when they can pull into themselves like turtles in a shell, and reclaim their bodies for themselves.

Furthermore, female physiology almost seems to discourage sexual activity in the nursing mother. Because of her lower levels of estrogen (caused by the higher levels of prolactin in her body during lactation), her vaginal wall becomes thinner and more sensitive, and there is less vaginal lubrication. Many women find that their nipples and breasts are less sensitive to touch while they're lactating. Some women also find that their nipples lose their ability to become erect with stimulation, even though they still become elongated in the baby's mouth. (These responses may be nature's way of discouraging getting pregnant again too soon.)

No matter which camp you fall into—whether you're eager to resume sexual relations, can't imagine ever wanting to again, or are willing to go along at first for your partner's sake—you probably have questions about lovemaking. You wonder how soon you should go back to enjoying regular sexual relations—and whether you should restrict your activities in any way, for your own sake or for your baby's.

Resuming Sexual Activity

Men and women generally have different attitudes toward sex, especially during pregnancy and after childbirth. While sometimes the woman is more sexually eager than the man, the more common situation is for the man to want a resumption of sexual relations, especially intercourse, earlier than the woman. Some researchers suggest that women can accept disruptions in their sexual relationships more easily than men do and that they're more apt to dismiss the impact of child rearing as a temporary sexual inconvenience, while men seem more likely to feel that children interfere with sex. How much of this is physical and how much cultural? This is a hard question to answer, but there are some obvious physical reasons.

A man's body does not, of course, undergo the changes that a woman's does. His shape does not change; he is not uncomfortable in various positions;

he is not exhausted and sore after childbirth; he is not subject to bleeding for a couple of weeks after delivery. Nor do the hormones in his body change radically during pregnancy, after childbirth, and during lactation. All of these physiological differences affect women in various ways, one of which is often a reduced desire for sex. Furthermore, men often find emotional comfort in the sex act itself, while women are more likely to be comforted by being held and caressed. Still, women who may not be hungry for sex will often be ready to resume relations because they want that intimacy with their partners.

When to Begin

Most doctors advise women not to engage in sexual intercourse until after their first postpartum examination. This is to prevent the two biggest postpartum risks, infection and hemorrhage. Either one can result from the introduction of an object—any object—into the vagina before it is fully healed from childbirth. Before you are ready for intercourse, you want to be sure that any vaginal tears or episiotomy incisions have mended, that the tenderness in your perineal area is less severe, that the placental site (the place on your uterus where the placenta had been attached) has healed, and that your vaginal canal has again developed the microorganisms that protect it from infection. Generally, once soreness has gone, stitches have been absorbed, and bleeding has stopped, intercourse is safe.

This postpartum exam has traditionally taken place at about six weeks after delivery, but may occur any time between three and eight weeks postpartum, depending on your desires and your doctor's policy. If you want an earlier postpartum exam than your doctor customarily schedules, ask whether this is possible. It's also a good idea to ask your doctor to explain to both you and your partner together the reasons for abstinence before this exam. Men who understand these reasons are less likely to pressure new mothers to resume intercourse before the moms are ready. In fact, even if your doctor says you're ready, this doesn't mean that *you* feel you're ready.

How to Begin

Sexuality is not, of course, restricted to intercourse, and there are many other ways by which a couple can keep their sexual relationship alive. You can enjoy physical, sensual closeness by many other paths. You can, for example, bathe together and be naked in bed together. You can caress and fondle and stroke and massage each other. You can pleasure each other through oral or manual alternatives to intercourse.

The first time you resume sexual intercourse, you will probably find that you're still quite tender in the perineal area. Intercourse may be painful, and you may worry that it will always feel this way. Fortunately, this is only temporary: Life—and sex—do get better. If you had a cesarean delivery, you may feel abdominal discomfort. You may have both abdominal and vaginal pain

Pelvic Floor (Kegel) Exercises

You may have been doing these exercises to strengthen your pelvic floor while you were pregnant. It's a good idea for every woman to do them, whether or not she is expecting or has just had a child and whether she is young or old. Kegels help to keep her pelvic floor muscles (also known as the pubococcygeal, or perineal, muscles) well toned. These muscles support the uterus, the bladder, and the rectum—everything inside the pelvic cavity—and contract spontaneously during orgasm.

Named after Arnold Kegel, MD, the gynecologist who first developed the exercises, principally to control urinary leakage, these exercises speed healing from childbirth, minimize pain and swelling, and strengthen the perineal muscles. Well-toned pelvic floor muscles enhance the experience of sexual intercourse for both you and your partner and also help resolve any problems of minor incontinence.

To do them, contract and relax the group of muscles directly between your legs, which involve the urethra, the vagina, and to a lesser extent, the anus. Hold the contraction for five to ten seconds, as if you were holding back the flow of urine; then slowly release the tension and relax the muscles for a few seconds. When you first begin, you may have trouble holding the contractions, but with practice your muscles will become stronger. Right after delivery, these muscles may be numb and you may not feel the contractions, but the sensations will return. Try to do three sets of 20 repetitions every day.

You can do them sitting (in a chair or while driving), standing (while brushing your teeth or in line at the bank), or lying down (while nursing or watching TV), and no one else will be able to tell what you're doing. You can evaluate your progress if you do them while you're urinating; you'll see how much better you get at holding back and then releasing urine. You can also do the exercises during sexual intercourse, to the enhancement of both partners' pleasure. And you can continue doing them for the rest of your life, to maintain muscle tone and strength.

---

if you had an unexpected cesarean after a difficult labor. This is common and, again, is almost always only temporary.

Talk to your partner ahead of time, so that he understands how your body feels and how to help you to make this first time a good time. He needs to know that he can alleviate your discomfort by going slowly, and by performing manual or oral stimulation first until you are ready for penetration. Because of the reduced secretion of estrogen after you give birth, you may not have enough vaginal lubrication for comfortable intercourse. It will be helpful to use a vaginal lubricant (like K-Y jelly or liquid, Astroglide, or contraceptive jelly or cream) and a position that allows you to control the depth of penetration. You might try woman-on-top, lying on your sides face-to-face, or spooning. Any discomfort should go away soon after intercourse. If pain persists for seven to ten days after intercourse or after the first half-dozen times postdelivery, call your doctor. You should feel good (even if tired) after having had a baby; if you don't, your pain may signal a medical problem.

If you began doing Kegel exercises soon after delivery (see the box on page 279), you are likely to enjoy intercourse more when you do resume.

If any activities or positions are painful for you now, let your partner know. Being a martyr won't feel good for you—or for him. He'll sense your lack of enthusiasm for sex and may attribute it to problems with your feelings for him rather than to your physical discomfort. Meanwhile, as you let him know what does *not* feel good, be sure to show or tell him what *does* feel good.

One way to begin is to have a "physical conversation." This involves no talk, just touching between you and your partner for 30 minutes or so. A few of these conversations can make a stimulating and pleasurable reintroduction to a full sexual relationship.

Sex and Your Breasts

Many mothers who are nursing wonder whether their breasts belong to their baby during lactation and should therefore be off-limits to their partner. They need not be. You can be a sexual partner during the time you are nursing your baby, and you can share your breasts with both your baby and your partner. Your breasts do not have to stop performing their erotic function just because they are now performing their biological function.

There's no reason why your partner cannot stimulate your breasts both manually and orally during the time you're nursing, if you enjoy this. Furthermore, your child's father won't be stealing candy from his baby if he gets an occasional swallow of your sweet milk. (Some couples regularly include this in their lovemaking.) There is plenty more where that came from.

You may find, particularly in the first couple of months, that your breasts become hard and tender an hour or two after a feeding. At these times, intercourse in the man-on-top position is apt to be uncomfortable. You would probably be more comfortable in such positions as woman-on-top or rear-entry. This might be the perfect time to experiment with lovemaking positions that you have never tried. You may even discover something you like better than your former favorites. In any case, the tenderness of the newly lactating breast goes away soon. After a couple of months, it will not be a factor in how you do what you do.

Spurting of milk during and immediately after orgasm is fairly common among nursing women, with the milk usually flowing more slowly from the breast that has been suckled more recently. Many women feel happy about this show of excitement; the ones who want to avoid getting spots on the sheet find that making love right after a feeding helps. It's also possible to wear a bra during sex. (There are some very pretty lacy nursing bras.)

One woman told us, "When Joe and I first realized that every time I experienced orgasm my breasts would spurt milk, it was a big source of satisfaction for both of us. There was no doubt in his mind that I had reached a climax, and I loved being able to show it in one more way."

You and Your Relationship

The months following the birth of a first child constitute a major transition in a marriage or other kind of partnership. As with any other new experience, you are likely to welcome parenthood with mixed emotions. The birth of your first baby brings home to you and your partner more dramatically than any other event in your lives the realization that you are now adults, newly responsible for another human being.

Eager as you may be to grow into this phase of life, it's only natural that you feel anxious about what it will mean and what will be expected of you. If you and your mate have been able to communicate well before the arrival of your baby, you'll have a good base to help you adjust to parenthood. If not, it's especially important for you to make extra efforts now to let each other know exactly how you feel.

Like every other woman in the world, you have to learn to be a mother. It does not happen magically via labor and delivery. You need time and practice to feel at home in your new role.

Meanwhile, while you're worrying about your ability to be a good mother, your partner has his own conflicts to struggle with as he faces up to the responsibility of parenthood. Yet all too often, both husband and wife assume that their partners know how they feel, and neither one expresses his or her real concerns.

The experience of breastfeeding introduces other elements into this period of your life, since as a lactating woman, you're experiencing a powerful phase in the female cycle of sexuality (see the box on page 282 for more about these phases). The physiological changes that occur in your body in connection with pregnancy, childbirth, and lactation are likely to affect your emotions, your sexual desires, and your adult relationship. Breastfeeding dramatizes the physical and emotional ties in the new pairing (you and your child) that overlap with those in the preexisting couple (you and your partner). Furthermore, both of you are bound to respond in some way to the sexual connotation of the breasts in our society.

The Five Phases of Female Sexuality

Niles Newton, PhD, a psychologist and mother who pioneered in the study of female development, defined five interrelated phases of female sexuality: the menstrual cycle, orgasm from sexual stimulation, pregnancy, childbirth, and lactation. Through interviews with women at different stages of life and drawing from research on physiology, Dr. Newton described phenomena that are common to more than one phase of female sexuality and also demonstrated how outside pressures and emotions can influence all five phases.

Phenomena Common to More Than One Phase of Female Sexuality

✤ The breasts enlarge just before menstruation, during pregnancy, just before orgasm, and during lactation.

✤ The nipples become erect upon sexual stimulation, during childbirth, and during lactation.

✤ The uterus contracts during orgasm, childbirth, and lactation.

✤ Body temperature rises during ovulation, childbirth, orgasm, and lactation.

✤ A woman usually feels an urge to take care of one loved one (the baby) during pregnancy, after childbirth, and during lactation, and the other (her partner) in a fulfilling sexual relationship.

✤ The hormone oxytocin surges through a woman's body during orgasm, during childbirth, and during lactation. This hormone causes the uterus to contract and the nipples to become erect. Oxytocin is also the stimulus for the milk-ejection reflex and probably the reason why milk sometimes spurts from the breasts of a woman in orgasm.

Female Sexuality

Historically, sexuality has been discussed mostly in terms of male-female genital intercourse. People have been considered fulfilled sexual beings if they have been able to reach orgasm through intercourse. This definition tends to focus on men, either ignoring women's needs for sexual gratification or assuming that they should achieve gratification in the same way men do.

Today, though, we recognize the distinctly female sexual experience. With this awareness, we have developed a more global definition of sexuality, keying it more into sensuality and to the many pleasurable sensations that can be attained through a wide range of activities, which may include, but are not limited to, intercourse. By thinking of sexuality in this way, we expand the

How Outside Pressures and Emotions Can Influence All Five Phases

✤ The menstrual cycle: The most regular cycle can be disrupted by excitement or anxiety. Many a bride, for example, has carefully set the date for her marriage—and yet still menstruated on her wedding day. And the tension of a job or family crisis often brings on or suspends a woman's period.

✤ Orgasm from sexual stimulation: The tremendous impact of outside influences on sexual interaction is obvious to anyone (male or female) who can't get in the mood for sex because of the distractions of financial, family, job, or health problems. People at the brink of orgasm may be abruptly turned off by a piercing yell from the nursery, by a ringing telephone, or by a fear that their privacy is about to be invaded.

✤ Pregnancy: Conception itself may be affected by emotional influences.

Studies in animal and human reproduction suggest that stress may affect hormone production in a way that interferes with ovulation.

✤ Childbirth: Outside events also influence childbirth. An emotional or physical shock can bring on premature labor, and the mother's anticipation of childbirth often seems related to the ease and duration of labor and delivery. A woman who's frightened of giving birth is apt to have a more difficult delivery than one who understands the physiology of childbirth.

✤ Lactation: Mothers and midwives have long known that a woman's ability to give milk to her baby is influenced by pain, embarrassment, and emotional conflict. Drs. Michael and Niles Newton confirmed this observation in the laboratory, when they showed that a nursing mother will give significantly less milk when she's distracted during feedings by discomfort and by various annoyances.

possibility of sexual fulfillment to include the later years of life, as well as those times in earlier years when intercourse may not be possible, advisable, or desirable, such as the weeks just before and just after the birth of a baby.

Both men and women can and do derive great pleasure from such noncoital activities as kissing, stroking, touching, cuddling, massage, and oral and manual genital stimulation. In addition, women's sexuality is even more wide-ranging, since it's closely tied to the five phases of the female reproductive capacity.

All five of these phases are controlled to a great extent by the interaction of hormones released inside a woman's body. Estrogen, progesterone, testosterone, follicle-stimulating hormone (FSH), luteinizing hormone (LH), oxytocin, and prolactin are among the hormones that help to make a woman a sexual being. Some of them manage the course of the menstrual cycle, causing ovulation and fertility.

Some dominate during pregnancy. Others signal the onset of labor, the production and release of milk, and the climax of orgasm. Most of these hormones have more than one function. While some are more active during one phase of the female cycle than are others, the interaction among them is responsible for some remarkable similarities in the various sexual phases, as shown in the box on page 282.

Female sexuality, then, involves a complex series of responses that carry over from a woman's reproductive capacity to her maternal functions. Yet in our society, woman's interest in sexual intercourse—in achieving her own orgasm and in helping her partner to achieve it, too—has been stressed, while those elements of sexuality related to childbirth and lactation have been virtually ignored.

The late Alice Rossi, PhD, a sociology professor at the University of Massachusetts, suggested that our "male dominant family and political systems have imposed a wedge between maternalism on the one hand, and female sexuality on the other. We define maternity in culturally narrow ways, clearly differentiate it from sexuality, and require that women deny the evidence of their senses by repressing the component of sexuality in the maternal role."

Fortunately, this attitude is being overcome, partly due to the women's movement and partly due to greater acceptance of sexuality in general. The groundbreaking work of sex researchers William H. Masters and Virginia E. Johnson (see facing page) continues to have an enormous influence on the ways in which people think about sex. In the past several decades, we have learned a great deal about the physiological mechanisms related to sexual activities and responses. We have felt freer to communicate with our sexual partners about how we feel and what we like, and many couples have found that their sexual rapport flourishes in such an open climate. The same can happen when we are open and understanding about aspects of sexuality in the maternal role.

The Sensuous Nature of Breastfeeding

Nursing is supposed to be enjoyable for both mother and baby. If it were not, our species might never have survived the thousands of years when no substitute for human milk was available. Some researchers have concluded that when women are encouraged to accept and enjoy the sexual pleasure breastfeeding can offer, they give more milk. This makes sense, since the let-down reflex is highly subject to emotional influences. Indeed, the good feelings associated with breastfeeding may be built into our natures to strengthen the bond between mother and baby in the early months of life.

Masters and Johnson's 1966 book, *Human Sexual Response,* reported on their pioneering research. The book included the results of interviews with 111 women during and after their pregnancies. These women talked about their sexual behavior, feelings, and responses during pregnancy and immediately following childbirth. Of this group, only 24 women nursed their babies (a reflection of the low popularity of breastfeeding at the time). Of course, the results of a similar study today might be quite different, with increased rates of breastfeeding and increased focus on sexuality.

Some of these nursing mothers reported experiencing sexual arousal while suckling their babies. Several felt guilty about this and worried that they were perverted. Some women did not breastfeed because they were afraid that they might be sexually stimulated from the suckling. (Only three of the women in the Masters and Johnson study reported incidents of orgasm while nursing.)

It shouldn't be surprising that breastfeeding has its sensual components. For many women, their breasts are highly erogenous zones, sensitive to the slightest touch and capable of sending messages of excitement throughout the body. In fact, some women reach orgasm from having their breasts fondled. The nerve pathways from the nipple to the brain are the same, no matter what the stimulation is. During lactation, of course, the breasts are constantly stimulated both by the mother's own handling and by the baby's frequent suckling and sometimes stroking.

As one mother told us, "There is something very earthy about nursing a child that can pleasantly affect the husband-wife relationship. I also feel that a good breastfeeding experience makes you more open and womanly."

Furthermore, since our society has eroticized the breast even beyond its own intrinsic nature, most nursing mothers are very conscious of their breasts as sexual symbols as well as sources of nutrition and comfort for their babies. (This, of course, is why so many women are reluctant to breastfeed in public. Even if they don't see the act as sexually provocative, they know that some others will.)

Unfortunately, many women who experience the normal sexual arousal while nursing their babies are apt to feel guilty—so guilty that they may wean their babies early and refuse to nurse future children. In our society, sexual feelings are supposed to stay in their place—to come out of hiding only when a culturally determined suitable partner is present. Yet we are sexual beings, and our sexual feelings spin a thread that runs through the fabric of our entire lives.

Most women do not experience sexual sensations from breastfeeding; those who don't needn't feel that they are repressed or inhibited. They simply have a different, but just as normal, experience. In his landmark book, *Sexual Behavior in the Human Female,* Dr. Alfred C. Kinsey stated that only half of all women seem to derive any satisfaction from having their breasts fondled—and that both oral and manual stimulation of the female breasts are often more exciting to the man who touches than to the woman who is touched. A woman whose breasts are not normally erogenous is not likely to become erotically stimulated by the suckling of her infant. And even a woman whose breasts ordinarily respond to her partner's loving touch or kiss may find that during lactation, they become almost insensitive to touch—the partner's as well as the baby's. Kinsey's basic findings are still pertinent today.

Also, it's been said many times that the most powerful sex organ in the human body is the brain. Situations that we think about as sexual are more arousing than those that we don't imbue with sexual connotations. Thus, a woman may be concentrating so fully on feeding and interacting with her baby that she isn't even aware of physical sensations that in other circumstances might be very erotic.

In sum, there's no right or wrong way for you to respond sexually to the nursing experience. You can be a successful nursing mother if you do become erotically aroused by breastfeeding—or if such feelings are the farthest thing from your mind.

Birth Control

As a nursing mother, you're less likely to become pregnant than women who are not exclusively breastfeeding. Based on records in societies where long-term nursing is the rule, and on studies of exclusively nursing, partially nursing, and bottle-feeding mothers in this country, there's considerable evidence that breastfeeding postpones pregnancy. However, lactation is not a foolproof method of contraception, especially as your baby grows.

If your baby is being fully or almost fully nursed, that is, is receiving no supplemental bottles or solid food and is being breastfed at least two or three times during the night as well as every four hours or more often during the day, the hormonal balance in your body will very likely prevent ovulation and therefore pregnancy for three to six months, or even longer. This is because the increased levels of prolactin in your body during lactation delay the return of ovulation and of your menstrual periods.

If you're exclusively breastfeeding, you may have one sterile menstrual period before you begin to ovulate again. But you can't depend on it, plus you can't be certain whether it's sterile or not. Many women do ovulate before their first postpartum period, and women have become pregnant while fully lactating or before their periods have resumed. If you don't want to conceive right away, you'll want to use some form of contraception. Since there are so many choices, discuss the possibilities with your doctor.

What Kind of Contraception Should You Use?

The Lactational Amenorrhea Method (LAM): One of the most dramatic research findings in recent years has been the proven effectiveness of exclusive or nearly exclusive breastfeeding coupled with the absence of menstrual periods as a means of delaying pregnancy for up to six months. Even though folk wisdom and society-wide statistics have for many years attested that women were less likely to conceive while they were breastfeeding, only during the past couple of decades have scientific investigations confirmed this. LAM draws on these studies, which have been conducted in several different countries.

LAM is effective if you can answer yes to all of the following questions:

1. Are you still not menstruating, not even spotting?

2. Are you nursing your baby at least two to three times during the night and every four hours or more often during the day? Is he receiving breast milk exclusively—no formula or solid foods? Does he receive less than 10 percent of his feedings in the form of bottled breast milk? Is all his suckling done at the breast, instead of on pacifiers or thumbs?

3. Is your baby less than six months old?

If you meet *all* of these conditions, your chance of conceiving is less than 2 percent, a rate that compares very favorably with most forms of birth control. But when any one of these circumstances changes, it's time to begin an alternative method of family planning if you want to be sure of healthy spacing between pregnancies.

The big advantage of LAM is that, as an introductory method effective in the first few months after childbirth, it gives you some time to decide on the method of contraception you'll use on a regular basis. Meanwhile, your body isn't taking in any hormones and you don't have to buy any special paraphernalia. You're just relying on your own body's ability to prevent pregnancy.

When LAM No Longer Applies: When you no longer meet the above conditions, and don't want to conceive right away, you'll need to adopt another method of birth control. You'll have to weigh the pros and cons of each choice and decide upon the method that best suits your own physiology, personality, and lifestyle—as well as those of your partner.

When you wish to start another method, the best kind of contraceptive is the nonhormonal kind (see discussion of hormonal contraceptives on page 229 and comparison of birth control methods on pages 288–291). If you took birth control pills or used an IUD, patch, ring, or implant before getting pregnant, it may be hard to adjust to one of the preferred barrier methods (diaphragm, condom, and/or spermicide), because they're closely tied to the time of intercourse. While these methods may at first seem intrusive and a nuisance, many couples make inserting the diaphragm or putting on the condom a part of their sexual foreplay and consider doing it together an act of shared love and responsibility.

Contraception for the Nursing Mother

For each method, the first percentage number given is the effectiveness rate for the method as typically used. The second number represents the effectiveness rate when the method is used correctly and consistently (most couples don't use contraception correctly and consistently). The information here is accurate at the time of writing. Consult your doctor before you begin any form of contraception.

Recommended during Lactation

METHOD	COMMENTS
Lactational Amenorrhea Method (LAM)	Supports breastfeeding and baby health. Should begin right after birth. About 98 percent effective for up to six months, and maybe longer if woman continues to breastfeed often, day and night, and is still not menstruating. Requires frequent breastfeeding around the clock; not effective if mother and baby are regularly separated for more than four to six hours. Expressing or pumping milk instead of actually breastfeeding will not maintain the effectiveness of LAM.
Male condom	No effect on lactation or baby. About 85 to 98 percent effective; more effective when used with a spermicide. Can be used three weeks after delivery; before this time there's a risk of introducing bacteria into the partially healed uterus. Polyurethane condoms seem to allow more sensation during sex than latex condoms because they conduct heat well. Lubricated condoms help to make up for vaginal dryness caused by the mother's changed hormonal balance.
Diaphragm	No effect on lactation or baby. Wait six weeks after delivery to minimize discomfort, assure proper fit, and minimize the risk of infection. Woman needs to be fitted after each birth. About 84 to 94 percent effective. Used with spermicide, which provides lubrication. Must be inserted no more than six hours before intercourse and left in place for six hours afterward. May be irritating to nursing mother if her lower estrogen levels cause vaginal dryness, and may be dislodged in certain positions if vagina is relaxed after childbirth.
Female condom	No effect on lactation or baby. Can be used six weeks after delivery and inserted up to 8 hours before intercourse. About 80 to 95 percent effective.
Sponge	No effect on lactation or baby. Can be started six weeks after delivery. Insert before intercourse, protects for up to 24 hours. Leave in 6 to 30 hours, then discard. Has higher failure rates among women who have had a baby, even if inserted perfectly. About 68 to 80 percent effective.

Spermicide (foam, jelly, cream, film, tablet, or suppository)	No effect on lactation; virtually none transmitted through milk, and no reports of absorption or ill effects on baby. Can be begun three weeks after delivery. Must be applied within five to ten minutes before each act of intercourse. About 71 to 82 percent effective; may complement LAM, diaphragm, and condoms. Some people are allergic.
Copper intrauterine device (IUD), e.g. ParaGard	No effect on lactation or baby. Can be inserted immediately, within 48 hours of delivery, or four to six weeks afterward. About 99 percent effective. Nursing women report fewer complaints of pain, bleeding, and insertion problems than do other women. Problems of uterine perforation can be minimized by careful assessment of uterine size; uterus may be smaller during lactation.
Sterilization	If you're absolutely sure that you don't want more children, either you or your partner can choose surgical sterilization. Female sterilization (tubal ligation) can be performed at time of delivery or within 48 hours. Doing it right away is best for nursing mothers, since one study found that women sterilized four to six days postpartum produced less milk for as long as two weeks. Immediate sterilization has no effect on lactation. If not done within 48 hours, it should be delayed for four to six weeks. About 99 percent effective. Male sterilization (vasectomy) can be performed at any time and is about 99 percent effective by three months after surgery. Both should be considered irreversible.

Conditionally Recommended during Lactation

The World Health Organization (WHO) recommends that women delay using any of the following methods until at least six weeks after delivery, due to concern that newborns, whose liver and kidneys are still immature, may be negatively affected by hormones. In addition, by six weeks the vagina and perineal area are likely to be healed from the birth.

Minipill (progestin-only contraceptive pill)	No effect on lactation or baby reported in research literature, but some anecdotal reports from moms suggest that milk supply may be affected. Best to wait until six weeks after delivery. Should be taken same time every day. About 97 percent effective.
Intrauterine device (IUD) with levonorgestrel (LNG); e.g., Mirena	Female hormone, has no effect on lactation and may even increase milk volume. No effects reported on child growth and development. Contains progestin. About 99 percent effective.

Injectable progestin-only contraceptive (Depo-Provera, others)	May produce slight difference in milk composition (more protein, less fat). Steroid in breast milk can be transmitted to baby. No reported effect on children up to age ten. About 97 to 99 percent effective. May begin six weeks after delivery. Injection required every three months. Return of fertility delayed four to nine months after last dose. Cannot easily be reversed.
Progestin-only implant (Implanon)	Implanon is the only product available in the U.S. Can be used for three years. Nearly 100 percent effective.
Natural family planning (rhythm or fertility awareness method)	The various natural methods may require long periods of abstinence, but most have rules that can be applied during lactation. They are harder to use efficiently during breastfeeding, since they depend on regularity of periods, body temperature, and mucus patterns, all of which are irregular in nursing women and cannot predict ovulation. (For example, basal body temperature can't be measured unless a woman has at least six hours of uninterrupted sleep—a distant goal for most new moms.) However, the natural protection of nursing may compensate somewhat, and the use of these less effective methods remains a personal choice. For nonnursing women and their partners, effectiveness rates may exceed 90 percent when used perfectly; however, perfect use is difficult for many couples.
Coitus interruptus (withdrawal)	No effect on lactation or baby. Unreliable in preventing pregnancy since some leakage of semen often occurs before full orgasm. Usually sexually unfulfilling for both partners. About 73 to 95 percent effective.
NuvaRing	A flexible colorless ring made of a polymer, inserted once every four weeks (removed for one week). Contains estrogen and progestin (lower doses than other combined hormonal contraceptives). May diminish milk supply so should not be used until milk supply is fully established, or at least six weeks after delivery. About 92 to 99 percent effective. Cannot be used with diaphragm.

Emergency contraception pill (ECP, the "day-after" pill)	Use of birth control pills containing higher-than-usual doses of hormones, to be taken ideally within 72 hours after unprotected intercourse, is considered safe for lactating women. Using them once will probably not affect either the quantity or quality of breast milk. Although some hormones may be passed on through the milk, a nursing child is not likely to experience any adverse effects. If you meet the conditions for LAM, you might not need to use an ECP if you had sex that would otherwise put you at risk for getting pregnant. But if you're also feeding your baby formula or other food, your baby is more than six months old, or you have gotten your period since your baby was born, you could become pregnant. To limit your baby's exposure to hormones, discontinue nursing for at least 8 hours but no more than 24 hours after taking an ECP. Discard pumped milk.
Birth control pill with estrogen and progestin	There is some evidence that combined hormonal methods reduce amount of breast milk and may affect its composition. Steroids in breast milk may be passed on to baby; however, no long-term effects reported on children up to age 8; no effect on growth up to age 17. Should not be begun for at least six weeks after delivery, preferably not for six months, and ideally not at all while nursing. If used, should be taken at beginning of longest interval between feedings. Mother should offer extra suckling time and nurse more frequently to rebuild milk supply. About 93 to 99 percent effective.
Skin patch (Ortho Evra)	Contains combination of hormones estrogen and progestin, a synthetic form of progesterone used in many medications. Works similarly to the estrogen-and-progesterone combination pill, with comparable effects on baby and milk supply. Therefore should not be used before milk supply is fully established, at least six weeks after delivery. Women using this patch receive 60 percent more estrogen than from a typical combo birth control pill, with a higher risk of blood clots. About 92 to 99 percent effective.

Your Partner
Is Still Your Lover

Yes, this can be a trying time in the life of a marriage or other partnership. You may find, as you struggle in the morass of diapers and colic and nursing, that you would like to be a little girl again and have someone else care for both you and your baby. Meanwhile, your partner, who's awed by the competent way you feed, bathe, and diaper your baby, sees only your outer shell of self-assurance. You may seem so capable in carrying out your maternal responsibilities that he underestimates your need for him. He may feel left out of the tight little circle around you and your baby. (Besides making special efforts to invite your partner into the parenting picture, you may want to suggest that he or she read the next chapter, "Especially for Dad or Partner.")

At the same time, this new responsibility of caring for a baby often reawakens a new father's own dependency needs. One study found that expectant fathers' heightened needs for mothering showed up in an increased frequency of requests to their own parents for stories about their own birth and infancy.

Suppose that your baby is a few months old now, and your partner says, "You never want to make love anymore! How long is this going to last?" You may be agreeably surprised to find that once things get started, you find your own interest rising.

St. Louis sex therapist Beverly Hotchner uses a food analogy when one partner is more interested in sex than the other: "Let's assume that your partner is really enormously hungry and you're not hungry at all. Wouldn't you be willing to sit down and have a cup of coffee just to be sociable? Sometimes when you do this, the food starts to look pretty good and you take a little nibble and your saliva starts flowing, and suddenly you think, 'Hey, I think I'm going to have some.' You don't have to have a whole course—you can have just dessert.

"It's the same with sex. If you're tired and don't feel aroused, you can masturbate your partner or hold him tenderly while he masturbates. Or you can take a bath together, which is very sensual. What people really hunger for is affection and closeness and warmth and relaxing fun together. And they have thousands of ways to get that. They don't have to limit themselves to intercourse."

The birth of a first baby often signals a low point in a couple's sexual relationship. As one husband told us, "My wife and I had had a very good sex life, but when our two children were small, both the quality and the quantity of sex went way down. We were both tired most of the time, we couldn't be spontaneous, and we never felt as if we had any privacy. We thought we had been prepared for this—but we were prepared in our minds, not in our hearts—or elsewhere in our bodies. But we never gave up—and finally it got better." The key is never to give up.

Talk, Talk, Talk

It's often difficult to talk about both sex and feelings, but since neither of you can read the other's mind, you need to share your thoughts. You might schedule regular talking times—a couple of times a week to take a short walk together, or even 15 minutes at the end of every day—when you can tell each other how each of you feels about the change in your lives, how you feel about your own relationship, and what each of you would like from the other.

At this time, your partner needs your reassurance that he has not completely fallen off your priority list. While he recognizes intellectually that your baby requires a great deal of your time and energy, he may not be able to help resenting all the attention lavished on the newborn—attention that was formerly his alone. In addition, he sees you sharing with your baby not only your time, energy, attention, and affection, but also the breasts that were formerly revealed only to him. Is it any wonder that he might be a little jealous of the new baby?

Such feelings are natural, but many men are ashamed of feeling this way and won't admit them. Others express them quite openly. This is one of those times when clear communication is essential.

Meanwhile, you need to explore your own feelings. Are you sensing some conflict between your role as a mother and your role as a sexual partner? Think about the attitudes you grew up with—whether you had the sense that your mother enjoyed sex, whether you absorbed a feeling that once a woman became a mother, she wasn't sexy anymore, or that the changes in a woman's body in pregnancy and childbirth signal the end of her attractiveness. If you can talk about these feelings with your partner or with a friend—or both—you may find that you're more responsive to the idea of making love again.

It's most important for each of you to let the other know how you feel emotionally and physically. You might tell your partner how much you value the intimacy between you—but that right now you're often too tired to act on it. Let him know that your lack of interest in making love is not a lack of love for him. Suppose you love the back rubs he gives you—but he considers them a prelude to intercourse, which you're not always ready for. You need to tell him—in a loving way—how you feel. And you need to ask him what you can do to help him feel valued and loved.

You can show your partner in many ways that he's still very important to you and that your love for him has not diminished because of your love for his baby. It's hard to have to think of one more thing at a time when you're facing so many new demands, but it's important to make extra efforts to preserve and enhance your connection with your partner. You can adjust to being a mother without forgetting that you are still in a committed adult relationship. The suggestions in the next section might help you both over some rough spots.

Keeping Romance Center Stage

❖ Make at-home dates ahead of time with your partner. These are evenings when you take your phone off the hook or let your voice mail pick up, when you set aside time just for each other. You need this relaxed time together, whether you use it for talking, for a massage or hot bath, or for an evening of watching a special TV show or maybe an erotic DVD.

These evenings at home can, of course, be wonderful times for making love. While planning ahead for love-making may seem unromantic at first, it's worth noting that in our society marriage is the only structure that demands spontaneous sex. Dating couples know they have to plan ahead to see each other—and they usually find the planning itself erotic. Married couples can have an "affair" with each other, too.

❖ Phone, text, or e-mail each other during the day, or leave romantic notes where your partner will see them.

❖ Invite your partner to enjoy the sensuousness of parenting by bringing him into bed, bare-chested, while you're nursing the baby, and following feeding sessions with three-way cuddling, or by taking family baths together. This brings the father into the family circle and enables you as sensitive parents to transmit warmth and comfort to your baby.

❖ Be flexible. If before the baby arrived, you usually made love at bedtime, planning your day differently now may help you get together more happily. Some couples like to make love in the early morning after the baby's first nursing of the day. Some partners are able to get home for lunch while their babies conveniently take a nap.

One husband who had felt ignored because his wife was always asleep by the time he got into bed with her after the 11 o'clock news finally realized that he could get into bed with her at about 8:30, snuggle for a while, and make love. Then, after she went to sleep, he would get out of bed to watch the news.

❖ Even though you're nursing, you can still leave your baby for short periods of time. Once the course of breast-feeding has been established, many couples plan an evening out once a week so that they can enjoy each other's company in a more carefree way. This needn't be anything more elaborate than a walk or a movie or a trip to an ice cream shop—but can, if you're feeling extravagant, include a few hours at a local hotel.

It's best if you can plan to go out at a time when your baby usually sleeps, but if there is no "usually," you can nurse your baby just before you leave and then leave her with a competent sitter. Once your milk supply is well established (usually by the end of the second month), you should be able to be away from your baby during feeding time by leaving a bottle that contains your own milk, which you've either hand-expressed or pumped earlier in the day.

While you and your partner are renewing your relationship, your baby can be learning to trust people other than the two of you. As the anthropologist Margaret Mead told Sally Olds, babies are most likely to develop into well-adjusted human beings when they are cared for "by many warm, friendly people"—as long as most of these loved people remain in the infants' lives.

❖ You can minimize disruptions of the dinner hour by waiting to prepare dinner until right after a feeding. Then if you and your partner pitch in together, you might be able to cook and eat dinner before your baby needs you again. Or Dad may take over dinner preparations for a while, even if his "taking over" means getting take-out.

No matter how much of a gourmet you may have been before your baby's arrival, be prepared for drastic changes in your eating habits, at least for the first few months, when the baby's schedule is apt to be irregular. The best kind of meal for now is one that involves a minimum amount of preparation—a casserole that can be put together whenever one of you has the time, fish that can be broiled quickly, or a salad or stew that won't mind waiting. If you have access to good, nutritious take-out food and can afford the extra expense (along with paper plates), this is the time to splurge.

❖ The simplest meal can take on a romantic aura if you eat by candlelight on your good china (which is no harder to wash than everyday ware).

❖ If you're used to having an occasional drink before or with dinner with your partner, you don't need to give it up entirely. It's probably best to time your cocktail hour to come soon after a feeding. You can enjoy a quiet interlude for the two of you over an occasional glass of wine while you're catching up with each other on the events of your days. (See Chapter 10 for suggestions about alcohol consumption.)

❖ If your baby sleeps in the same bed with you, you need to show a little ingenuity. Bed isn't the only place to make love. Why else was the rug in front of the fireplace invented? Or you might slip quietly out to a guest bed, a living room couch, or any other welcoming surface while your baby sleeps.

One couple whose two-year-old daughter continued to fall asleep in their bed every night would wait until she was sleeping and then tiptoe out and make love in another room. They would sometimes put on music before their daughter went to sleep and let it continue to play to drown out any sounds they might make. In these child-rearing years some parents who work hard at finding the time and the place to make love get an added excitement from the illicit feeling that reminds them of their teenage years, when they would make out beyond their parents' sight.

❖ Pay attention to yourself. Your baby will think you're beautiful no matter what, but you'll feel better about yourself and show your partner that you care about his opinion if you can do a little grooming shortly before you expect him home. You might expend the energy to run a comb through your hair and put on a shirt that doesn't carry that unmistakable perfume of spit-up milk.

If you're ordinarily small-breasted, you might enjoy dressing seductively during the time you're nursing, when you've got more cleavage than you've ever had before. If you're less thrilled about your added pounds and curves, you'll feel and look more attractive if you buy one or two flattering outfits to fit your current figure (see Chapter 9).

❖ If you're eager to resume sexual relations, don't be shy about letting your partner know. He may be waiting for a signal from you. If you couldn't care less, you may want to give it a try out of love for him. Reaching orgasm is often less important than the physical closeness of sex. While women more often seem to be comforted by being held lovingly, men tend to find genitally oriented sexual activity comforting and life-enhancing.

One of the most important things you can do for your partner—and your children—is to make him feel part of the family circle as early as possible. This decision can help your children forge a close relationship with both parents and can help them feel good about themselves throughout their lives. If your partner is interested in doing things for his baby, don't limit him to fetching and carrying. And don't criticize the way he does things—what difference does it make if he puts a shirt on backward? Encourage him to hold, play with, and bathe the baby.

Remember: You're not the only person who can do the right thing for your child. Also remember: The stronger your child bonds with both her parents, the better off she will be. However, if your partner is not terribly interested in doing a great deal with your young infant, it's better not to push him but to wait for his attitude to change—as it probably will the first time the baby smiles at him.

If you're with a person you love, you are lucky, indeed. You have the opportunity to give of yourself and to be physically close to your baby—and to your partner. You have fulfilled your birthright—that cycle of sexuality that only a woman can know.

CHAPTER FOURTEEN

Especially for Dad or Partner

*"Having children made me realize what
breasts are really for and in my eyes it made them
that much more beautiful."*

DAVID R. MARKS, MD Weston, Connecticut

W hy, you may wonder, should we have a chapter for spouses and partners in a book about breastfeeding? The answer is easy: Because you, as a father, are a vital part of the nursing experience; because it will enrich your life as well as those of your wife and baby; and because your support and help are needed as much now as they will ever be in your family's life. (If you're not married to the mother of your baby, you can just mentally substitute the word *partner* wherever we have written *wife*.) As a father, you're in the unique position of providing a source of strength and balance for your entire family—and to grow through the challenges and opportunities your new role as father affords you.

As a new father, you have embarked upon a new adventure. Like most adventures, it will have its times of exhilaration—and its times of anxiety. Both are normal.

Throughout history most men have yearned to father children and have taken their parenting seriously. Today, however, men in our society seem to have an even deeper involvement in bringing up their children than many did in times past. Our new society-wide appreciation of the father's role in his children's lives acknowledges that his participation in their care is at least as important as his traditional responsibility as family breadwinner—or even more so, especially when Mom shares breadwinning.

There are some interesting signs of this new appreciation. In public places, we see men out alone with their small children. In baby supply stores, we see strollers with longer handles and diaper bags with fewer frills. In television commercials, we see fathers diapering and bathing their children. In airports, we see diapering tables in the men's restroom. This newfound appreciation for fathering is bound to enrich the lives of these men, as well as those of their families.

Breastfeeding's Benefits for You, the Father

As the father of a breastfed child, you can appreciate the advantages that nursing confers on both your baby and your wife (described in Chapter 1). You can also find benefits for yourself, such as the following:

❖ You don't have to worry about running out of formula at an inconvenient time and dashing around trying to find an open store.

❖ Breastfeeding costs less than formula-feeding.

❖ When you go places with your baby, you have less to lug—no bottles or cans of formula, no sterilizing equipment. Since the father is usually the one who carries all the paraphernalia required by a new baby, you'll appreciate this lightening of your load when you go on vacation, visiting, or on family errands.

❖ Changing your baby's diapers is much pleasanter, since the bowel movements of a breastfed baby have a much milder smell than those of a formula-fed baby.

❖ You can get to know and appreciate a new aspect of your wife's womanliness and a new dimension of the parent-child bond.

Becoming a Father

Before a baby is born, we have a warm fuzzy feeling about the delights of parenthood. And yes, parenthood is wonderful and no one who has never been a parent can truly appreciate that special depth of feeling you can have for a child.

But being the father of a new baby is not unalloyed bliss. There will be mornings when your adorable baby will not look at all adorable to your bleary-eyed gaze, after you have been up with him all night. The very helplessness of an infant means that your wife will need to be more attuned to your baby's needs than yours. But even though you know intellectually that you are an adult who can wait for gratification, while your baby cannot, you may not feel so adult emotionally.

Listen to what one new father has said about what he calls, with some embarrassment, spousling rivalry: "I feel like a big baby, jealous of my own son. I love the baby, sure, but I miss having a wife who cares about me. She goes on and on about him, which I can understand, but occasionally it would be nice if I got the feeling that she cared how I am."

Most new fathers are apt to feel somewhat shut out of the family circle, no matter how their babies are fed. Some men can accept these feelings more easily than others—but virtually every new father has them to some degree. You're not abnormal; you're not a selfish brute; you're not immature for

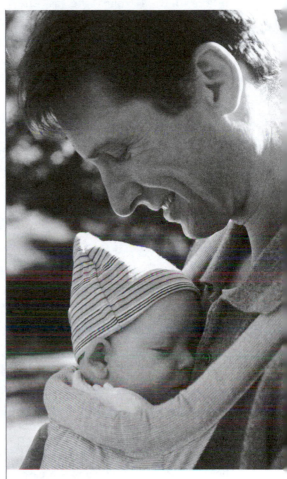

The father who spends time with and cares for his baby develops a very special attachment that will enrich both their lives.

experiencing twinges of jealousy and hurt after the birth of your baby.

Remember that this is a time of transition. Your familiar household routines are completely disrupted. You and your wife have to learn how to carry out your roles as parents. You have to take into account the needs and wants of a very noisy addition to your family. You have new responsibilities toward your wife as she recuperates from the physical demands of pregnancy and childbirth and copes with the hormonal changes accompanying these events. You may feel sexually frustrated, since lovemaking has already taken a hiatus for a while, and even when it resumes it will probably take some time to get back to the sex life you enjoyed previously. Your older children are especially needy now. Your social life is disrupted, and you may worry that you'll never again have the freedom and the fun you and your wife used to have together. In addition, you have new financial strains, especially if your wife had been making a substantial contribution to the family income and is now taking an extended maternity leave. You not only have to cut back to living on one income, you have all the added expenses brought by the baby.

But you need to remember that these early days hold excitement and thrills, as well as concerns, and that you and your wife have embarked on an inspiring adventure. The more involved you get, the more gratifying it will be.

The Father's Importance in the Family

A common refrain of many happy breastfeeding mothers is: "I couldn't have done it without my husband's help." While some expectant fathers are afraid they'll feel like a fifth wheel in the family after a baby is born—especially if the baby is breastfed—the reality is far different. You are needed.

Your emotional support and encouragement are even more important to your breastfeeding partner than they would be if she had chosen to bottle-feed. This is because a woman's ability to give milk is so strongly influenced by her emotional state. If she's feeling your love and support, her let-down reflex is more likely to function well. As a result, your baby feels satisfied, your wife feels gratified, and you can bask in both of their happy states of mind and body.

You have a vital role to play in the lives of your wife, your new baby, and your other children. A strong, supportive, helpful partner can often make the difference between breastfeeding success and failure and between family harmony and discord. Let's talk about the different ways—both emotional and practical—by which you can show this support.

Encouraging Your Partner to Breastfeed

Your opinions on breastfeeding are important to your wife, and your encouragement is vital to her success in this endeavor. Study after study has found that a father's favorable attitude toward breastfeeding is the most important factor in a mother's decision to nurse. You're more important in this regard than a doctor, a nurse, or a lactation consultant.

Before you can encourage your wife to breastfeed your child, however, you have to be convinced of the value of nursing for both mother and baby. You may have some worries about your wife's becoming a nursing mother— worries that you can allay by learning more. You'll want to read Chapter 1 in this book, which discusses the benefits of breastfeeding for both mother and baby; Chapter 2, which addresses such common concerns as a woman's fears of losing her figure and of being tied down; and Chapter 13, which talks about a nursing woman's sexuality. You may also want to browse in some of the other chapters in this book, like those that consider the social and work lives of the breastfeeding mother.

A major reason to support your wife's decision to breastfeed is because you want to do everything you can for her well-being. The longer a woman breastfeeds, the more she is protected from various conditions, including breast cancer at any age and hip fractures (an all too common consequence of osteoporosis) in later life.

If your baby has not yet arrived, you can learn a great deal about breastfeeding and other issues related to the arrival of your baby by attending prenatal classes for expectant parents. Even if you're not going to be in the delivery room, it will still help you to learn about childbirth ahead of time. Prenatal courses usually discuss breastfeeding and the postpartum period, as well. Another advantage to enrolling in one of these classes is the chance to see that you're not alone, that other men share your concerns and possible confusion.

After your baby is on the scene, you might enjoy attending a special meeting for fathers held by a local chapter of an organization such as the International Childbirth Education Association, La Leche League, Boot Camp for New Dads (see page 302), or by your pediatrician, where you can ask your questions and receive authoritative answers. Or you may want to take your questions to your wife's doctor or midwife, to your parents, to your brother or sister, or perhaps to a friend whose own wife breastfed her children.

Being Your Wife's Strongest Ally

Even today, when most people accept— or at least give lip service to—the benefits of breastfeeding, your wife may encounter discouragement from relatives, neighbors, her employer, or even her doctor. If you wholeheartedly support her desire to breastfeed, she will be better able to handle any outside opposition.

You can support your wife most effectively if you're really convinced that breastfeeding is best for baby and mother. But even if you aren't 100 percent convinced, you can appreciate the fact that she is and you can show

Boot Camp for New Dads

In 1990, Greg Bishop, a father of four in California, started a workshop to help expectant and new fathers develop skills and confidence so they could connect with their children in a meaningful way right from the start. Fathers of two- to four-month-old babies join fathers-to-be in the classes, and the man-to-man orientation (no women over two feet tall allowed!) helps men feel comfortable asking questions and getting answers. Since then, Boot Camps for New Dads have been held all over the United States and are now expanding internationally. More than 300 fathers coach workshops in 42 states, in hospitals, churches, synagogues, and Head Start programs and on military bases, and more than 200,000 men have graduated from the programs. To find a nearby workshop, go to www.bcnd.org and click on "Locations" in the left-hand column.

Meanwhile, you can get a good start with information from the organization's free magazine, *Dads Adventure,* which is distributed through doctors' offices and childbirth education classes, and can also be downloaded from www.dadsadventure.com. Also on the website is a resource guide organized by subject, which refers fathers to helpful organizations and books. Dads Adventure has also published two books for fathers: *Hit the Ground Crawling: Lessons from 150,000 New Fathers* (which has information on how dads can help breastfeeding moms) and *Crash Course for New Dads: Tools, Checklists & Cheat-Sheets,* a workbook with lists, charts, and tear-out tools. Both these books are oriented more toward expectant fathers, but also have good information for new dads. Royalties from the books support the nonprofit Boot Camp for New Dads.

your love by helping her as much as possible. What can you do?

❖ Let her know that you're happy with her choice.

❖ Let everyone else know that you stand behind her decision.

❖ Speak to the doctors—your wife's and your baby's—to tell them you'll help her in any way you can.

❖ Arrange to take one or two weeks off from work after your baby's birth, so that you can be on hand to help your wife and bond with your baby.

❖ Answer the phone and doorbell to let your wife rest or breastfeed without distraction.

❖ Fix her a snack or bring her a drink while she's nursing.

❖ Speak to well-meaning friends and relatives who may be showing their disapproval of breastfeeding or doubting your wife's ability to nurse. Be her buffer and defend her against their subtle (and not-so-subtle) disparaging remarks. If you make it plain that she is not to be discouraged from nursing, people will probably take their cues from your attitude and will keep any negative opinions to themselves.

❖ Agree with the new mom on a secret sign that means it's time for guests to go. Or say something like, "Sara is looking pretty tired. Excuse me for a minute while I get her and the baby settled in the bedroom."

❖ Remember that your wife is probably busier and more wrapped up in her daily schedule (especially if this is her first baby) than she ever has been before and ever will be again; that the hectic pace of these first few weeks does abate; and that with a little time, she'll become calmer and less anxious about her new responsibilities.

❖ In a good relationship, you need to feel free to express your worries as well as your joys, your anger as well as your happiness. But because of the effect the emotions have on the course of breastfeeding, if you can put off giving voice to your more negative feelings at least for the first few weeks after your baby's birth, you'll be giving a great gift to your baby, as well as to your wife. Try to understand why she may be more irritable than usual, why she forgets to do things, and why she sometimes seems distracted when you're talking to her.

As important as your role is in your baby's nursing, don't stifle all your feelings. But do try to deal with them in as adult a way as possible so you can spare the new mom, at least in the first few weeks after your baby's birth, as much emotional upset as possible. The calmer and more relaxed a woman is, the better able she is to produce and give milk.

In the especially sensitive early days after childbirth, a woman flourishes from being lovingly cared for. Even the simplest gestures—like bringing her a glass of juice while she's nursing, tucking a pillow behind her back, bringing home a small gift, or offering to go to the store—can go far to make her feel appreciated and to alleviate the down-in-the-dumps feeling that often follows childbirth.

Learning How to Cope

What do other fathers do? How do they deal with the challenges of parenting the breastfed baby, supporting the breastfeeding mother, and meeting their own needs as well? According to one study, fathers of happily breastfed babies developed five coping techniques:

1. They were realistic about the sometimes inconvenient ways breastfeeding affected their lives as well as their wives'.

2. They accepted the situation, often by reminding themselves that breastfeeding was best for their children, and that it would not last forever.

3. They focused on the benefits breastfeeding held for them—like not having to get up at night. (Many a father whose baby did not sleep in the family bed did get up to bring the baby to his wife, but then he'd roll over and go back to sleep until it was time to take the baby back to her own bed.)

4. They did other things for their babies—bathed them, diapered them, held them, walked with them, put them to sleep.

5. By playing an active role in their children's lives, both during the nursing days and after weaning, they forged close attachments with their children that were comparable to the bonds their wives and children shared.

Your Baby's Mother Is Still Your Lover

One of the most important ways you can boost your wife's morale is to keep showing your interest in her as a woman. You have a relationship that includes more than shared parenthood. She needs to know that you still consider her interesting and attractive, that you still value her opinions, and that you still share interests besides the baby.

As we point out in Chapter 13, some women find that the sensuality of lactation makes them more interested in sex, while others find this a time of diminished sexual interest. Even if your wife is in the latter group and isn't interested in resuming sexual relations as soon as you are (which is no reflection of her feelings for you), she still needs to be reassured of your love. This reassurance can take such physical forms as cuddling and kissing even when it doesn't include sexual intercourse.

One study of 194 couples found that the first sexual experience after childbirth was considered satisfying by more than two-thirds of the new fathers, but by fewer than half of the mothers. Pain and fatigue are major factors in many new mothers' more negative experience of sex.

Another major factor in the less satisfying sexual experiences of some women is their feeling about their own attractiveness. Women who don't like the way they look—because they're heavier than usual, because they have stretch marks, or because they feel top-heavy—don't feel like desirable sexual partners. As a result, they may withdraw from sex.

It's clear, then, that there are things you can do with regard to all these factors. In Chapter 13, we talked about ways to lessen the discomfort of renewed sexual activity. It's important to realize that for some women, sex after childbirth causes pain, and to be patient as well as flexible in your sexual techniques.

One happily married father of adolescents recalls the period just after their births as a time of "less sex and lower-quality sex." His advice to other men: "After childbirth and breastfeeding, you go back to square zero. You're almost starting out all over again. You don't know how you and your wife will relate to each other. You don't know what you'll be doing in bed. You may not do some things you used to do, but you may be doing some new things. And then the hardest thing: Try not to be anxious. And when you are anxious, just accept your anxiety as something you'll both get beyond. Just relax and concentrate on having pleasure."

You can help your wife feel better about her desirability by letting her know that you like the way she looks. If you can value her curviness throughout pregnancy and new motherhood as signs of her fertility and her ability to nurture, you'll be helping her to accept herself, too. One way to show her that you think she's beautiful is to tell her so; another is to take photographs of her, especially while she's nursing the baby. Other ways are to surprise her with an occasional appearance-related gift, such as a piece of jewelry or a pretty item of clothing she can wear right now. You might even go shopping

together, enjoying the outing as well as the gift.

Of course, as always, it's important to talk. Sharing thoughts and feelings is the cornerstone of a close relationship, and the timing and manner in which you talk to each other go far in determining the quality of your communication.

As Susan, a mother of three small children, told us, "We didn't do a lot of talking, of sharing our gut feelings until this past year. I never said to Bill right after our first child was born, 'I really love you, but I need some space now for me.'" Her husband added, "And I never said anything to her about how deprived and left out I was feeling. What we did do was fight. I found a lot to criticize in Susan—the house was a mess; the kids were dirty; I didn't have any clean socks."

Now, after they've begun talking more, Susan says, "Now I realize that it wasn't the socks—it was the sex. Or rather, the lack of it. Now I can let the house go, and I don't get those complaints. In fact, he pitches in and does more himself. As hard as it is, we manage to find time and energy for each other—for talking and for sex."

Rolling Up Your Sleeves

While the kind of emotional support we've just been talking about can be enormously helpful to your wife, she's sure to appreciate more practical kinds of help, too. Fortunately, these days there's much

less distinction between work that's appropriate for either sex.

Every woman benefits from as much rest as she can get after giving birth. Her body has to recover its strength, even while her sleep is

How a "Breastfeeding" Father Can Nurture a Baby

❖ Change diapers, either before or after a feeding, or during the mid-feeding break.

❖ Take your baby out of the crib at any time of the day or night to carry her to her mother for feedings.

❖ "Wear" your baby (see page 149). Walk around with your baby, carrying her in a baby carrier to feel her soft warmth next to you and to let her enjoy your presence.

❖ Give your baby a soothing massage (see the Resource Appendix to find instructors).

❖ Work through some baby exercises.

❖ Rock or walk your baby when she's unhappy, or soothe her some other way (as suggested in the box on page 152).

❖ Enjoy a fun-filled parenting activity for anyone who likes to play in water: Give your baby a bath.

❖ In a warm room or under a blanket, hold your baby, clad only in a diaper, against your bare chest, where she can hear your heartbeat and feel your warm (and maybe fuzzy) skin. Your baby can hear your heartbeat louder than she can Mom's, since men have a thinner fat layer to muffle sound. You can bond through that wonderful skin-to-skin contact, and you can give your baby a different tactile experience from the one she has with her mother.

❖ Hold and stroke your baby and show how gentle and loving your touch can be.

❖ Lie down on the floor and let your (older) baby crawl over you. You'll be getting rest while you're close to your baby.

❖ Do the "daddy neck nuzzle": Skin to skin, place your baby against your chest with her head under your chin. Cover both of you if the room is cool. Talk, hum, or sing so your baby can feel your vocal cords vibrating against her scalp.

❖ Sing or talk to her even when you're not snuggling—she could be in her high chair, stroller, or in Mom's arms, but she'll love hearing your voice.

With these last two activities, you'll not only be establishing a relationship—you'll also be furthering language development, an important contribution to your child's cognitive growth.

---

constantly being disturbed. Although a tired, run-down nursing mother can still produce milk, the effort will take its toll on her own health and on the quality of care she can give to her baby and to the rest of her family. The more rest she gets, the better off everyone in the family (including you) will be.

One of the most important things you can do as the father of a breastfed baby is to be available to your wife and baby in the crucial early days after your baby's birth. The success of breast-feeding often hinges on what happens in the first week or two.

A valuable gift for your wife is helping her get the rest she needs at night. This helps you become closer to your baby, too. When he awakens during the night, you become the one on call. If your baby is sleeping in a separate bed, you become the one who gets up out of bed, gets the baby, brings him to your wife, and helps her get into a comfortable nursing position. After the feeding, you diaper the baby, if necessary, and put him back to bed. Or you can welcome your baby into your bed (for suggestions for safe co-sleeping and bed-sharing, see Chapter 7); he will cry less often and wake you less often, since his mother will be able to nurse him at his first stirrings.

By being on night duty this way, you'll be helping your wife to conserve her energy so that she'll be better able to breastfeed—and better able to get through the day. There's no way to overestimate the psychological as well as the practical benefits of this help.

Another way to help the new mother conserve her energy is to hire someone to come in to help with the housework for a while if your budget permits. Your investment will pay off in everyone's good spirits and in the time both you and your mate can devote to each other. If this is out of the question, pitch in yourself. You can shop, cook, vacuum, do laundry, bring home take-out food, and take care of the baby and any older children.

One father told us, "The more I do in the house, the better our relationship gets—especially our sex life. My wife isn't so tired, she feels good about herself, and she feels good about me. Besides, it's satisfying to know that I can do things I'd never done before, like whip up a pretty good meal."

You Can Be a Complete Father

One common worry among partners of women who plan to breastfeed is that they won't be able to care for the baby. While this fear is very real to men who want to be actively involved in their babies' lives, it has to bring a smile to the face of any experienced parent. There's so much more to taking care of new infants besides feeding them! Babies look to Dad to fulfill different needs.

You and Your Baby

If you want to be close to your baby, you can be. Just because your baby's mother went through nine months of pregnancy, bore your child, and is now nursing, this doesn't mean that she's the only person who can care for your baby. You can be just as tender with your baby as any woman might be—with no loss to your masculinity.

Many men are finding the nurturing sides of themselves and are forging close attachments with their children, right from infancy.

What can you do to become close to your baby? A lot, as shown in the box on page 306.

You'll want to have time alone with your baby. This isn't babysitting, which by definition involves taking care of someone else's baby. This is parenting. This is taking care of your own child. This is an activity that knows no gender limitations.

You can do your one-on-one parenting between feedings at first, giving your wife a chance to rest or go out while you and your baby enjoy each other's company. Or you can take the baby out in carrier or carriage. As Mom's milk supply becomes well enough established to miss an occasional feeding (after the first several weeks), you may be giving your baby an occasional bottle or cup, either of expressed breast milk or of formula. For tips on bottle- and cup-feeding, see Chapter 12.

At home with your family, you can take off that protective shell you may wear all day at work. You can free yourself to express those warm, tender emotions that are yours to give. A man who can freely give and take loving feelings can know completion as a human being.

You and Your Older Children

If you have older children, one of the most meaningful things you can do for them, for your partner, and for yourself is to lavish extra time and attention on them after your wife comes home with the new baby. If you as an adult feel pushed to one side, imagine how they feel.

Plan outings with them so they can have your undivided attention. Offer special treats to show them how important they are to you. The extra time you spend with your older children will mean as much to your wife as to the children themselves, since her mind will be more at ease, knowing that they're happy while she's taking care of the new baby. They'll also provide extra benefits to you as you get to know your children better and reap more of the rewards of parenthood.

As David Stewart, PhD, has written in his wise little pamphlet *Fathering and Career: A Healthy Balance,* "Careers are fickle, but parenthood is forever." As this father points out, while many things in life can wait, the growth of a child is not one of them. "To enjoy a two-year-old," he says, "you must do it when he or she is two."

You can create extra time for your children by waking up earlier or by setting aside time when you come home in the evening. In some families, fathers enjoy taking over the bathtime and bedtime routines, and these become their special times with their children.

If possible, declare a temporary moratorium on overtime, travel, and weekend work. It's a question of priorities: If you consider time with your children a necessity, you'll find time for it. And you'll use this time to build precious memories and powerful bonds.

Getting Support for Yourself

t sounds as if a great deal is being asked of you at this time. You're right. That's why you'll benefit from having someone that you can turn to for comfort. New fathers need special helpers, too—caregivers who, as described in Chapter 4, can offer friendship, reassurance, and both practical and emotional support.

At a time when you have to be more giving to both your wife and your baby, you may feel like being taken care of yourself. Both you and your wife are likely to have mixed-up feelings, and each of you needs a lot of moral and practical support.

Many men consider their wives their best friends. This may work at most times in their lives, but when they have an issue they can't talk to their wives about, these men have no one to go to. Often, men are unable to talk to another man about their most deeply felt feelings for fear of appearing vulnerable. Yet sharing ourselves, including the selves we usually don't show to the outside world, is often a bridge to intimacy with another person, who can then share something of himself.

This may be an ideal time in your life to seek out a man you feel you can trust (if you don't already have such a friend in your life). Your father, brother, brother-in-law, or clergyman may be good candidates. Or you might approach a coworker or tennis partner with whom you're friendly. You'll probably get the best kind of understanding and possibly even practical advice from someone who's already been through this stage in his life, but if you can't find someone like that, you can at least find someone who can lend a sympathetic ear and just listen.

In one recent study of hundreds of expectant fathers, every man interviewed said that the researcher was the first person to ask about the father's experience and stick around to listen to his response! Often, other people don't know how to talk to an expectant or new father and instead ask only how the mother and baby are doing. You can take an active role in training a few close friends and relatives to talk to you about your feelings and the changes in your life.

The role of fathers in their babies' lives has become a research interest for contemporary psychologists. They have found that attachments and close ties form between fathers and their children during the first year of the children's lives and that the fathers then go on to exert a strong influence over all aspects of their offspring's development. Anyone who plays a large part in a baby's day-to-day life will have an important influence on that life. After the birth of your baby, you can justifiably feel proud of the major contribution you're making to the lives of your wife and your children.

CHAPTER FIFTEEN

Preventing and Treating Nursing-Related Problems

"I nursed my first two daughters with no problem. But then, when my third daughter wasn't gaining weight fast enough, I worked with several very patient and gentle lactation consultants and pumped for 2½ weeks until I finally got my baby back to the breast. I'm so glad we managed to push through."

KIM Weston, Connecticut

You may not encounter problems while breastfeeding your baby, but if you should run into any, this chapter can help you resolve a number of possible situations. If your questions are not answered here, call your doctor, nurse, midwife, childbirth educator, lactation consultant, or local La Leche League leader.

If you ran into a breastfeeding problem with a previous baby, don't assume that it will occur again. Breastfeeding history does not necessarily repeat itself. Each nursing situation is unique, and now that you're more experienced, breastfeeding is likely to go more smoothly. On the other hand, this is a different baby, and each baby brings his own personality, habits, and feeding patterns to the table (make that "to the breast"), sometimes with problems as a result. Don't blame yourself or your baby if something doesn't seem right. Just look at the situation as it is and see what you can do about it.

When you come across the lists of suggestions in this chapter, remember that you don't need to follow every suggestion listed to resolve a particular problem. Try one or two ideas and see what happens. If the situation doesn't improve very soon, try one of the other ideas. If nothing works within a couple of days, call a practitioner. It's important to treat problems promptly so they don't become worse. This chapter represents the most current thinking about the issues covered here, but your practitioner may advise you to do something differently. If that happens and you agree, fine. But suppose you don't agree?

Disagreement with Your Doctor

Suppose the physician taking care of you or your baby gives you advice that contradicts other information you've received. You may be advised to stop or suspend nursing, you may be told to feed your baby formula or solid foods when you want to offer only breast milk, or you may be told to nurse your baby less frequently than you think necessary. What do you do?

First, find out why the doctor is giving you this advice—is it a consequence of a specific problem that has arisen with either you or your baby?

✤ Are you having a problem, perhaps with painful or infected breasts or nipples?

✤ Is your baby jaundiced?

✤ Is your baby not gaining weight at the rate the doctor feels is appropriate?

In this chapter, we discuss some of these and other problems that may give rise to conflicting advice, and we present the most current remedies for them. Some of these solutions may be at odds with the advice you're receiving. Because each case is unique, however, your own physician is in the best position to evaluate your situation and make recommendations. If your baby is sick or not thriving or has any special problem, it can be dangerous to disregard medical advice. If you don't have confidence in what your doctor says, find another competent doctor and get a second opinion (see Chapter 4).

But if your baby is healthy and you're well informed, discuss your differences with your doctor. Some doctors routinely recommend supplemental bottles of formula, early weaning, or early feeding of solids for all their patients, either because of long-established practice or because of their own opinions about desirable lifestyles, which may be different from yours. You need to separate medical advice from personal opinion, and talking with your doctor may help you clarify the difference.

One mother approaches such situations by saying, "I'm not comfortable with that. Can you suggest something else?" Another has found this way effective: "I use the words *I feel* when I disagree with my doctor. If you *think* or *insist,* he won't like it. But if you *feel* you would like to do or not do something, this is a gentle way to open the discussion, because nobody wants to step on your feelings."

Another mother who ran into a disagreement with her doctor over breastfeeding her jaundiced baby showed him professional literature supporting her position and said, "I don't know whether you saw this recent research recommending that mothers of jaundiced babies continue to nurse them. Can you read this and tell me what you think of it?" Still another mother, who bolstered her argument with her knowledge about breastfeeding, found that her doctor was won over not only by the information she presented, but by her strong commitment to nursing her baby.

You might also want to check with La Leche League to see whether the league or any members of its Health Advisory Council have published materials on the topic or can suggest other sources to consult.

How you approach this situation depends on your personality and your sense of your doctor, as well as the specific issue under discussion.

Engorgement (Hard, Swollen Breasts)

Your breasts will normally become larger, heavier, and somewhat tender about two to five days after childbirth. The combination of the swelling of the tissues, the increased circulation of blood in the breasts, and the pressure of the newly produced milk can sometimes make them feel hard, tight, and uncomfortable. The skin on your breasts may be shiny and your nipples flat or distended; these are signs of engorgement. Although this is common for the first few days, it is not inevitable and can usually be avoided.

The best way to relieve, minimize, or even prevent engorgement is to nurse your baby as soon after birth as possible and very often from then on. Instead of waiting for your baby to cry, which is a late sign of hunger, feed her whenever

Ways to Relieve Engorgement

The most important and effective way to relieve engorgement is to remove as much milk as possible from both breasts, as frequently as possible, either by nursing your baby often or by using a good breast pump. Some of the following remedies may help.

❖ Feed your baby frequently, 8 to 12 times in a 24-hour period in the first few days after birth, even if you have to wake him to nurse.

❖ Express or pump a little bit of milk just before feedings to soften your breasts and make the nipple easier for your baby to latch on to.

❖ The technique of reverse pressure softening—using gentle pressure to relieve some of the congestion in the breasts—is sometimes helpful in the first two weeks postpartum. Ask your lactation specialist to teach you how to do this.

❖ If your breasts are severely engorged, massage them once or twice a day before feeding, starting gently at the outer edges with your fingertips and going toward the nipple area. A mild cream may make the process easier, but don't get any on the areola, because that would make it harder for you to express milk. It may help to do the massage in the shower.

❖ Apply warm, moist compresses about 10 or 15 minutes before a feeding (and before a massage). Between feedings, apply cold compresses. The warm compresses aid the let-down reflex, and the cold packs relieve swelling and pain. Apply cold using an ice pack, a bag of frozen vegetables, or a blue freezer pack wrapped in a thin towel. Apply heat using a moist-heating pad, a small hot-water bottle wrapped in a towel, a towel soaked in hot water, or in a hot shower. If you use a heating pad, be very careful not to burn your skin.

❖ Wear a firm bra for support. Be sure it's not too tight, since this can make you more uncomfortable and also cause other problems. If you use breast shields (see top of next page), wear a bra that has enough room to insert the shields. Try taking off your bra while you're nursing, to be sure it's not constricting your milk ducts.

❖ Apply fresh cabbage leaves to your breasts. This simple home remedy seems to help some women. Pull two outer leaves from an ordinary head of cabbage and strip out the large vein in each leaf. Then cut holes for your nipples and wash the leaves to get rid of any chemical residue. Chill them for about ten minutes if you want to. Then wrap the leaves around the irritated areas of your breasts. They're convenient, cheap, safe, and disposable, and some women report that they relieve pain. You might try it if you don't mind staining your bra—and smelling like dinner.

continued on next page

continued from previous page

❖ Wear a silicone breast shield (also known as a milk cup, breast shell, or Woolwich shield) inside your bra for 30 minutes before feedings to soften your areola and bring out your nipple.

❖ If you cannot breastfeed right after childbirth, express or pump your milk until you'll be able to nurse your baby. An electric pump is easiest and most efficient (see Chapter 11).

❖ Take a pain reliever—either one of the over-the-counter agents listed in the box on page 224, or something your doctor can prescribe that will not affect your baby or your milk.

❖ If only one breast is engorged because your baby is consistently refusing to suckle from it, it may be a sign of a possibly serious medical problem (see page 115). To rule this out, see your obstetrician.

she shows such early signs as sucking her fist, making sucking motions with her mouth, moving around, looking more alert, and so forth. Women whose babies nurse vigorously and frequently right from the start rarely suffer from engorgement. If you should become engorged, the procedures listed in the box on page 313 and above should bring relief in a couple of days.

When the engorgement goes away—and it will—be assured that you still have plenty of milk. Once your milk supply is well established, your breasts become softer and stay that way most of the time.

Sudden Weaning

If you have to wean your baby abruptly, you run a high risk of engorgement. In this situation, your approach will be different from the procedures given in the box on page 313 and above, which you would follow if you were continuing to nurse. For suggestions on relieving the discomfort of abrupt weaning, see Chapter 17.

Sore Nipples

Many women experience a pulling sensation and a mild, temporary tenderness in the first few days after giving birth, and sometimes through the first week or two. If you're not in real pain and if your discomfort is relieved when your milk comes in and lets down for your baby, you don't need to do anything special. This initial tenderness usually goes away in a few days as your milk begins to let down. But if your nipples look red and chapped or cracked or if you feel severe pain during or after nursing, call your doctor or lactation consultant right away. Don't wait until the pain becomes unbearable, because that will make the problem much harder to clear up. Martyrs are not happy breastfeeders!

It's important for several reasons—aside from removing the "ouch" factor and making breastfeeding a happier experience—to resolve nipple problems early. A major medical reason lies in the fact that any break in the skin makes you more susceptible to infection. And a psychological reason for prompt treatment was brought out by research that found—to nobody's surprise—that women without nipple pain were much less likely to be depressed than were women whose nipples hurt. When nipple problems were cleared up, rates of depression decreased. What had looked like postpartum depression seemed in many cases to be the result of physical pain.

Not all women experience nipple discomfort during early nursing. If you have positioned your baby properly from the start, and if she has latched on well, you can usually prevent sore nipples. Some infants, though, have more trouble than others learning how to latch on and to suckle; as a result, their mothers' nipples begin to hurt. Proper positioning techniques almost always alleviate or completely eliminate sore nipples. So check the way you're holding the baby. Is she in a position that lets her get enough of your breast in her mouth without straining? If not, take another look at the pictures and text in Chapter 6 and reposition.

You may be doing everything right, but your baby may have a suckling problem. Some babies suck their tongues instead of the breast, or suck their lower lips along with the breast. Others thrust their tongues forward, or because of a tight frenulum (the membrane that attaches the tongue to the floor of the mouth) cannot grasp the nipple properly (see page 332). Ask your lactation consultant or a La Leche League leader to observe you and your baby while you're nursing. She may be able to pick up any suckling problems and advise you.

Even if some blood appears in cracks in your nipple, you can continue to nurse. You may even see this blood in your baby's spit-up. Your blood won't harm your baby. If you're bleeding, take immediate measures to heal your nipples. Aside from the pain you'll be feeling, cracks in the nipples can let in bacteria that can cause a breast infection (mastitis—see page 322).

Moist Wound Healing for Cracked Nipples

Moist wound healing involves putting a dressing on broken skin to increase the skin's moisture content from within. For example, if you have dry, chapped lips, you put on lip balm to restore their internal moisture and you avoid surface wetness by not licking your lips. The same principle applies to nipples. If your nipple cracks, moist wound healing can accelerate the healing process, eliminate scab formation, and provide pain relief. At the same time, you avoid surface wetness by not allowing milk to pool on your skin.

If your nipples are not too sore, you can express just a little bit of your breast milk and apply it to the affected areas. You will thus be taking advantage of the healing and antibacterial properties of human milk, as well as its moisturizing benefits. You don't need to wipe this small amount off your nipple before your baby nurses.

For more severely sore, cracked nipples, you can apply pure, medical-grade, anhydrous lanolin (Lansinoh HPA Lanolin), which is soothing and will also lubricate the skin and help it retain its internal moisture. Pure lanolin is hypoallergenic and does not need to be wiped off before feedings. Lansinoh HPA Lanolin can be purchased from your local pharmacy or supermarket, or online. Your doctor or lactation consultant may recommend a topical balm or antibiotic that they have had good results with. If the nipple cream you're using has steroids in it, wipe it off before you nurse and don't use it for more than two days. Be very cautious about using other over-the-counter nipple creams; one widely marketed cream was recently taken off the market after the FDA determined that it contained ingredients that could harm babies.

While some moisture is good, too much is not. Too moist an environment can promote bacterial growth, leading to an infection. Therefore, change your breast pads or your bra often enough so that your nipples don't remain wet.

Treating Sore Nipples

✤ Since so many nipple problems are caused by incorrect latch-on, go back to the positioning advice in Chapter 6, and make sure your baby is properly positioned for nursing. His chest should be facing yours, his face and nose facing your breast, and his mouth covering all or part of your areola. Be sure that your nipple is well into your baby's mouth and that his gums are compressing the milk ducts under the areola.

If he is not properly positioned, carefully take him off the breast (breaking the suction with your finger in the corner of his mouth) and bring him back to it. If you are in any doubt about your nursing technique, consult a lactation specialist.

✤ Some babies latch on well but then slip down on the breast during the feeding, getting out of position and causing nipple pain. Keep checking the distance between your baby's nose and your breast during the feeding, and if it increases, take him off and have him latch on again.

✤ Never let your baby chew on your nipple. If you feel this happening, carefully take him off the breast as above and bring him back. If he keeps doing it, end this feeding session.

✤ Express a little milk manually before putting your baby to the breast; this will start your milk flowing, help

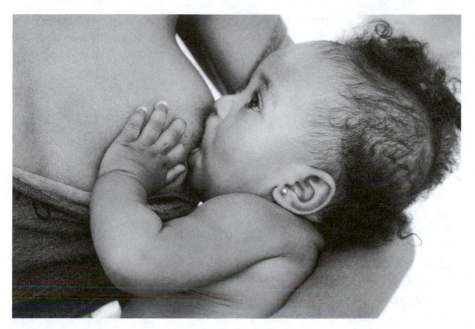

This baby is suckling well. She's taking enough of the breast into her mouth, has a good latch, and is obviously enjoying the experience. Her little hand feels good on Mom's breast.

your let-down reflex operate more quickly, and lubricate your nipple.

✤ Practice a relaxation technique just before nursing (see the box on page 145).

✤ Nurse your baby more frequently, but for shorter periods of time. Your breasts are less likely to overfill and your baby is more likely to suckle gently, since he'll be less hungry.

✤ Briefly apply an ice pack to your sore breast just before you bring your baby to it. This will help to make the breast numb.

✤ Offer the less sore breast first most of the time. This will give your milk a chance to let down from the sore nipple, and your baby won't be suckling as hard by the time he gets around to his second course.

✤ Change your position at each feeding. Lie down; sit up; hold your baby in different positions so that you can change the position of your baby's jaws on your breast. If you have a crack in your nipple, it's especially important to position your baby so his mouth clamps down elsewhere.

✤ If a scab forms on your nipple during early nursing, leave it alone. You can continue nursing.

✤ Avoid all irritating and drying substances. Never use soap, alcohol, tincture of benzoin, or witch hazel on your nipples.

❖ Don't wipe away a little bit of milk left on your breast after a nursing. As we said, you can express a few drops of your milk and rub that gently onto your nipples.

❖ Wear hydrogel pads (made up of water, moisturizer, and polyurethane) inside your bra, and keep them in the refrigerator or freezer when not in use. These pads provide cool, soothing relief. Prices vary considerably for the different brands, as do the amounts of time they can be worn. Popular brands include Ameda ComfortGel, Medela Tender Care, Soothies Gel Pads, Lily-Padz, and Blossumz. Pads with adhesive backing next to the skin should be used only for special occasions and only for a short time, since longer wear can irritate your skin.

❖ Ask a lactation consultant about the advisability of wearing an ultrathin silicone breast shield to help your baby latch on better, and use it only under her direction.

❖ If only one nipple is sore, breastfeed only on the other breast and pump (with an electric pump) from the sore breast. If nipples on both breasts are sore, consult with your lactation specialist. You may need to stop nursing completely for a couple of days, during which time you can pump or express your milk. (Using an electric pump is usually less irritating than your baby's suckling might be.)

❖ Be careful of excessive suction or vigor from the breast pump. An electric pump is the most nipple-friendly. Meanwhile, check for a good fit at the flange of the pump, the cup or funnel that is centered over the breast. Usually, pumping will not hurt, but if your nipple soreness seems related to pumping, call the pump's manufacturer for help (see the Resource Appendix). You can also hand-express your milk from the sore side. For instructions on how to do this, see page 242.

❖ Keep your nipples free of surface wetness (except for a few drops of expressed milk) to prevent skin breakdown or infection:

   ❖ If you wear breast pads to catch leaking milk, change them when they get wet. Don't use the kind with plastic liners.

   ❖ Wear an all-cotton bra, not one made of a synthetic fabric. Change it every day.

   ❖ If you wear breast shells (milk cups) to bring out inverted nipples, empty them often.

   ❖ Walk around the house with your nipples uncovered when you can. If the air in your home is very dry (as in an overheated apartment), use a humidifier or keep a pan of water on the radiator.

   ❖ If it's too painful to have clothing touch your nipples, apply a light coating of lanolin and insert into your bra small mesh tea strainers from which you have removed the handles. Or you can use plastic breast shells that have holes in them to allow for air circulation.

✤ If your nipples are tender after showering, apply a coating of lanolin before you take your shower.

✤ Try seashells. Seashells? Yes, Scandinavian mothers have worn them over their nipples between feedings for thousands of years. If you can't go beachcombing yourself, you can buy them online. Air-dry your nipple area before you put seashells over your nipples, and boil them between uses. One mom said she liked the idea of using "this potent feminine energy" from nature on her breasts. (We have no direct experience with treating sore nipples this way, but you can find enthusiastic testimonials to this method online.)

✤ Occasionally take a mild pain reliever to ease your discomfort. See Chapter 10 to learn which medications are safe for your baby.

✤ Thrush is sometimes the cause of sore nipples. This fungus infection may be affecting both you and your baby. See the next section.

✤ If, as happens in rare cases, your soreness worsens until your nipple cracks and bleeds and is absolutely too painful to nurse from, take your baby off the affected nipple for 24 to 48 hours. Nurse him often on the other breast. If necessary, give him expressed milk or formula. Pump your milk from the affected breast every three hours, or every time you would ordinarily be nursing. If pumping is painful, hand-express.

Gradually resume nursing on the breast with the sore nipple, starting twice a day. Continue to pump or express from the sore breast at other feeding times until your nipple is healed enough to work up to the full nursing schedule. Apply pure lanolin to heal the nipple fissures. If both nipples are sore, stop nursing temporarily and express as much milk as you can, either by pump or by hand, until your nipples are healed enough to resume nursing. Following a schedule like this, many women are able to work through their nipple problems and go on to a happy breastfeeding experience.

✤ If you have a persistent rash around your nipples that does not clear up, see your own doctor to rule out any underlying problem.

Thrush

Thrush, a yeast infection caused by the fungus *Candida albicans,* loves milk and places where milk goes. It isn't serious, but it can be very painful. If your baby has it in her mouth, it may hurt her to nurse. If you have it on your nipples, it may hurt you to breastfeed. If one of you has it, you'll probably pass it to the other.

To check your baby, look inside her mouth for milky white spots or a whitish coating on her tongue, gums, or the insides of her cheeks. She may also have a diaper rash. Or she may have no symptoms at all. You may have bright pink, flaky, crusty, itchy, or burning nipples; a burning pain inside your breasts during or soon after feedings (which signals an infection in the milk ducts); and you may also have a vaginal yeast infection. Thrush sometimes develops after antibiotic treatment in mother or baby; also, women with diabetes are more prone to develop thrush. If you suspect thrush, see the suggestions below.

❧ Continue to breastfeed, in short, frequent feedings, on the less sore side first. Be sure to break the suction of baby's mouth before taking her off the breast.

❧ Call your doctor, who will probably prescribe either nystatin or fluconazole (Diflucan). Since nystatin is less expensive and may be more readily available in some areas, some doctors recommend this first. The baby gets a liquid form for her mouth, and you may get the same formulation for your nipples, which does not have to be wiped off. Or you may get a cream to put on your nipples, which must be gently wiped off.

If you started with nystatin but it doesn't work, you'll probably get a prescription for fluconazole, which is given orally to both mom and baby.

❧ Follow the treatment for both of you for two weeks or longer, even though your symptoms may clear up in a couple of days. Some women need to take Diflucan for as long as a month or more, in a high dose (higher than for a vaginal yeast infection).

❧ While your baby's infection is clearing up, wash your nipples after every nursing with a solution of 1 teaspoon of baking soda to 1 cup of warm boiled water. Dry them gently.

❧ Try probiotics (which provide good bacteria—see page 228), like yogurt with active cultures, or supplements of *Lactobacillus acidophilus*, like Culturelle, especially if you have recently taken or are currently taking antibiotics.

❧ If you're especially susceptible to this kind of infection because you're diabetic or have an immune system dysfunction, limit your intake of sugars. Do this in conjunction with the treatment your doctor ordered. OTC or alternative remedies sometimes do nothing for a yeast infection and can even make it worse. Don't diagnose and self-prescribe a treatment unless you have previously been diagnosed and treated by a professional for a yeast infection, and then only if you're certain about your symptoms.

❧ To prevent reinfection, wash your hands and your baby's hands often, and dry them with soft paper towels that you discard after one use.

❧ Don't give your baby any milk expressed and frozen while you have a thrush infection.

❧ Thoroughly wash anything that goes into your baby's mouth. Boil rubber nipples, pacifiers, teethers, and toys for 20 minutes once a day and discard them after a week to prevent a recurrence. Boil breast pump parts. Wash nonboilable toys and breast pump parts thoroughly with warm soapy water. Sterilize bottles after every use.

❖ After the bout of thrush clears up, buy new rubber nipples, pacifiers, and toys that your baby is likely to mouth.

❖ Change your nursing pads after each feeding, and wear a clean bra every day.

❖ If thrush recurs after two courses of treatment, include all family members in the treatment plan. Thrush can be transmitted during sexual relations. Siblings who are both nursing or sharing toys can pass it to one another.

Clogged Duct (Plugged Duct, "Caked" Breasts)

In this condition, which can occur any time during nursing, one or more milk ducts are blocked so that the milk cannot pass through them. If you develop a clogged duct, you're likely to find a small reddened lump on your breast that's painful to touch. If not treated, this condition can lead to a breast infection, so take immediate measures, as suggested below.

❖ First, continue to nurse. If you stop suddenly, your breast is likely to get too full, the condition will worsen, and infection may result.

❖ Be sure your bra (or other clothing, like a T-shirt or sweater) is not so tight that it's pressing on the milk ducts. Try a bra in the next larger size. Or try going without one, at least while you're nursing. Also check other items that may be putting too much pressure on your breasts, like a baby carrier or a shoulder bag.

❖ Breastfeed more often and for a longer period of time, so that your baby can help you empty the breast, release the blockage, and unclog the duct.

❖ Change your position with every feeding, so that the pressure of your baby's suckling will be felt in different places on your breast, exerting pressure on different ducts.

❖ Express or pump milk from the affected breast after each feeding if your baby has not nursed long and vigorously, to get out as much milk as possible.

❖ If dried secretions seem to be covering your nipple openings, wash them off very gently after each nursing with a piece of cotton saturated with warm water.

❖ Offer your sore breast first, so that your baby will drain it more thoroughly.

❖ Apply moist heat several times a day with a moist-heating pad, a hot-water bottle, hot wet towel or washcloth, disposable diaper filled with hot water and squeezed out, or tub bath or shower. Be careful not to burn yourself!

❖ Gently massage the area of the clogged duct, stroking toward the nipple, especially after moist-heat treatment.

❖ Try ultrasound at a physical therapy office or sports medicine clinic for one or two consecutive days. Sometimes spontaneous milk ejection occurs while the treatment is being given, especially if the breast is full of milk or the device used in the procedure stimulates the nipple, triggering the release of oxytocin. If the therapist is not familiar with this use of ultrasound, ask your lactation consultant to recommend the dosage.

❖ Rest as much as you can.

❖ Don't wear a nipple shield, which will make it harder for your baby to drain your breast adequately.

❖ Don't sleep on your stomach, which puts pressure on your breasts.

❖ If your baby refuses to nurse on the breast with the clogged duct, see your obstetrician. The milk from that breast may have changed in taste, which may be a sign of an infection or other problem.

❖ If a lump remains for more than three days, see your obstetrician. While the lump is probably related to breastfeeding, it may not be and must be looked at promptly.

❖ If you repeatedly suffer from clogged ducts, consult a lactation specialist to reevaluate the way you're holding your baby or the way your baby is suckling.

Breast Infection (Mastitis)

When breast infections occur, they usually show up between two and six weeks after birth, but they may appear earlier or much later.

A breast infection may be a complication of a clogged duct or the result of an infection carried from the baby to the mother or picked up elsewhere. The risk of infection is increased by broken skin on the nipple. Symptoms tend to appear suddenly and may include some of the following: headache; an intense localized pain; a lump that may or may not feel sore; engorgement, with the breast hot and tender to the touch; redness; fever; a cracked nipple that looks infected; red streaks on the breast; the appearance of blood or pus in your milk; and a generally sick, achy, flulike feeling. If you have any of these symptoms, call your doctor right away.

Mothers with breast infections

used to be told to stop nursing immediately. We now know that breast infections clear up more quickly and with fewer complications when the mother continues to nurse, and nurses frequently, from the affected breast since breast milk itself confers immunity to various organisms. There's no danger of the baby's becoming ill from nursing at an infected breast; he probably harbors the same germs in his mouth and nose that may have caused the breast problem. Occasionally, a baby may not nurse well at an infected breast because the milk tastes salty. If this happens, nurse from the uninfected breast and pump and discard the milk from the infected one.

Treat a breast infection right away. With treatment, the fever should drop within 36 to 48 hours, and the soreness and hardness will go away soon afterward. The usual treatment for mastitis is an antibiotic for 10 to 14 days, plus other measures like those below. The antibiotic will be safe to take while you continue to nurse. It should be taken for the full course, even if your symptoms have gone away before then.

❖ Go to bed and stay there as long as you can. If you can't stay in bed, rest as much as possible.

❖ Apply moist heat to the infected breast with one or more of the following: moist-heating pad, hot-water bottle, or hot wet towel. Or soak your breast in a basin of warm water, or take a warm shower or bath. Nurse soon after application of heat.

❖ Nurse frequently, as often as every two hours around the clock. This will keep your milk flowing, will avoid engorgement, and will drain the infected area of the breast. Be sure your baby is well positioned, and change positions so your baby is not always putting pressure at the same spot on your breast.

❖ Offer the sore breast first at each nursing so that it can be drained more completely.

❖ Be sure your bra is not too tight. Try one in the next larger size. Or try going without one, at least while you're nursing. Also check other items that may be putting too much pressure on your breasts, like a baby carrier or a shoulder bag.

❖ Drink plenty of fluids.

❖ Don't wean suddenly if you can help it, since this can contribute to an abscess, a serious and painful infection. An abscess is a localized collection of pus surrounded by swelling, which is usually treated with antibiotics and warm soaks, but may require surgery.

❖ If you suffer from repeated breast infections, see your doctor, especially if a lump is not reduced in size even after three days of treatment, if the mastitis keeps reappearing at the same place on your breast, and/or if you have dimpling on the breast. Breast cancer is extremely rare in lactating women, but it does occasionally occur and you must have it ruled out.

Galactocele (Milk-Retention Cyst)

Occasionally, a nursing mother develops a nontender lump in her breast. If you find a lump in your breast and if it doesn't change or go away within three days, see a gynecologist who's knowledgeable about lactating breasts.

The lump may be a galactocele, a benign cyst that contains milk. It is caused by blockage of a milk duct, and it does not become infected. Galactoceles can be diagnosed in two ways, by performing either an ultrasound test or a needle aspiration (in which a sample of fluid and cells is removed through a needle and tested) to determine whether the cystlike structure contains milk.

If you have a galactocele, you probably won't need surgery, and you don't need to wean your baby. Although you may need to treat the clogged duct, the galactocele will go away when you stop nursing.

Sudden Increase in Baby's Demand

Your baby may have seemed happy with a nursing schedule that the two of you have worked out, but then, just as soon as you think you've settled into a routine, she begins to want more. You wonder what happened, and you worry that you don't have enough milk. This is a fairly common occurrence and nothing to worry about. It can occur for a number of reasons and is usually easy to resolve. All you have to do in most cases is nurse more frequently for several days. This will build up your milk supply and get your baby over the transition.

One reason this sometimes happens has to do with the baby's growth. Babies grow irregularly. During periods of particularly fast growth, sometimes called growth spurts, they need more fuel. A baby's need for nourishment frequently increases around three weeks, six weeks, three months, and six months of age. While you're nursing more frequently, you may also be able to increase your milk supply in other ways (see Chapter 7). When your baby reaches four to six months of age and still seems hungry no matter how often you nurse her, she may be ready to start eating solid foods.

Another reason for what seems like a sudden increase in your baby's appetite may lie with you. Nursing and motherhood may have become so routine and manageable that you forgot to mother yourself. You work more, you go out more, you do more, and you forget about resting enough and eating right. As a result, your milk supply may diminish. This is easy to remedy. Take a look at your life and cut back on outside involvements while you take better care of yourself.

The Baby Who Gains Too Slowly

Typically, babies lose up to 7 percent of their birth weight within the first week of life, and then by two or three weeks are back up to birth weight. But occasionally, a baby two or three weeks of age will still be below birth weight. Sometimes a baby has begun to gain and then for no apparent reason hits a plateau. The baby may be crying constantly, obviously hungry all the time. Or he may sleep for several hours at a stretch, seem to nurse well, and seem happy. Either way, it's worrisome. Is the baby sick? Or not getting enough to eat?

Any baby who doesn't gain or seems unhappy much of the time should be examined by a physician. See the box on page 130 for signs that your baby should be evaluated right away. A sick baby won't do well at either breast or bottle until his condition is dealt with. If your doctor does not find any medical problem, see a lactation consultant, who may be able to help your baby become a more efficient nurser and who can check to see how much milk the baby is getting at a feeding. Also, take a look at your own health. Are you feeling good, eating enough, and getting enough rest? Are you taking any drugs that could interfere with your milk production?

If, as is usually the case, no physical problem is found with either you or your baby, you can take steps to encourage weight gain and normal growth, as suggested in the box on page 326. One technique developed by Jack Newman, MD, is breast compression, which can help your milk to flow and your baby to nurse actively. Your lactation consultant may teach you, or you can go to www.drjacknewman.com/help/breast-compression.asp for instructions.

Helping the Slow-Gaining Infant

Look at Your Breastfeeding Patterns

✤ Is your baby nursing only every three or four hours, either because she sleeps for several hours at a stretch and doesn't "ask" to nurse, or because you've been encouraging her to go longer between feedings? If so, nurse every hour or two, even if it means waking your baby up every couple of hours during the day.

Helping the Older Baby Who Isn't Gaining

Sometimes there's a sudden weight loss or a failure to gain weight in a baby several months old who has been doing fine up until now. If this happens, look for the following:

❖ Is your baby teething? If he's drooling a lot and trying to put everything into his mouth, he may be teething and finding nursing uncomfortable. Whenever you see him sucking his fist or fingers, pick him up and nurse him. More frequent short nursings will provide him with the nutrients he needs, while lessening his discomfort. Before nursings you can massage his gums, and after nursings you can give him ice-chilled teething rings until he seems more comfortable. If he seems extremely uncomfortable, ask your doctor for suggestions.

❖ Has he become so efficient at nursing that he zips through his feedings and is ready to stop after five minutes? If so, he may not be getting enough milk. Burp him and switch breasts several times during a session; the new surge of milk after a second let-down may interest him in staying at the breast.

❖ Has your baby been sleeping more than six hours at night before 8 to 12 weeks of age? If so, wake her every four hours at night.

❖ Have you been timing feeding sessions, removing your baby after only 20 or 30 minutes? If the baby is swallowing frequently (no more than two sucks to a swallow), let sessions run for at least 45 minutes, or until the baby comes off by herself with a "drunken sailor" look.

❖ Has your baby been taking only one breast at a feeding? If so, nurse from both. If she falls asleep after one, burp her and change her and then nurse on the other side. Switch breasts more than once during a feeding. This encourages multiple let-downs and, as a result, more milk.

❖ Is your baby using a pacifier to fill her sucking needs? If so, take away the pacifier and offer your breast; this way she will get nutrition along with suckling.

❖ Is your baby getting milk or water from bottles? If so, your breasts may not be getting enough stimulation, or your baby may be experiencing nipple confusion. Eliminate the water. If your baby needs supplemental formula, consider using a nursing supplementer (see the box on page 328), an eyedropper, a teaspoon, or a cup. Even some premature babies can drink from a cup.

Remember, though, that this last suggestion doesn't help the baby learn how to suckle correctly. Furthermore, you need to be very careful if you use the eyedropper approach or a cup, since there is the risk of putting more

❖ Are you doing too much? Cut back as much as possible on your activities for a while. Rest more, eat and drink more, and take better care of yourself so that your body has more energy to increase your milk supply and to fight infection.

❖ Is he easily distracted? Does he break away from the breast to look around and see what's going on? Breastfeed in a quiet, dimly lit room.

❖ Does he spend many happy hours with a pacifier, or sitting in a swing? Devices like these can be wonderful helpers for a busy mom, but if your baby is losing weight or not gaining as fast as he should, put them aside for a while and have him spend more time nursing. When he's once again gaining well, you can reintroduce the other pleasures.

❖ Does your baby begin to nurse, then reject the breast? If so, see "Temporary Rejection of the Breast" (page 331).

❖ Work with your baby's doctor, who can help you determine why the baby isn't gaining weight and suggest ways to promote weight gain. If she or he determines it's breastfeeding-related, contact a lactation consultant or a La Leche League leader.

---

fluid into the baby's mouth than she is able to swallow easily, possibly causing her to aspirate it into her lungs.

Look at Your Baby

❖ Does your baby arch his back during nursing? If so, he may not get enough of your breast in his mouth. Hold him in the clutch (football) hold with his feet up behind you so that he can't push against anything. (In some cases, arching the back may be a sign of gastroesophageal reflux, or GER; see page 155.)

❖ Is your baby so excitable that he keeps losing the breast? Try swaddling him in a blanket.

❖ Some babies become frustrated if the milk does not flow freely. Express a little bit before you begin to nurse.

What to Do Now

❖ Suppose you're already doing everything suggested above. If so, the first thing to do now is to make extra efforts to build up your production of milk. The best way is to nurse more frequently, as often as every hour or two. Other suggestions, given in Chapter 7, may also help.

❖ If, after one or two days of this frequent-feeding regimen, your baby is still not gaining weight, seek the advice of your doctor or lactation specialist, who may help you and your baby to overcome whatever obstacles have been keeping your baby from gaining.

❖ The lactation consultant will look closely at your baby's suckling technique, as explained in the following

Nursing Supplementers

These devices are used by women who want to increase their milk supply while supplementing their breast milk with formula, women who want to nurse an adopted child, or women who want to initiate breastfeeding after not having nursed for some time. Nursing supplementers deliver milk to a baby while the baby is suckling at the mother's breast. He thus gets a mouthful of breast milk along with a mouthful of formula.

The two most commonly used methods are the Supplemental Nursing System (SNS) made by Medela, Inc., and the Lact-Aid Nursing Trainer System. Whichever one you choose should be used only under the supervision of an experienced lactation specialist, and your baby must be closely monitored for healthy weight gain. These devices are helpful to a baby who is latching on well; if there is a latch problem, you need to seek a different solution.

With the Medela SNS, a thin plastic tube runs from a plastic bottle hung upside down (to take advantage of gravity) from a strap around the mother's neck. The end of the tube is placed at the edge of the mother's nipple and held there with surgical tape. Or you can place a small Band-Aid on your breast and run the tube under the gauze square to avoid taping and retaping the tube. As the baby nurses at his mother's breast, he simultaneously suckles the tip of the nursing tube and the mother's nipple, and his efforts are rewarded by the flow of milk through the tube. Bottles come in different sizes to accommodate premature babies and those with cleft palates or other feeding problems.

The Lact-Aid Nursing Trainer System consists of a soft, presterilized plastic bag that contains milk. The bag is attached to a plug that, in turn, is attached to a slender nursing tube. The filled and assembled supplementer is worn on an adjustable neck strap in the mother's nursing bra between her breasts.

In both these systems, the baby suckles the breast and the tube simultaneously, receiving milk as soon as he starts to nurse. Because of the way the system delivers fluid, letting

---

section, and/or may suggest that you supplement breastfeeding with formula or pumped breast milk.

Checking Your Baby's Technique

Before you consult a specialist to have your baby's suckling evaluated, you can do a little detective work on your own.

First, test your baby's suckling technique using the Marmet Suck Assessment. Trim the fingernail on your index finger, wash and rinse your hands, stroke your baby's cheek toward her lips, and when her mouth opens, insert your finger with the nail down. If your baby is sucking correctly, the following will occur:

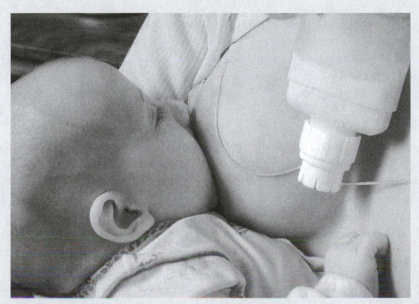

A nursing supplementer delivers milk to a baby while the baby suckles at the mother's breast. It's helpful to babies whose mothers don't seem to have enough milk to foster normal weight gain and to those who need help mastering efficient suckling techniques.

the baby suckle breast and tube at the same time, it encourages a type of oral patterning that helps to improve or train the baby's suckling skill and coordination. Meanwhile, the device helps to increase the mother's milk supply, since the baby is stimulating her breasts. Throughout, the baby is getting the nourishment he needs, and both mother and baby are able to enjoy the experience of nursing at the breast, with all the warmth and intimacy that are such a rewarding part of breastfeeding.

For information on obtaining nursing supplementers, see the Resource Appendix.

❖ The sides of her tongue will curve around your finger.

❖ Her tongue will cover her lower gum ridge.

❖ You'll feel a sucking motion starting at the tip of her tongue and rolling back with a wavelike motion.

❖ She'll suck your finger far back into her mouth.

❖ Your finger pad will touch her soft palate, and she won't gag.

❖ She'll suck rhythmically, occasionally taking a rest without breaking the suction.

If your baby's suckling does not feel like this, she may have a suckling problem that a trained lactation specialist may help you correct. Other ways to catch a suckling problem involve asking a friend or family member to help you check the following:

✤ Does your baby seem to be sucking her lower lip along with your breast? If so, take her off the breast and start her over again to see if she latches well this time. If she still sucks her lip after you put her back on the breast, gently pull out her lip.

✤ If your nipple tends to point down, point it up into your baby's mouth by pressing down on the top of your breast with your thumb. Or let the nipple fall where it may, and before teasing your baby's mouth open for the latch, aim your nipple at her nose.

✤ If your baby seems to clench her jaws and clamp the end of your nipple, gently pull down on her jaw with your index finger, and when she begins to suck properly, release the pressure.

✤ Gently pull down your baby's lower lip while she's nursing. Either you or a helper can use a small mirror and see whether you can see the underside of her tongue between her lower gum and your breast. If not, she may be sucking her tongue. Imagine a hot dog in a roll: Your nipple should be the hot dog and your baby's tongue should be the roll. If you cannot see your baby's tongue, remove her from your breast.

✤ Put your index finger on your baby's chin, pressing it down a little, and let her use her rooting reflex to find your nipple and take it into her mouth.

✤ Or put your finger in her mouth, flatten her tongue, and insert your nipple on top. You'll need a helper for this. Repeat until she's doing it right.

If none of these techniques works, ask your baby's doctor or a lactation consultant to look at your baby's tongue; occasionally, the membrane attaching it to the floor of the mouth (the frenulum) needs to be clipped (see illustration page 332).

The Baby Who Gains Too Fast

While we used to think it was impossible to overfeed a breast-fed baby, an occasional totally breastfed baby seems to be extremely heavy. This is a baby who is gaining so much weight that he weighs in the top 5 percent for a baby of his length and is considered fat by your pediatrician. Although it was once thought that a fat baby is a healthy baby, we now know that too much fat is not good in infancy, and it may lead to obesity later in life.

However, nursing babies are rarely overweight. They benefit from the basically self-regulating system of breastfeeding, and most heavy breast-fed babies slim down when they begin to crawl and move around more.

This is usually not an issue during the first year of your nursing baby's life. Continue to feed your baby frequently enough to satisfy his hunger.

Meanwhile, at your baby's regular checkups, your pediatrician will follow his growth curve to make sure his growth is on track. So don't restrict your baby's intake unless your pediatrician recommends it. Meanwhile, while continuing to breastfeed, try also to meet your baby's emotional needs in a variety of ways that don't involve feeding him.

Temporary Rejection of the Breast ("Nursing Strike")

There are two kinds of breast refusal—that by a newborn who does not even begin to nurse, and that by a baby who has been nursing well and then decides to go on strike and refuses to take the breast. In either case, you can almost always figure out why this is happening and help your baby nurse happily.

If your baby consistently refuses only one breast, see your own doctor, since sometimes a medical problem will make a woman's milk taste different. If your doctor says that everything is fine with you, don't worry about the fact that your baby is not nursing from that breast. If the unpopular breast fills up with milk and becomes uncomfortable, hand-express a little milk, just to relieve the discomfort. Every now and then, offer this breast again to your baby. If she keeps refusing it, one breast may become larger than the other, so you may want to pad your bra on the smaller side so you'll look even on both sides. The size difference will go away after you wean your baby.

If Your Baby Has Not Nursed at All

If your baby rejects the breast almost from birth, check the following possibilities:

❖ He may have been suctioned too vigorously just after delivery and may be showing aversion to putting anything in his mouth.

❖ He may be reacting to someone's having held the back of his head and pushed him onto the breast.

❖ He may be having a problem latching on. Check the way you're holding him and experiment with other positions. If you're engorged, relieving that condition (see the box on page

313) may make it easier for him to take your breast.

❧ Your baby may be "tongue-tied." Some infants have a tight frenulum. This is the stringy fibrous membrane that connects the lower part of the tongue to the floor of the mouth. If it's too tight, the baby cannot extend his tongue far enough to take hold of the nipple and latch on. A lactation consultant can sometimes spot what appears to be a short frenulum. If your doctor confirms this diagnosis, you can ask the doctor to clip the frenulum, a quick, safe, and painless procedure that may be performed in the office if done soon after birth. Or you may need to go to a specialist. There may be a small amount of bleeding for a minute or so; as soon as this stops, your baby can and should be put to your breast.

❧ Some infants, right from birth, fight being held and fight being nursed. You're not doing anything wrong; you just have a baby whose personality makes it hard for him to settle into your arms and onto your breast. You need to experiment with ways to calm your baby and to find a position that he will accept. You also need to remember that your baby is not rejecting you and that you are not to blame. You may need to express your milk for a while and feed it to your baby by cup, eyedropper, bottle, or nursing supplementer, until he feels comfortable in the nursing situation. One mother finally got her baby to nurse by leaning over him and dangling her breast into his mouth.

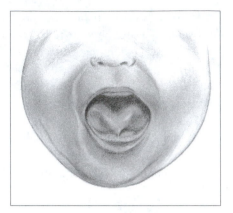

In this drawing, a tight frenulum, which can make it difficult for a baby to latch on correctly, is slightly exaggerated in order to show the condition clearly.

The Older Nursing Baby on Strike

Sometimes in the first few weeks after birth, but more often between four and ten months of age, a baby will nurse for a couple of minutes, then arch her back and cry. Nothing the mother can do will induce her to go back, and yet it's obvious that she wants something. What's wrong? And what can you do about it? As with so many other child-rearing issues, you have to look closely at your own baby and see what is going on in her life. The following suggestions have worked for some mothers, and the box on the facing page lists several possible causes, along with some specific solutions.

❧ If you want to continue nursing, don't substitute bottle-feeding for the times you would ordinarily nurse. Doing that may make the problem worse. Chances are that this nursing

When an Older Baby Refuses the Breast

Explore the following possibilities, one by one.

❖ The taste of your milk may have changed because of a cream you're using on your breasts, a new food you're eating, a new medicine you're taking, a strenuous exercise program, a breast infection, or because you're pregnant or have resumed menstruating.

❖ Keep a log of what you eat and how your baby reacts, so you can identify and eliminate an offending food. Schedule nursing sessions before exercise sessions. If you feel a lump in your breast, first treat it as a clogged duct; if it has not healed in three days, see your obstetrician.

❖ If your baby's gums are tender from the pressure of new teeth coming in, it may hurt him to nurse. If he bit you, he may have been startled by your cry of pain and be afraid to nurse again. (See the box about biting on page 168.)

❖ If your baby is wildly hungry and can't seem to wait for the milk to let down, pick him up about 15 minutes before you would ordinarily feed him, or express a little milk first to give your let-down a chance to work.

❖ If your baby has a cold and is having trouble breathing through his nose, use a humidifier in the room where he sleeps, ask your doctor whether nose drops would help, and use an aspirator (a syringe with a rubber bulb) to suction mucus out of his nose. Get careful directions on how to use the aspirator before using it on your baby.

❖ If you suspect thrush, call your doctor and treat it immediately, both to relieve your baby and to prevent the infection from spreading to you.

❖ Ask your pediatrician to evaluate your baby for a possible earache.

❖ Check your baby for signs of gastroesophageal reflux (GER; see page 155.)

❖ If you're going through a particularly difficult time emotionally, your baby may sense your feelings and become too upset to nurse. Make a conscious effort to forget about your cares, at least while you're nursing. You'll enjoy these oases in your life and your baby may be calmer, too. See the box on page 145 for suggestions to help you relax.

strike may last only a day or two, and your baby will then go back to being an eager nurser.

❖ If your baby has begun to eat solid foods, increase her portions of these for a few days to tide her over. Also, add some of your pumped breast milk to her cereal. If she has been eating large amounts of solids, however, this may be causing the problem. She may be too full of food to be interested in nursing.

❖ Express or pump your milk and give it to her until she resumes taking the breast.

❖ Keep offering your breast. The most effective time to do this is to pick her up while she's asleep or very sleepy; she won't remember to reject the breast, and once she's back in the routine of nursing, she may decide it's pretty good, after all.

❖ Vary your nursing positions. Your baby might prefer one you haven't used yet.

❖ Nurse in motion—in a rocking chair or walking around.

❖ Give your baby a bottle with just a small amount of milk (ideally your pumped breast milk) first—and then put her to the breast.

If none of the possible reasons listed in the box on page 333 to explain why your baby might be refusing your breast seem to apply to your situation, if none of the suggested remedies works, if after a couple of weeks she's still refusing to nurse, and if she's more than six months old, you can pump your milk and feed it in a cup or a bottle. You may also want to contact a lactation consultant to try to persuade the baby to continue nursing a while longer. While some children want to nurse long after their mothers had thought they would, others surprise and disappoint a mom by wanting to give up the breast earlier than she wants to stop nursing. For suggestions for how to make the weaning process as physically comfortable as possible, and with the least amount of emotional upset for both mother and baby, see Chapter 17.

CHAPTER SIXTEEN

Special Situations

"I really feel that breastfeeding my baby while she was sick in the hospital helped us both. It calmed her down and soothed her during our time away from home and it made me feel that I was doing all that I could to help her through a somewhat scary ordeal. Breastfeeding is instant comfort to my baby and I feel that she was in better spirits during her hospital stay because of the consistent physical closeness. Plus, I love the fact that I am giving her my antibodies through my breast milk."

MEGAN Westport, Connecticut

A number of situations involving a mother or baby—or both—can affect the course of breastfeeding. What if your baby is born early? What if you or your baby gets sick? What if you have had breast surgery? What if you want to nurse more than one baby? And what if you began to feed your baby formula and then decided to breastfeed? Most women don't encounter these situations. But if you do, you'll have special questions, which we address in this chapter. You'll want to know how your situation is related to your ability to nurse your baby. One thing you need to know is that in many such instances, you and your baby will both benefit from breastfeeding.

If you need more information about any of the topics discussed in this chapter, call your doctor, lactation consultant, or local La Leche League leader. Or look for answers to your questions in one of the books listed in the Resource Appendix.

Breastfeeding Your Preterm (Premature) Infant

The normal gestation period for human babies ranges between 37 and 41 weeks, and a birth that comes before 37 weeks is often a frightening event, especially if a baby is born very early (before 34 weeks) and/or is very small. However, medical technology has advanced so dramatically that even the tiniest babies have an excellent chance of growing up healthy and normal.

In your desire to do as much as possible for your baby, you're likely to feel disappointed if she can't nurse right away, as you had intended. However, you will still have colostrum and milk for her. You can express your milk for her immediately after birth and either supply it to hospital staff or freeze it for later use. Then, as soon as your baby is able to suckle at your breast, you'll have the milk to offer her.

Whether your baby gets your own breast milk right from the beginning or not until she has achieved a certain size and strength, you will be able to breastfeed her. Remember that prematurity is a temporary condition, but that breastfeeding can continue for many months. In either case, you can help your baby's development by giving her kangaroo care (see page 344).

Many women express or pump their milk for the first several weeks of their babies' lives. This milk is fed to the baby in the neonatal intensive care unit (NICU) either by tube or by bottle, helping to assure a good start in life, often in combination with a specially fortified formula. Sometimes the breast milk itself is fortified. After the baby has become stronger, mother and baby have gone on to forge a fulfilling, satisfying nursing relationship. As one mother said, "Breastfeeding a premature baby means a few weeks of uncertainty and inconvenience, followed by many months of blissful happiness, contentment, and satisfaction."

This route is eminently doable—but it does take time, effort, patience, persistence, and most of all, determination. Many women are grateful that they persisted through the early difficult times until they were able to establish a normal breastfeeding relationship. Research shows that the breast milk preterm babies received in their first days or weeks of life gave them a better start than they would have had without it. Some women who decided against breastfeeding at the beginning changed their minds later and were able to relactate, a process described on page 359.

How and What Will Your Preterm Baby Eat?

Procedures for feeding a baby born before term vary, depending on the infant's size, gestational age, strength, and special needs. Your baby may be technically classified as preterm, but be strong and lack only a few ounces to be considered of normal weight. In this case, you can probably start to nurse immediately.

Very tiny infants, however, are often not able to suck; they may have to be fed by gavage (via a tube that goes from the nose into the stomach) for several weeks until they become strong enough to nurse. Ideally, the doctor in your hospital's preterm unit will graduate your baby directly from gavage to breast. In the United States, this often happens when an infant reaches a weight between three and four pounds. Some hospitals, however, still require preterm babies to suck first from a bottle to demonstrate their ability to feed; only when they're taking a bottle

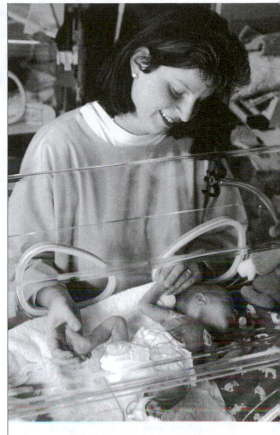

A preterm baby in an incubator can thrive on his mother's milk, which is especially suited to his growth needs. It's also vital for mothers to touch their tiny babies, as this mother is doing.

at every feeding are they permitted to nurse at the breast.

Because of the protective factors in breast milk, it is best for preterm babies, too, *if* the mother can produce enough milk either to nurse her baby directly or to pump milk that will be fed by bottle or gavage. However, very small preterm infants who are receiving pumped breast milk may need

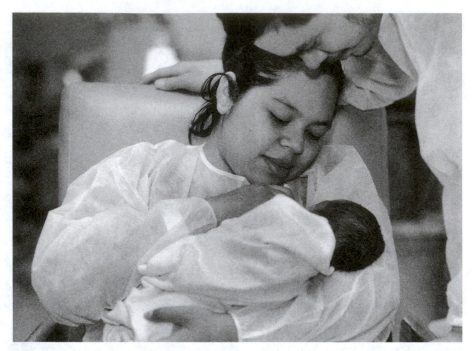

When parents can spend time with an infant in the NICU, it helps them to bond with the baby and to look forward to the day when the baby can come home to be a full-time member of the family.

more nutrients than the milk can provide. These babies often receive a supplement added to breast milk called human milk fortifier (HMF), which is rich in calcium and protein. Your doctor may want your baby to continue to receive extra calcium and protein along with your breast milk for some months after discharge from the hospital. Since HMF is available only in hospitals, these nutrients may come from specially fortified formula given in addition to breast milk.

Whether your baby will be fed your own breast milk or formula or both depends on many variables, including your baby's size and strength, as well as the philosophy of your doctor and the hospital's medical staff. Using the knowledge you gather from this book and other sources, you may want to educate your health-care providers on the benefits of breast milk for preterm babies.

Why Your Milk Is Best

Your milk is better for your baby than the milk he could get from a milk bank, which pools the milk from different women (usually mothers who produce more than their own full-term babies need). It's also better for a preterm baby than a standard formula. As we said, however, if your baby is very tiny, a specially fortified formula may be required in addition to breast milk until he gains some weight.

Compared to the milk of a mother of a full-term baby, a preterm baby's mother's milk is easier to digest and better constituted for developing the preterm baby's brain and nervous system. Milk from mothers of preemies has higher levels of nitrogen, protein, sodium, and chloride, and lower lactose content than full-term milk. It provides more energy for the preterm infant's growth needs than mature milk. It also has a high level of lipase, an enzyme that aids in fat digestion.

One way of helping low-birthweight babies gain weight on breast milk involves having the mother divide her milk into fore milk and hind milk. The fore milk, which is expressed first, is frozen for later use, while the baby gets the hind milk, which is three to four times higher in fat and thus also higher in calories.

If your baby won't be able to receive your breast milk right away—whether for a few days or several weeks—begin expressing your milk as soon as possible after the baby's birth. Arrange to rent a hospital-grade electric pump so you can continue frequent pumping after you go home. This will let you build up your milk supply until the day your baby will be able to nurse, and will provide a supply of breast milk to be given to your baby either now or as supplemental feedings in the future. See Chapter 11 for suggestions on pumping your milk.

Why Breastfeeding Is Good for You, Too

Parents of preterm babies experience a jumble of upsetting emotions. You're likely to be disappointed, worried, confused, exhausted, and possibly guilt-ridden until the day you feel your baby is out of danger and will survive, healthy and happy. All these feelings are normal. It will be easier for you to get through these early, difficult times if you get as much support as you can, take as good care of yourself as you can, remind yourself that medicine can do more today for preterm babies than ever before, and look forward to the day when your baby will have made up for his hurry to come into this world.

For many women, offering their milk to their babies makes them feel that they really are mothers even though they can't bring their babies home yet. You don't need to make a long-term commitment to breastfeed. Even if your preterm baby gets breast milk for only a week or two, he will benefit, and you will know that you contributed something very special to this small life. All the time, keep your ultimate goal in mind—mothering a healthy, happy baby and enjoying the relationship.

If you want to breastfeed, tell your baby's doctor right away and ask for help in doing it. She or he is the one who makes arrangements for your baby to receive your expressed milk or for you to come in to nurse your baby. The two of you will be in close touch about your baby's daily progress. You'll find it easier to nurse your preterm baby if you follow the guidelines given below.

Link Up with a Support System

As soon as possible, contact your childbirth educator, an organization for parents of babies with special needs, a local La Leche League leader, or another mother who has breastfed a preterm baby. Your doctor or nurse may be able to put you in touch with a support person.

Let your family and friends know that you plan to breastfeed your baby. Surround yourself with people who will help and encourage you, and stay as far away as you can from those who question and doubt.

Before Your Baby Is Able to Nurse

Ask hospital personnel what arrangements can be made to feed your baby your own expressed milk—where and how you should bring it and how it will be stored, both at home and in the hospital.

❖ Rent an automatic, hospital-grade electric breast pump that allows you to pump both breasts at the same time, the most efficient and comfortable way to express milk (see Chapter 11 for suggestions for pumping and storing breast milk).

❖ Begin to pump milk within a day or two of your baby's birth. Even though your mature milk will not yet be in, your colostrum will be, with its special immunity-boosting properties.

❖ Pumping every two to three hours around the clock (at least eight sessions in 24 hours) will build up your milk production now and in the future. Freeze any extra milk for use later on. If you're supplying most or all of your baby's milk, pump more often, about ten times in 24 hours.

❖ If the hospital is feeding your baby a special fortified formula and you're expressing only to maintain your milk supply until he'll be able to nurse, a pumping frequency of every four hours may be enough. You can freeze this milk for use later on.

❖ Find out your own best way to manage nighttime expression. Some women produce more milk if they sleep longer at night, while others do better if they wake up once or twice during the night to pump.

❖ You need to remember that pumping will rarely produce as much milk as a nursing baby will, so don't be discouraged. Once your baby begins to nurse, he'll stimulate your breasts to help you make more. Meanwhile, you're giving him precious antibodies, nutrients, and enzymes.

One mother of a baby who weighed only four pounds at birth told us, "I pumped for five weeks, and no amount of pumping would produce more than half an ounce at a time, so I thought that was all I had. But then once Emma latched on, my body responded and made so much milk that I actually leaked!"

❖ Don't be alarmed about ups and downs in your milk supply. Every woman has them; women who express their milk are more aware of the variations.

❖ Expect a drop in your milk supply if you're still pumping after several weeks, because no pump stimulates the breasts the way a baby does. Your production will rise again once your baby begins to nurse.

❖ If your baby is being fed by bottle, he should be sucking on the kind of soft rubber nipple made especially for preterm babies.

❖ You may begin to ovulate and menstruate during the time you're pumping your breasts. Exclusive breastfeeding often delays ovulation and menstruation, but pumping does not stimulate the breasts as much as a baby's suckling. Once your baby is nursing regularly, your periods may stop again, not to resume for several months. Either way, it's possible to get pregnant at this time (see Chapter 13 for a discussion of birth control).

Breastfeeding Your Preterm Baby in the Hospital

Nursing your preemie is not that different from nursing a baby delivered at term, although you may need to adjust your nursing positions to accommodate her small size and to help her a little more than you would if she were bigger.

If your hospital won't let your baby leave the nursery to breastfeed, ask whether there's a special place where you can nurse in private. Many hospitals have separate rooms for this purpose; ideally, this place will shield the baby from distracting sounds, lights, and activity. Others provide screens in the nursery.

❖ Choose a time when your baby is awake and alert but not yet crying from hunger. It's also best if she hasn't just come from a stressful and tiring experience like having blood drawn.

❖ Ask for a comfortable armchair, with support for your back, arms, and feet.

❖ Get into a comfortable position. Put one or two pillows on your lap to raise your baby to breast height.

❖ Make an effort to relax, paying special attention to relaxing your face, neck, shoulders, and arms. Take a few slow, deep breaths before you begin.

❖ Ask a nurse or lactation consultant to help you position your baby and to sit with you the first few times.

❖ Experiment with different positions (described and pictured on pages 105–110). You'll need to support your baby's entire body, and especially her head. The clutch hold is good for tiny babies. Another good position for pree-mies is the cross-cradle or transition position.

A good sitting position involves extending your arm (the one opposite the breast you're nursing from) under your baby's back and neck and holding her head steady with your hand. Then gently move her to a half-upright posi-tion. Her body should not be flexed; her spine should be straight so she can breathe easily. Her body is now facing you, her chest next to your midsection, her back, neck, and head supported by your arm and hand.

❖ Make your nipple as easy as possi-ble to grasp, pinching it to make it longer. (If necessary, wear ultrathin sili-cone breast shells before the feeding to draw out your nipples.) Consult a lactation specialist to advise you.

❖ Use your thumb and forefinger to keep the breast away from your baby's nose and to support your breast.

❖ If you're not sure whether your baby can suck and swallow well enough, offer a breast from which milk has just been expressed so that the flow of liquid into your baby's mouth won't be too rapid.

❖ Express a few drops of milk into your baby's mouth to whet her appetite.

❖ If your preterm baby is getting most of her nutrition from bottles of specially fortified formula or your pumped breast milk, she can take a

little time to learn how to nurse at the breast. Consider the first few nursings practice feeds, and give her plenty of time to develop her suckling skills. If she does no more than lick the nipple a few times, count this as a good begin-ning. Even full-term babies often take a while to learn how to suck; preterm babies need extra time. While your preemie is learning to nurse, be sure that your pediatrician monitors her weight gain.

❖ If your baby falls asleep at your breast, burp her and switch to the other breast. Or offer the other breast after an hour or two.

❖ Expect the first few feedings to be short, possibly only two or three minutes, since a small baby tires easily. Feeding activity is likely to vary from day to day, and if your baby doesn't nurse long, use the rest of your time together to hold her and be available if she does express interest in nursing more.

❖ If you are discharged from the hospital before your baby, push to stay with her as much as possible. If the hospital is far from your home, look for temporary lodging nearby so you can visit frequently every day. This will also give you more opportunities to give your baby that energizing, growth-enhancing special ingredient—your loving touch.

❖ If your baby has to stay in the hos-pital for a long time, ask for permission to stay overnight for a few nights just before her discharge. This will help you learn her rhythms and begin to establish breastfeeding while you still have the nurses to help you. If there are no rooms set aside for parents, ask to sleep on a portable cot or a reclining chair in a room not used in the evening and night.

❖ A growing number of hospitals are letting parents stay with their babies, either before initial discharge or upon a child's later admission to the hospital. If this is impossible, you may still be able to visit several times a day and nurse your baby at those times, and pump or express your milk at the times of any missed feedings.

When Your Preterm or Vulnerable Baby Comes Home

This is an exciting—and often scary—day, especially if the two of you have been separated for some time. Remember, though, that the hospital would not have discharged your baby if the doctors who were caring for him didn't believe he was ready to go home. He'll have some catch-up growing to do, and you can help him do this in your own home. You can do a number of things to make this period easier:

❖ Keep your rented hospital-grade breast pump for at least a month after the homecoming, and maybe longer. If your baby still has too weak a suck to stimulate your breasts enough, pumping after feedings will help you build

your milk production. It will also give you additional milk to supplement nursings if you need to.

❖ Nurse frequently—every one-and-a-half or two hours for at least the first day or two, then every two to three hours (eight to ten times a day).

❖ See a lactation specialist for careful assessment of your baby's abilities.

❖ Because preterm and other vulnerable babies often don't have the strength to nurse efficiently and get the calories they need, a mother is sometimes told to give her baby bottles of either formula or expressed breast milk. Some lactation specialists who work with these small babies have evolved different feeding sequences.

1. One sequence involves breastfeeding first and then topping off with the bottle, doing this for a couple of days, and keeping track of how much milk the baby takes from the bottle after the nursing. If the baby gains weight and becomes stronger and takes relatively small amounts of milk from the bottle, the bottle can gradually be eliminated.

2. The second sequence involves offering the bottle first. Ask your pediatrician how much milk to put in the bottle. Then offer the breast to finish the feed and give the baby the feeling of fullness at the breast, thus encouraging him to associate that feeling of satiety with the breast and making him want to nurse. Gradually the supplementary bottles are eliminated.

This is very much a trial-and-error procedure, and the amount of milk a baby takes from either breast or bottle may vary day-to-day and at different feedings within the same day. There's no one approach that will help all babies. Your doctor or lactation consultant will be able to help you tailor your baby's feeding pattern to his individual situation.

❖ If you need to supplement, use a bottle with a special nipple for a small baby, a nursing supplementer (see Chapter 15), or some alternative feeding method like a cup or syringe (see Chapter 12).

❖ Take good care of yourself. Sleep when your baby does; get as much help as possible with the housework; take as long a leave from work as you can. Concentrate on feeding your baby until he's stronger and breastfeeding is well established (which may not be until your baby's actual due date, or later).

❖ Be patient. As your baby gets closer to his original due date or to a weight considered healthy for a full-term baby, he'll become a more eager and efficient nurser. When this happens, you'll be able to stop supplementing and pumping.

Kangaroo Care

Over the past couple of decades, research has shown that more and more preterm infants have benefited from a kind of care that's physically and psychologically sound—and simple and cost-free. This care involves skin-to-skin contact between baby and parent in a position similar to that of the baby kangaroo in its mother's pouch. In kangaroo care, an infant, clad only in diaper and hat, is held against her mother's bare skin. The baby's body and the mother's exposed skin are covered by a blanket or loose-fitting shirt or gown to maintain body heat.

In the most complete version of this care, the mother serves as the infant's incubator, as well as her main source of food and stimulation. She keeps her baby for many hours a day in an upright position, skin-to-skin against her chest, until the baby shows she wants to move by crying and moving her arms and legs.

This kind of care produces almost magical results, especially with regard to breastfeeding and infant development. Mothers produce more milk and breastfeed longer, and babies have more oxygen in their blood, are calmer, and breathe better. Studies by Dr. Nils Bergman also show that this kind of care (which he calls skin-to-skin contact) in the neonatal intensive care unit improves survival rates in premature babies. Although much of the attention to kangaroo care has involved preterm babies, the bonding and closeness that result from this intimate contact are good for babies of any size.

More and more hospitals are integrating some form of kangaroo care for their preterm babies, and fathers often participate as well. As Dr. David Marks said, "When my first son came home he weighed less than five pounds.

When I was asked to 'kangaroo' him to keep his body temperature up, it sounded difficult. Little did I know that the time spent snuggling up and bonding with him would be one of the most wonderful times of my life."

Late-Preterm and Near-Term Infants

In recent years, the number of babies born between 34 and 36 weeks' gestation has risen steadily, partly due to miscalculated early inductions or elective cesarean deliveries. These babies, known as late preterm or near-term infants, now account for nearly three-quarters of all preterm births in the United States. Their needs are very similar to those of babies born even earlier. They have a higher risk for medical problems than do babies born at term, especially if their mothers have any medical problems. They're more likely than full-term babies to become dehydrated or jaundiced, conditions that carry complications for the course of breastfeeding.

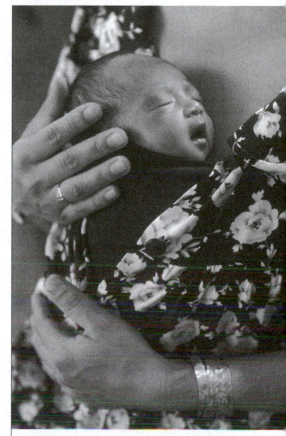

With the skin-to-skin contact permitted by kangaroo care, preterm babies breastfeed better and also enjoy other health benefits.

These immature infants are often sleepier than full-term babies and have less stamina; are more likely to have problems latching on, suckling, and swallowing; are more susceptible to infection and respiratory problems; and have a harder time maintaining body temperature. Some are physically large and therefore assumed to be more mature than they actually are and are sent home too early from the hospital. Their mothers' milk often doesn't come in soon enough for vigorous breastfeeding to begin. It's important to keep track of these babies' health and breastfeeding progress both in the hospital and in the first days after discharge.

Everyone involved in these babies' care—mother, father, partner, doctors, nurses, lactation consultant—needs to be aware of their special needs. The babies may benefit from much of the same kind of care that preterm babies get, depending on their individual situations. Some of them, like some preterm infants, benefit from the mother's using an ultrathin silicone nipple shield to help the baby latch on and get enough breast milk. Nipple shield use needs to be supervised by a professional knowledgeable in lactation and in the needs of these vulnerable infants.

If mother and baby leave the hospital within 72 hours, the baby should be seen by his doctor within two days of discharge to be sure he has not lost too much weight and that he is not at high risk for jaundice. He should also see the doctor at five to seven days of age. Until these babies grow and develop some more, it's not advisable to carry them in a baby sling because their bodies may flex too much. An infant wrap is a good idea to keep them in a more upright position.

Separation of Mother and Baby

Preterm and near-preterm births are not the only times when mother and baby may be apart for a while. Occasionally, emergencies occur that separate a breastfeeding mother and her baby for a period of days or weeks. If you want to continue nursing past this separation, you may well be able to. During the separation, pump or express your milk at about the times that your baby would ordinarily be nursing. When you and your baby get together again, it may take a week or more before you resume the kind of schedule you had before. You may need to nurse more frequently for a while to build up your supply and comfort your baby. If you want to wean your baby before the separation, plan ahead, if possible, so that you can do it gradually.

If Your Baby Gets Sick

In most cases, breastfeeding is the best thing you can do for your sick baby. For one thing, it will provide her with protective antibodies. Because breast milk is extremely digestible, it's the ideal nutritional substance for a baby with a gastrointestinal disorder. Breast milk is probably the best fluid to give a baby with diarrhea, since the fat, carbohydrates, and proteins in your milk can be easily broken down in your infant's digestive tract, and its nutrients and antibodies are quickly absorbed into your infant's bloodstream.

If your baby has a cold, nurse her more frequently. If she can breathe comfortably, don't treat her stuffy or runny nose. But if she's having trouble breathing through her nose, and therefore having trouble breast-feeding, you can use nasal saline solution and a syringe to suction out mucus. Be sure to squeeze out the air in the bulb before putting it into the baby's nostril so that it doesn't shoot air into her nose. A humidifier may help a baby breathe more easily, and so can elevating her head by sliding a towel, blanket, or wedge under the head of the mattress (not directly under your baby's head). Do not give your under-two-year-old over-the-counter cold remedies (see box on page 227).

If your baby has to be hospitalized, ask for permission to stay with her and nurse her in the hospital. If she needs surgery, you should be able to nurse her up to three hours before the operation. If it will be impossible for you to nurse your baby, and if she'll be in the hospital longer than a week or two, rent a hospital-grade electric pump so that you can express your milk and resume breastfeeding when she returns home. See Chapter 11 for suggestions for pumping and feeding breast milk.

If your baby needs to be in the neonatal intensive care unit right after birth, many of the suggestions given for preterm babies in this chapter may apply.

If You Get Sick

If you catch a cold or come down with the flu, pneumonia, a urinary tract or respiratory tract infection, or intestinal upset, you can continue to nurse. In fact, doing so helps to protect your baby from the bacteria or virus that made you sick. By the time you showed symptoms, your baby had already been exposed to those organisms, and you had already begun to make the antibodies to fight them, and you passed them on in your milk. Be careful about any cold remedies you take, since some can be dangerous to your nursing baby (see Chapter 10).

If you have a condition that raises questions about your ability to nurse, or the advisability of your nursing, ask your doctor and your baby's doctor if it's safe to breastfeed. Also check with La Leche League (see the Resource Appendix), which is apt to have the most current information on medical issues. At this printing, recommendations are that you should not breastfeed if:

✤ You have active untreated tuberculosis (TB). You can start nursing once you have been on anti-TB medicine for one to two weeks.

✤ You have contracted chicken pox within two days before childbirth to five days afterward. You can start to nurse once your lesions have developed scabs.

✤ You have HIV or AIDS (see page 349).

✤ You are taking any medications or drugs that would not be safe for your baby (see Chapter 10).

If you must be hospitalized and your condition permits, you may be able to have your baby come to stay with you in your room or at least visit you. If this is impossible, ask your doctor to leave orders and make arrangements so you can pump your breasts regularly during your hospital stay. Meanwhile, your baby can be fed with the breast milk that you have previously expressed and frozen or with formula.

The following are some current recommendations for breastfeeding mothers with certain conditions.

Herpes

Two kinds of herpes virus that can be passed from mother to baby during vaginal delivery are cytomegalovirus (CMV) and herpes simplex virus (HSV). CMV, the commoner, less harmful kind, can also be transmitted through breast milk. This does not pose a problem to the typical full-term newborn; in fact, it may help the baby develop antibodies to the virus. However, CMV can pose a problem for preterm infants.

HSV, which carries more risks for an infant, does not seem to be transmitted through breast milk, but it can be passed to a baby who comes into direct contact with a herpes sore on the mother's body. HSV can cause cold sores or fever blisters on the lips, face, mouth, hands, or breast, or the same type of sore in the genital area. The virus can be spread through sexual relations with someone who has an active infection, or by contact with an infected person's open sore.

While much research still needs to be done on this condition, at this time the following guidelines seem useful:

❖ If you don't have herpes, don't have sexual relations with anyone in an active stage of the disease, especially while you're pregnant or breastfeeding.

❖ If you have already contracted herpes, get periodic exams and cultures before delivery.

❖ If you have an active outbreak before you give birth, or are in the stage just before sores are apt to break out, tell your doctor. It may be safest for you to have a cesarean birth.

❖ If you have an active outbreak after your baby is born, you may breastfeed if you do not have sores on your breast. See that your baby does not come into contact with any sores anywhere on your body or with clothing that has been worn over them. Wash your hands very carefully after you use the toilet, after you touch your sores, and before you hold your baby. When you hold your baby, drape a clean towel or robe over your lap. You don't need to wear gloves while you nurse.

❖ Consult your doctor and watch your baby closely for any symptoms that might indicate HSV infection.

❖ If you have sores on your breast, postpone nursing your newborn on that breast until the sores are fully healed. Until then, express or pump your milk to maintain your supply, and throw away milk pumped during your outbreak. Meanwhile, feed your baby on the other breast or by bottle or cup.

❖ If you have a sore on your mouth, don't kiss your baby—or anyone else.

❖ Your doctor may prescribe an antiviral drug like acyclovir or vidarabine. Continue to nurse while taking either of these—provided you don't have active lesions on your breast.

Hepatitis B

This virus appears in breast milk, but there's no evidence that it has ever been passed to a nursing infant. Therefore, there's no reason for mothers who carry this virus not to breastfeed. Chances are that the baby of a mother who has hepatitis B will have already been exposed to the virus during pregnancy or delivery.

All newborns now should receive immunization against hepatitis B immediately after birth. The baby of a hepatitis B carrier should receive both the active vaccine and the passive hepatitis B hyperimmune globulin. Even if the infant was not immunized, there's no reason for a mother who is a carrier not to breastfeed. Since each case is different, however, if you suspect or know that you have been exposed to hepatitis B, discuss your situation with your baby's doctor.

Hepatitis C

This virus may begin with a mild infection and flulike symptoms, or it may carry no symptoms at all for years. Then a person carrying the infection may begin to feel tired all the time, lose his or her appetite, become jaundiced, and suffer abdominal pain, nausea, and/or vomiting. Breastfed babies of mothers with hepatitis C have about the same incidence of the virus as do formula-fed infants. There's no evidence that breastfeeding increases the risk of an infant's acquiring the infection from the mother; those infants who have developed hepatitis C seem to have contracted it during pregnancy or childbirth.

Human Immunodeficiency Virus (HIV) or Acquired Immune Deficiency Syndrome (AIDS)

A mother who is HIV-positive—that is, who has been infected with the virus that can cause AIDS—or has AIDS can pass the virus to her child through her milk. Most public health advocates (including the American Academy of Pediatrics, the World Health Organization, and the U.S. Centers for Disease Control and Prevention) advise against breastfeeding by a mother with an AIDS or HIV infection. In developing countries, however, where clean water or safe formula are not available, exclusive breastfeeding is still the best option, and recent regimens of anti-HIV medications given to babies during the first 14 weeks of life have made this safer.

Diabetes

Breastfeeding is not only safe for diabetic mothers, it is recommended, since breastfeeding will help to protect their babies from developing diabetes themselves later in life.

If you use insulin, you'll probably use less while you're nursing, and in any case insulin use by the mother is safe for the nursing baby. You do need to be aware that you may be more susceptible to developing skin infections and mastitis, and your baby may be more likely to develop jaundice. Both these conditions are very treatable.

Stay in close touch with your obstetrician, your endocrinologist, and your baby's pediatrician to monitor your medicines, as well as your hormone levels and blood sugars, and your baby's progress.

Breast Cancer

As we've noted, breastfeeding tends to protect both mother and baby from developing breast cancer. Women who breastfeed are less likely to develop breast cancer before menopause. In China, where women routinely breastfeed for three years, breast cancer is also less common among older, postmenopausal women who nursed their babies.

Fortunately, breast cancer rarely occurs in pregnant or nursing women. In the rare event that a malignant tumor is found in a pregnant or lactating woman, its surgical removal should be carried out immediately. Waiting can be dangerous for the mother.

Fortunately, there's no evidence that women transmit any cancer-causing factors to their babies through breast milk.

❖ Breastfeeding can safely continue through most diagnostic tests—including mammogram, ultrasound, and biopsy. However, if radioactive isotope testing is performed, nursing has to be interrupted (see Chapter 10). The mother needs to express her milk and discard it until the radioactive elements are gone from her body. If a biopsy needs to be performed, the mother should ask her surgeon to avoid cutting the milk ducts.

❖ It's harder to get a good image in a mammogram during lactation and for four to six weeks after weaning because lactating breasts are quite dense. However, a skilled radiologist trained in reading exams given to breastfeeding women can often achieve good results. If your doctor urges you to wean your child so you can get a mammogram or a Mammotome (vacuum-assisted biopsy), you have a decision to make.

If there's a sound medical reason (for example, if you have a suspicious lump on your breast), you'll want to wean, or at least interrupt, breastfeeding. However, if your doctor just wants you to have a baseline mammogram because of your age or family history, consider your child's readiness for weaning or need for continued nursing, and discuss this with your doctor so that you can reach the wisest decision for you and your child.

❖ A woman who has had a breast surgically removed because of a diagnosis of breast cancer may continue to nurse from the other breast, with no apparent risk to her child. However, if she's receiving chemotherapy, she'll have to wean the baby, since the drugs used in this treatment may be dangerous for the baby.

At one time, physicians advised women who had breast cancer not to get pregnant and not to breastfeed, because both these activities were thought to stimulate hormones that seemed to activate cancer cells. Now these recommendations are rarely made, however, since several large studies have shown that pregnancy after diagnosis of breast cancer does not increase the chance of the cancer's recurrence and does not affect the woman's chance of survival.

✥ Although breast cancer is extremely rare in nursing women, it can happen. Missing a diagnosis of breast cancer during lactation can occur because lumps in the breast may be attributed to nursing-related causes and may not be sufficiently investigated. It's important to see a physician about any lump that remains unchanged for more than three days.

✥ A lump isn't the only symptom that can act as a warning signal.

One very rare but aggressive cancer is called inflammatory breast cancer because its main symptoms are swelling and redness of the breast. It's sometimes treated as an infection, and only when symptoms don't improve after taking antibiotics is the cancer diagnosed.

Another rare cancer is Paget's disease of the nipple, which first shows up as redness or crusting. If you have this kind of skin irritation on a nipple and it does not respond to treatment, see your doctor, who will probably be able to rule out Paget's disease.

Timely treatment is important for both these cancer types. This is why it's important to act quickly whenever you experience any symptoms.

✥ A galactocele, or milk-retention cyst (see page 324), is benign and does not require surgery.

If You Have Had Breast Surgery

If you have had surgery on one or both breasts for any reason, you may be able to breastfeed, depending on what kind of surgery you had and how it was done. If you had a mastectomy, you'll probably be able to nurse from the other breast. For specific information on this or any other breast surgery, ask your surgeon.

Even if you're doubtful, go ahead and try to breastfeed, unless you're undergoing chemotherapy. Lactation may well proceed normally. If it doesn't, you can always switch to formula. Meanwhile, watch your baby very closely to be sure he's getting enough milk and gaining weight appropriately, and to know whether you need to supplement breastfeeding. If you're currently considering any kind of elective breast surgery, wait until after your childbearing years if you want to be sure you can nurse your babies, since any kind of breast surgery can interfere with your production of milk.

Breast Augmentation

If you had silicone or saline implants to make your breasts larger, contact your surgeon before your baby's birth to say you want to breastfeed and ask for ways to minimize the effects of the surgery. If the implants don't come into contact with mammary tissue—and most do not—and if the duct system in your breasts remains intact after the surgery, you may be able to breastfeed.

Some augmentation techniques are less likely than others to damage the milk ducts. If the incision is made under the fold of the breast and the implant is placed beneath the mammary gland and under the muscle, the implant is less likely to interfere with breastfeeding. Women whose implants were inserted through an incision in the nipple area are more likely to have an inadequate milk supply.

There has been very little research into the safety of breast milk from women with implants of either kind. No objective scientific studies of the effects of implants on breastfed

children's health have been conducted. Some doctors believe that since infant formula contains *silicon,* any *silicone* in breast milk is unlikely to harm a baby. However, the silicone in implants is a manufactured compound and not identical to the chemical element silicon, which is in infant formula. In addition, small amounts of other chemicals and substances have been found in the milk of women who have silicone gel breast implants. One peer-reviewed published report found small but potentially dangerous levels of platinum in such women, and some of the women in the study reported health problems for themselves and for their breastfed babies.

Silicone breast implants are rubbery shells of silicone that are filled with silicone gel, and saline implants are rubbery shells of silicone filled with salt water. Either kind can rupture, usually after seven to twelve years or from unusual pressure. The FDA recommends that patients with silicone implants get magnetic resonance imaging (MRI) exams on a regular basis to check for any ruptures. If one is found, the implant should be removed. (Breast MRIs cost about $2,000 on average and are not covered by insurance if done because of cosmetic surgery.) Ask your surgeon what kind of implants you received, who manufactured them and when, and whether any complications have shown up with this type.

At this time, there is no clear evidence one way or the other about the safety of breast milk from women with implants. Although it is likely that nursing is safe for most babies of mothers with implants, research is needed to determine whether there are risks to some babies or risks with certain types of implants.

Some herbal remedies are marketed to increase breast size. These are unproven and possibly unsafe, and especially worrisome for pregnant or nursing women. Avoid them.

Breast Reduction

If you had surgery to make your breasts smaller and if the nipple/areola complex was not severed during the operation, you can probably breastfeed. While the newer procedures are more likely to permit breastfeeding than previous techniques did, there's still a chance that breast reduction may interfere with your ability to nurse. If, for example, your nipple has been removed and replaced on the reconstructed breast, the milk ducts and nerves will have been cut and breastfeeding may be impossible. You can try nursing, while monitoring your baby very closely to be sure she's getting enough milk.

Piercing and Tattooing

If you have had one or both nipples pierced, you should still be able to breastfeed. There might, however, be a problem if there was any scarring, either internal or external, or if an infection occurred at the time of piercing or during the initial healing. Occasionally, some milk leaks through the site of the piercing, but since the hole is usually small, this shouldn't interfere with nursing. If there's any question about whether your baby is nursing well (for signs of suckling and adequate milk intake, see Chapter 6), consult a lactation specialist.

If you wear a nipple ring, remove it while you're breastfeeding. This is especially important if the ring is large, since a large ring can prevent a baby from being able to get his mouth around the nipple and areola as fully as he needs to to latch on properly.

Removal of even a smaller ring will make nursing easier for your baby, and of course will eliminate any possibility of your baby choking on the ring or swallowing it. Also, body jewelry can hurt your baby's soft gums, tongue, and palate if left in during nursing. It's best to put it away throughout lactation, since constantly removing it and putting it in can introduce germs.

Tattoos on one or both breasts shouldn't pose an obstacle to breastfeeding, either, especially if you got them more than a year before you gave birth and didn't have any problems right afterward. The pigment isn't a problem; it's the risk of the procedure, which could predispose you to infectious disease, especially HIV and hepatitis.

If you're thinking about piercing or tattooing, play it safe and wait until after you have weaned your baby. Either procedure can provide a gateway to infection, and you don't want to expose your baby to any risk. You'll have plenty of time in your life to decorate your body, but the opportunity to nurse your baby is precious and time-limited.

Twins and More

When Bobbi McCaughey told the doctors caring for her septuplets that she wanted to provide breast milk for them, the neonatalogist in charge said, "We are committed to providing as much milk as she is able to come up with to all of the babies." This indeed showed confidence in the benefits of breast milk! Even though it would be a major challenge for this mother to breastfeed all seven babies, whatever breast milk these tiny babies received would be a bonus.

But what about twins? Movie star Angelina Jolie's determination to nurse her newborn babies attracted attention—but that was more because of her fame, not the feat of feeding twins. If you deliver two babies, one question is moot: You don't have to wonder if you should offer one or both breasts at a feeding. You have been designed for just this possibility. Furthermore, since your breasts operate on a supply-and-demand principle, they will produce ample supplies of milk for both babies. Since babies born in multiples are likely to be small, they derive special benefits from breast milk.

A common chorus from mothers of multiples is that getting through the first few weeks is hard, but it does get easier. As with other new moms, if you can get help with your other duties so you can spend much of your time nursing, life will be much easier. One popular accessory for these moms is a breastfeeding pillow; another is a hospital-grade pump.

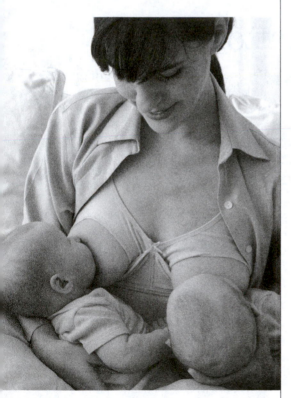

A combination of positions, like this mix of cradle and clutch, sometimes works for mom and babies.

Many moms, like Jolie, try nursing both babies simultaneously for most early feedings. The actress studied books that taught her positioning techniques, like the double football hold. After she weaned the twins, she said of simultaneous nursing, "You think, *Ah, if anybody can do that, I can do that.* [But] it's a lot harder than it looks in the books. I did that a few times, [but mostly] I would take turns. It just takes a long time."

Another nursing mom found it easier to transition from separate to simultaneous nursing. "At first I nursed my twin boys separately," Ellen said. "This gave me a chance to spend time alone with each of them and create a special bond. Later, when all three of us became latch experts, I nursed them at the same time. I would still be able to look both of them in the eyes and talk or sing to them, and I spent half as much time nursing."

Others can't even imagine feeding two at once. In any case, you'll want to nurse them individually occasionally, so that each one will have a chance from time to time to enjoy your undivided attention. Then there will be times when one twin is desperately hungry—and the other sound asleep. As a general rule, let the hungrier twin set the pattern. When you're about to feed her, wake her twin at the same time. This works best, of course, if both babies are about the same size.

Try to alternate breasts and babies, so that the same twin doesn't always drink at the same fount. This way, if one baby nurses more vigorously than the other, both your breasts will be

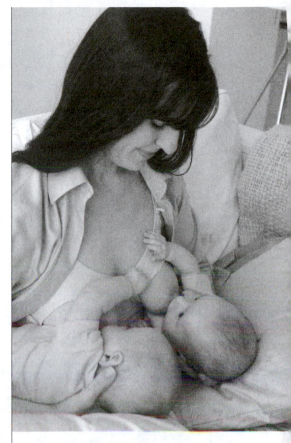

Some mothers prefer to nurse twins at the same time. This mom is nursing both babies in the clutch hold.

stimulated more or less equally. Says our friend Leslie, "I kept a chart to keep track of which baby fed on which side first, when, and for how long."

You'll work out your own individual schedule. Some mothers nurse twins or even triplets totally, never giving any of the babies a bottle. Others alternate bottles of formula right from the start, rotating between breast and formula. Thus, baby A gets the breast at one feeding, baby B the bottle; they switch at the next feeding. You need to weigh the benefits of breast milk for your babies with the demands on your own energy and time, and do what's best. For a special source of help for mothers of multiples, see the Resource Appendix.

You'll see, too, how long you want to continue nursing. Early in her pregnancy, Ellen planned to breastfeed until her babies were six months old, when she would have to return to work. "Now that the boys are five months old, I'm rethinking my plan," she says. "Breastfeeding has created such a unique and special bond with my boys that I'm not ready to stop quite yet."

Nursing Two Babies at the Same Time

When breastfeeding two babies simultaneously, position is everything. The first few times you nurse, ask someone to help you get the babies set in one of the positions described below. Experiment until you and the babies are comfortable. Find a comfortable armchair and a couple of firm pillows. Then try one of these:

❖ Half-recline and lay each baby on his side or stomach lengthwise along your body.

❖ Sit up and tuck each baby under an arm, heads resting on firm pillows on your lap and feet by your back (the clutch hold).

❖ Hold baby A on your lap and criss-cross baby B across baby A's body.

❖ Hold baby A on your lap and tuck baby B under your arm.

Nursing Through a Pregnancy and Tandem Nursing Afterward

If you become pregnant while you're nursing, your baby may decide to wean, either because your milk tastes different or because there's less of it. Or you may take the initiative in weaning your nursling because of breast or nipple pain, because you're tired, or because you're uncomfortable with the idea. Around the world, a new pregnancy is among the most common reasons for weaning. Some women do, however, continue to breastfeed throughout pregnancy. In 2002, the American Academy of Family Physicians said, "Breastfeeding during a subsequent pregnancy is not unusual. If the pregnancy is normal and the mother is healthy, breastfeeding during pregnancy is the mother's decision."

Some moms continue to nurse both the older child and the newborn infant afterward. This practice is known as tandem nursing. Why do mothers do this? They cite the continued needs of the older child, whose emotional need for nursing is heightened by the arrival of the new baby. The mothers themselves sometimes don't feel ready to sever the nursing tie with the older child. Still, tandem nursing mothers often have ambivalent feelings, sometimes resenting the older child, questioning the wisdom of what they're doing, and dealing with the doubled demands on their bodies.

Some of the challenges facing the mother include the need for extra nutrition and extra rest, which she needs first because of the pregnancy and then because of the nursing infant. While pregnant, she needs to find comfortable nursing positions and maternity clothes compatible with nursing. Women with a history of miscarriage are often advised to wean their nursing babies before becoming pregnant again, since some reports have indicated that nipple stimulation can induce labor.

In an effort to increase the milk supply that may have lessened during pregnancy, some women are tempted to take herbal or pharmaceutical agents. However, these are controversial for any nursing mother and are generally not recommended in pregnancy. What the mom needs to do is to continue taking her prenatal/postnatal vitamins and eat a healthy diet.

After the new baby is born, if you decide to tandem nurse, you need to ensure that the new baby gets his rightful share of the colostrum and milk. Be aware of the danger of cross-infection between the children (thrush, for instance, can be passed back and forth between tandem nursers). Most women who nurse a baby and a toddler nurse the infant first. Some use explanations, agreements, and delaying tactics to reduce the number of times the older child nurses. (Some of these are suggested in Chapter 17.)

Tandem nursing isn't a decision to be undertaken lightly, and it isn't for everyone. There's no evidence, however, that the practice is harmful to the new baby, either while in the womb or after birth, if his needs are kept paramount.

Milk Banks

When babies cannot get enough, or any, of their own mother's milk, and formula cannot provide the nutrition they need, these babies are sometimes nurtured with breast milk from a milk bank. These banks carefully screen volunteer donors; collect and process milk; and dispense it to infants and children in need, usually only upon receiving a doctor's prescription for the milk. Donor milk is transported frozen, and then the milk from several donors is pooled and pasteurized (heat-treated to kill bacteria and viruses). After processing, the milk is refrozen, a sample is tested for bacteria growth, and the batch is then shipped frozen by overnight express to hospitals or homes.

Donors are not paid and recipients are charged only a processing fee (about three dollars an ounce), but no one is denied milk if they can't pay. Rarely, insurance companies pick up some of the cost. The reasons for babies' receiving donor milk include the following: prematurity, failure to thrive, immunologic deficiency, allergy to formula, infectious diseases, and some inborn disorders such as phenylketonuria (PKU). In addition, some adoptive parents seek, and sometimes receive prescriptions for, donor milk.

Lactating women who want to donate their extra milk are screened for health behaviors and communicable diseases—like tuberculosis, HIV, hepatitis, and venereal diseases—to make sure their milk is safe. They must be nonsmokers, not use drugs or certain medicines, and not consume alcohol or certain excluded medications within a specified period. As of this writing, there are only ten milk banks in the United States and Canada, according to the Human Milk Banking Association of North America. To request or donate milk, contact your closest milk bank (see the Resource Appendix).

Breastfeeding Another Woman's Baby

Giving an infant milk from a woman who is not her mother is a practice that has gone on for millennia and is documented as far back as 2250 B.C. in Babylonia when the Code of Hammurabi specified the qualities needed for a good wet nurse, a woman paid to nurse another woman's infant. In eras when many women died in childbirth, wet nursing was sometimes the only way to keep babies alive, and it's still fairly common in developing countries. Also, wet nurses were employed for centuries by women who could not, or did not want to, breastfeed their own babies.

Early in the twentieth century, with the development of safe, convenient artificial baby milk and the awareness that disease can be transmitted to babies through breastfeeding, wet nursing fell out of favor in developed countries. In recent years, as more women have become convinced of the benefits of breast milk, another trend has come to the fore—that of cross-nursing, in which women nurse the babies of friends or relatives with no money changing hands. Other women and some businesses advertise breast milk for sale on the Internet, sometimes for one or two dollars an ounce.

Although cross-nursing's advocates describe it as a way of helping friends and family, the practice carries serious risks for babies of any age. No matter how well you may know your friend or even your sister, you don't want to run the risk of harming your baby, and so if you want to go this route, you need to be sure that anyone who might be nursing your baby is carefully screened for all the conditions that the milk banks scrutinize for.

Relactation and Nursing an Adopted Baby

Sometimes a woman decides, or is advised, not to breastfeed her newborn infant; or she begins to nurse and then stops for one reason or another. Then, as soon as one week or as late as several months later, she wants to nurse—either because her baby has grown stronger and is now able to nurse, because he has a digestive or allergic problem that makes it difficult for him to take formula, or for some other reason. In such a case, it is often possible to initiate or reinitiate breastfeeding. This process is known as relactation.

In other cases, women who have adopted babies have been able to lactate, even if they have never been pregnant or haven't been pregnant for years. This process is called induced lactation.

Neither of these endeavors is easy. As Elizabeth Hormann, an adoptive breastfeeding mother and a lactation consultant, writes in *Breastfeeding an Adopted Baby and Relactation,* "It requires time, strong commitment, a good bit of patience, and as much support as you can muster." Both also require very close observation of the baby to be sure he is gaining weight properly.

It's quite likely that you won't be able to fulfill all of your baby's needs for milk. Many women who have made the effort, however, have been happy with their decision, especially if they look at it not for its value as a feeding method, but for the ways in which it can enhance the mother-baby relationship.

One mom talks about the "psychological calories" she has given her baby, which is the most important aspect of this kind of nursing. If you hold up quantifiable measures like the amount of milk you produce or the length of time you nurse your baby, you may be disappointed and frustrated. Based on several studies of women who have done this, the guidelines given in the box on pages 360–361 should help you and your baby to achieve a happy nursing relationship. You may want to talk to your obstetrician or a lactation consultant, as well.

Succeeding at Induced Lactation or Relactation

❖ Ask yourself whether you'll be happy with the experience of nurturing your baby at your breast, and not necessarily completely nourishing her from your breast. If so, you're likely to have a more positive experience than if you have your heart set on providing a set amount of milk. It's rare in Western countries for all of an adoped baby's nutritional needs to be met with induced lactation and it may even be difficult for biological mothers to relactate.

❖ Be prepared for a stressful first few weeks, during which time your baby may resist suckling at the breast, your milk may be slow in coming in, and you'll be nursing almost around the clock and supplementing your baby's diet with formula.

❖ Find a support system, consisting of people who will encourage and help you through the difficult days. These people can include your husband or partner, doctor, lactation consultant, La Leche League leader, and, ideally, another woman who either relactated or nursed an adopted baby. You can find some of this support online.

❖ You'll find it easiest to relactate or induce lactation if your baby is under three months old.

❖ Expect initial resistance from your baby, who's used to getting milk some other way. It may take ten days or longer for her to nurse well, but after that she's very likely to become an avid nurser.

❖ If your baby resists strongly, feed her another way and try again another time.

❖ Nurse your baby frequently, whenever she shows any signs of hunger. Don't wait until your baby begins to cry, which is a late sign of hunger and is likely to result in her rejecting the breast.

In one study, most of the relactating babies nursed eight times a day, at intervals of two to three hours, with two night feedings. (This is an average; some babies need to nurse more often than this at the beginning.) The average duration of each feeding was about 20 to 25 minutes.

❖ Nipple stimulation is the most important mechanism for bringing in your milk. The best kind of stimulation is your baby's suckling. Other techniques include breast massage and breast pumps or hand-expression.

✤ The most popular form of supplementing the baby's diet is the use of a nursing supplementer (see Chapter 15 and the Resource Appendix) during efforts to induce lactation. This assures your baby of adequate nutrition while providing stimulation to your nipples. Many women who considered their experience highly successful continued to use a supplementer throughout the course of breastfeeding.

✤ Follow the same practices that encourage all breastfeeding: close contact (lots of it, skin to skin), frequent feedings, and rest and help for the mother. The success of induced lactation and relactation in developing countries rests on the expectation that all babies will be breastfed and on the practices that support nursing. While mothers in the West cannot duplicate the cultural milieus of other societies, we can adopt some of their practices.

✤ Monitor your baby very carefully for adequate weight gain. The suggestions given in the section beginning on page 123 will help you and the doctor assess whether your baby is being well nourished enough for healthy development.

Helpful Techniques

✤ Breastfeed frequently.

✤ Increase your fluid intake and the amount of protein in your diet.

✤ Rest as much as possible, and lie down to nurse when you can.

✤ Stroke your baby while she's nursing to help you relax and let down your milk.

✤ Provide as much skin contact as possible. (See the description of kangaroo care earlier in this chapter.)

✤ Put a little pumped breast milk or formula on your nipple and areola to lure your baby onto the breast by showing her how good it tastes.

✤ See the suggestions on page 333 for encouraging a baby who's gone on a nursing strike.

Techniques That Are Not Helpful

✤ Letting the baby go hungry to try to encourage her to nurse.

✤ For adoptive mothers, trying to stimulate the breasts with the nursing infants of friends (those babies usually refuse to suckle at a breast that's not producing milk).

Babies with Special Needs

It's acutely painful if your baby is born with a medical condition or physical limitation that will greatly impact the child's life. You need to deal with your grief over your baby's special circumstances and your deep disappointment at not being able to care for the baby in the ways you had expected to. In a case like this, both you and your partner will benefit from getting help both in coping with your feelings and taking care of your baby. Consulting a psychotherapist and making contact with other parents in similar situations are good steps to take.

If your baby's condition makes breastfeeding difficult or impossible, you can take comfort in knowing that even babies who can't get any or all of their nutrition from breastfeeding can usually receive the benefits of your good milk, which is even more important for these infants. Health professionals with expertise in your baby's condition can assist you with learning to care for your baby and, if possible, to breastfeed. Some helpful information is listed in the Resource and Website Appendixes, and a search on the Internet for a particular condition can yield resources from special-interest organizations that offer assistance to parents of babies with a variety of conditions. These groups can often refer parents to lactation consultants experienced in working with children with special needs. In many cases, the neonatologist caring for your baby will be able to refer you to other professionals for other kinds of help.

Cleft Lip or Palate

Some infants are born with a cleft, or opening, in which parts of the mouth did not fuse properly during prenatal development. This congenital condition is usually corrected with surgery at three to six months of age, or when the baby weighs at least ten pounds.

Until then, parents have to adapt their feeding methods to the baby's special needs. For a baby with a sizable cleft palate, in which the split is in the roof of the mouth, the opening between the mouth and the nasal cavity prevents the baby from creating the suction necessary to take in milk from the breast, or from an ordinary bottle. Although some of these babies can nurse from the breast to some extent, most of their nutrition usually needs to come from pumped breast milk or formula via specially designed bottles. However they're fed, they need to be held in a fairly upright position.

Babies with a cleft lip or gum or small clefts of the palate can often breastfeed, since the mother may be able to close the opening in the lip with her finger or her breast may be full enough to close off the space. Sometimes an obturator, a plastic plate that completes palate closure, is put in place to help a baby feed.

Down Syndrome

Babies born with this chromosomal disorder, which causes mental retardation and a number of health problems, can usually nurse at the breast. They benefit from breastfeeding, which employs the same motor skills used for speech and can help strengthen the jaw and facial muscles, and therefore help them to speak better in the future.

Down syndrome babies often need extra help because of their low muscle tone. Their lip, tongue, and cheek muscles may not move in a coordinated way, they sometimes have trouble getting a tight seal on the nipple, and they may have trouble swallowing. A lactation consultant, a speech therapist, or a feeding therapist can often suggest ways to help these babies nurse.

Hypoglycemia

When the rate at which the body *uses* glucose, the sugar in blood, is greater than the body's ability to *produce* glucose, hypoglycemia, or low blood sugar, can result. The condition is rare in healthy full-term babies and, except for babies at high risk for this condition, can usually be prevented by breastfeeding early and often. Babies at risk include very small or very large newborns, preterm and low-birthweight infants, those born to diabetic mothers, and babies who had a stressful birth or are sick. For these infants, their blood sugar levels are usually closely followed in the hospital nursery. Like the advice given to hypoglycemic adults—eating small, frequent, high-protein meals—the best approach for infants is to nurse ten to twelve times a day in the first few days after birth, so they receive bounteous amounts of colostrum.

Phenylketonuria (PKU)

As we noted in Chapter 5, newborns are routinely screened for this disorder in which the infant cannot produce the enzyme that lets the liver process phenylalanine, an amino acid essential for brain development. Babies who test positive should receive a followup test, and if this one is also positive, they should immediately be referred to a clinic whose practitioners are experienced in treating PKU. Infants with PKU can be breastfed, but they will also require one of the special PKU formulas that do not contain phenylalanine.

Galactosemia

Infants with this disorder lack an enzyme that allows their bodies to use lactose, the sugar in milk. Since breast milk is high in lactose, these babies cannot breastfeed and need a special formula. If a baby shows symptoms like vomiting, diarrhea, or failure to thrive, a test for galactosemia may be ordered. Since a false-positive reading sometimes shows up in warm weather, the baby should be tested at least two times. In fact, any positive test should be redone.

Heart Disease

Babies born with cardiac problems usually need extra nutrients and calories, so that they can gain enough weight. Their hearts may have to pump faster, and they may need to breathe more rapidly. Some of these babies can be exclusively breastfed, but others require extra nutrients in addition to breast milk. Feeding may be a problem because babies with heart problems often lack energy to suck efficiently, but once stabilized on medication they may develop a stronger suck.

Whether or not your special-needs baby can nurse at your breast, take comfort in knowing that you will do whatever you can to help him develop to his full potential.

Beyond Breastfeeding

*"Weaning from the breast happened so gradually
and naturally I hardly noticed when my child nursed for
the 'last' time. The relationship that was forged
during breastfeeding continues today—long past that
'final' nursing. To me, that's the legacy of breastfeeding."*

MELISSA Huntingdon, Tennessee

Y ou've known from the first time you nursed your beautiful newborn that breastfeeding would not last forever—even though
sometimes over these weeks, or months, or years, you may have
felt that it would. You've known that one day this child who at first depended
on you for all her nourishment and all her comforting would reach a stage
when she—and you—would leave your breastfeeding days behind.

As part of the weaning process, and while she's still breastfeeding, your child will be eating other foods and getting nutrition from other sources. Let's take a look at some of these other sources of nutrients.

Vitamins

Most of your child's vitamins will come through your milk, and later through the food he eats, rather than from vitamin drops or pills. Some vitamins, however, cannot always be obtained through diet. Some controversy exists in the medical community about the extent to which breastfed babies need vitamin supplementation, and you and your doctor may hold opinions different from ours. Our recommendations are summarized in the box on the facing page.

Vitamin D

During the first six months, your breastfed baby should receive a daily supplement of 200 IU (international units) of vitamin D. The only babies who do *not* need vitamin D supplementation are those drinking at least 17 ounces (500 ml) of vitamin D–fortified formula daily. Even if your breastfed baby does receive some supplementary bottles, she is probably not getting this much formula.

Vitamin D is especially important to help your child absorb calcium and phosphorus, essential elements for bone and tooth growth and development. Both you and your child need this vitamin, which appears in only tiny amounts in any food, including breast milk. Vitamin D is nicknamed the "sunshine" vitamin, since it's manufactured by our bodies through normal exposure to sunlight. Of course, with concerns about the risk of skin cancer, it's critical not to overdo the amount of sunlight exposure a baby gets (see pages 176–177 in Chapter 8). Talk to your baby's doctor about the precautions you should take to protect her from overexposure.

Some mothers and children get enough vitamin D from sunshine, but many do not. Dark-complexioned people don't absorb as much from the sun because of their deeper pigmentation. High levels of air pollution block transmission of vitamin D to residents of some urban areas, and mothers and babies who don't go out of doors often, or who are almost completely covered by clothing or sunscreen when they do, lessen their direct exposure to sunlight. If you're not in any of these categories, you probably don't need a vitamin D supplement, but again, taking it in the recommended dose can't hurt. The combination drops are harmless, inexpensive, and convenient. You need adequate vitamin D throughout pregnancy and lactation. If your baby's doctor recommends it for her, she can begin taking it from the seventh to tenth day of life. If your doctor doesn't mention vitamin D supplementation, ask him or her about it.

Recommended Vitamin and Mineral Supplementation for Breastfed Babies

This chart lists the vitamins and minerals that babies need at different stages of life.

CHILD'S AGE	MULTIVITAMIN/ MULTIMINERAL	VITAMIN D	IRON[1]	FLUORIDE[2]
Full-term Infant	No	Yes	No	No
Preterm Infant	Yes	Yes	Yes	No
Healthy Baby (over 6 months)[3]	No	Sometimes[4]	Sometimes[4]	Yes
High-risk Baby (over 6 months)[3]	Yes	Yes	Yes	Yes
Healthy Child (over 2 years)[3]	No	No	No	Yes
High-risk Child (over 2 years)[3]	Yes	No	Sometimes[4]	Yes

1. Iron-fortified cereal is the preferred form of supplementation except in the case of preterm infants, who can receive multivitamin drops with iron.

2. If your child drinks water with a fluoride content of more than 0.3 ppm (parts per million), supplementation is not needed.

3. These recommendations apply if the child is eating a well-balanced diet of solid foods at this time.

4. Ask your doctor whether your baby should receive the indicated supplement.

Fluoride

If your community's water supply contains less than 0.3 ppm (parts per million) of fluoride, your older baby (over six months) will benefit from a fluoride supplement. If he doesn't drink much water (and as a breastfed baby, he doesn't need water in the early months), a fluoride supplement may be beneficial even if your water contains a higher level than this. You can find out the level of fluoride in your water by calling your local health department. Then ask your doctor whether you should supplement. The fluoride in the water that a nursing mother drinks probably does not pass through her milk in amounts sufficient to help her child develop decay-resistant teeth. Since research has shown that children who get fluoride supplements (either in the water or in drops) develop fewer cavities, you'll want your child to have this advantage. However, too much is not good, since it can affect his tooth development. If you do give a fluoride supplement, it may be included in his vitamin drops and should be offered starting at six months of age.

Iron

Although breast milk contains little iron, what it does contain is present in a very easily absorbable form. This iron, plus the stores your baby is born with, will usually see her through her first six months. After this time, she'll probably need extra iron. If your baby's hemoglobin levels are low at the six-month checkup, the doctor may prescribe an iron supplement.

One way to provide extra iron to your baby is by feeding her an iron-fortified baby cereal, which is usually the first solid food your pediatrician will suggest. Babies absorb the iron in cereal better than the iron in drops. Because of the danger of choking, the American Academy of Pediatrics recommends that babies be fed cereal from a spoon and not from a bottle, except in cases of gastroesophageal reflux (GER; see discussion on page 155). Should your doctor recommend feeding cereal from a bottle, she or he will give you clear directions on how to do it. Basically, it involves making the cereal thinner and the nipple hole bigger.

After baby cereal, meats and other iron-rich foods can be added to your baby's diet. Your doctor will check for iron-deficiency anemia at six months and at twelve months and will tell you if you need to give your baby an iron supplement. If you do offer an iron supplement, it will be absorbed best if given with a fruit juice that's rich in vitamin C.

Weaning Your Child

Weaning can take many different forms, depending on when it's begun, how it's begun, and who initiates it—the mother or the child. This chapter is about making the transition of weaning as easy as possible for both of you.

What exactly is weaning? The most global definition involves the process by which your child stops depending on your milk for nourishment and eventually stops nursing at the breast completely. This process starts the minute you give your baby something besides your breast milk and ends when you are no longer nursing at all. The usual progression includes four phases: (1) accustoming your baby to small amounts of foods other than breast milk before they are needed for nutrition; (2) adding foods when breast milk can no longer meet all your child's nutritional needs; (3) replacing breast milk with other foods; and, finally, (4) stopping breastfeeding completely. (Sometimes this progression is cut short because of the need to wean abruptly, a situation we discuss on page 376.)

Weaning has an emotional meaning, too, one that's just as significant as the nutritional one. Weaning is one of the first steps in a child's becoming independent of his mother. It's hard to look at your infant or toddler, who still needs so much care, and think of his moving toward independence. But this is only the beginning of a long path that every child must take to achieve maturity. And it's a path that must be walked by every mother, too.

Many babies accept, or even drive, gradual weaning fairly easily. Sometimes it's harder for the mother to wean than it is for the child. Other babies love—or seem to need—nursing so much that they want to continue long past the time their mothers think it's time to stop.

The end of breastfeeding is bittersweet: Together with the relief and the freedom of not being tied to your child's nursing needs—which even the happiest nursing mother is apt to feel when she stops breastfeeding—comes the sadness you may experience from giving up this precious way of relating to your child and from no longer being needed in the same special way. But even as you feel the end of one era, you know that you are ushering in others, in which your relationship with your child will develop in innumerable ways. As a child gets older, nursing is more about a relationship than a food, and if that relationship has been forged through meeting the child's needs, then the relationship continues long after the official end of breastfeeding.

Now let's talk about the when and the how of weaning.

When Should You Wean Your Child from the Breast?

While you'll probably be asked "How long do you plan to breastfeed?" more times than you care to think about, there's no reason why you have to set an advance deadline for the end of breastfeeding, any more than you set a deadline for the length of time you plan to wheel your baby in a stroller. You'll stop nursing when the time seems right for both you and your child.

This is a topic on which many people have strong opinions (which they don't hesitate to voice), but few have any evidence to base them on. There's no single optimal time for weaning, as we can see from the great range of weaning ages in cultures around the world.

The AAP recommends nursing for at least a year and as long thereafter as mother and child want to continue. Both the World Health Organization and UNICEF recommend breastfeeding for at least two years. In many countries, babies are routinely nursed well into the second or third year of life. However, even if you cannot or do not want to nurse for many months, whatever breastfeeding you do offer your baby will go far to provide a good start in her life.

During the first couple of days after birth, infants get the immunological advantages of colostrum, and they continue to receive immunological benefits from breast milk at least through the toddler years. During roughly the first six months, babies can usually satisfy all their nutritional needs from breast milk; at some time after this, the combination of breast milk and various other foods will provide their essential nutrients. By nine months, they usually have enough teeth and the intestinal maturity to handle a wide variety of foods. They are still, of course, dependent on their parents for many of the essentials of life, but from a nutritional aspect, they need no longer be dependent solely on their mothers' milk.

The emotional benefits that a mother and child derive from breastfeeding are just as valid, however, at two months, six months, nine months, one year, or later. You are still maintaining a special intimate relationship with your child, still able to comfort her at your breast when she's sick, unhappy, or in an unfamiliar situation. You're still able to forget the cares of the day for those peaceful minutes while the two of you are a nursing couple.

If you want to continue nursing for emotional reasons rather than nutritional ones, there's no need to stop at any specified time. Your decision will depend on your own unique situation. If you have a challenging child who gets upset easily and nursing is the most reliable way to calm her; if she finds it hard to get to sleep; or if you have to be at work all day and want to offer her something that her caregiver can't give, you may want to nurse longer. If, on the other hand, you decide to or have to stop nursing before six months, you are still a successful nursing mother. Any breastfeeding is better than none at all.

Making the Decision to Wean

You and your child together constitute the nursing couple, and either one of

you may begin the weaning process. Under child-led weaning, you continue to nurse until your child loses interest. This may happen toward the end of the first year, or when your baby begins to walk, or later.

Babies sometimes reject the breast completely and refuse to nurse, no matter how hard you try to hold their interest. One may make a big joke of biting: He gets into a nursing position, laughs, and then bites the breast that feeds him. Another may nurse eagerly for a minute or two and then—just as soon as his mother's milk lets down—pull away and show no further interest. Or you may have a jolly gymnast on your hands (and your lap)—a baby who starts to stand up while nursing, then shows off some of his other acrobatic tricks.

If you think that your baby may be on a temporary nursing strike, try the suggestions in the box on page 333. If you've given it a fair trial and none of these work, if you have talked with a lactation consultant or a La Leche League leader, and if your baby is more than eight months old, he may be letting you know that he's ready to say good-bye to his nursing days.

But suppose that your baby or toddler has shown no signs of giving up the breast, but you are restless. Your child eagerly takes an occasional bottle, eats healthy portions of solid food, and drinks from a cup. You have gone back to work or school, are busy caring for older children, or have resumed other activities. You look at your nursling and, with some impatience, wonder, *Is he ever going to stop?* How, then, do you set a time for weaning?

At this point, you have options. You can continue to breastfeed, accepting the fact that your child still benefits from the experience and that this is one way to meet his needs.

But if you find yourself resenting your child's nursing, you may be doing both of you a favor by taking a gentle initiative toward weaning. Otherwise, your child will sense your annoyance. It seems a shame to spoil months of happy breastfeeding by continuing to nurse out of a sense of duty, when you can be a better mother if you feel happy and comfortable about what you're doing. It's better for a child to drink a bottle happily than to nurse at a grudging breast. Sometimes just knowing that you have begun the process of weaning will enable you to continue to nurse happily for another few months.

Extended Breastfeeding

On the other hand, suppose you would really like to continue breastfeeding past your child's first, second, or even third birthday, but are embarrassed by the idea. Somehow friends, relatives, and perfect strangers criticize a late nurser more than they do the toddler or preschooler of the same age who carries a bottle around. In our society, women who nurse babies older than a year are often "closet" nursers, who hide what they're doing to avoid

There's no "right age" to wean a baby; nursing is good as long as both mom and child want it to continue.

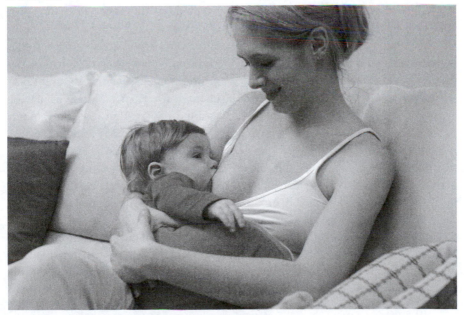

"When Are You Going to Stop Nursing?"

You can toss off this question with a good-natured smile and a light response. Some of our favorite answers among those we've heard:

❖ "Oh, in about five minutes."

❖ "When he can call to order takeout."

❖ "When she grows breasts of her own."

❖ "When he finds a pair he likes better than mine."

❖ "When his mustache gets in the way."

❖ "When she'd rather have a chocolate milkshake."

❖ "Till she starts dating."

❖ "Well, I plan to accompany him to college, so I can continue to breastfeed there—especially before his exams."

Then there's always:

❖ "Why do you want to know?"

having to defend the practice. Critics sometimes maintain that long-term nursing moms impose breastfeeding on their children, but one researcher who studied 114 breastfeeding children two years old or older found that the children actively sought breastfeeding. When asked why they breastfed and what they felt like when they breastfed, the children said it made them feel happy, good, or nice—and they liked the taste, with some pronouncing it "as good as chocolate" and "better than ice cream."

You may also wonder whether nursing beyond infancy harms your child psychologically. But there's no evidence that extended breastfeeding makes children more dependent on their parents or harms them in any other way. Some lactation experts phrase the question differently—whether *not* nursing beyond infancy may be a form of emotional deprivation. The AAP has stated, "There is no

upper limit to the duration of breast-feeding and no evidence of psychologic or developmental harm from breast-feeding into the third year of life or longer."

Although we haven't found any scientific research comparing children weaned at different ages, our own observations and those of many other child-care professionals suggest that children who were nursed as toddlers or preschoolers seem no different psychologically from children who were weaned earlier. Provided the mother-child relationship is warm and loving, the length of breastfeeding—or even the fact of breastfeeding itself—does not seem to be an all-important factor in a child's healthy psychological development.

One problem that your child may encounter if she is still nursing at a later age than is typical in our society is teasing or ridicule from relatives, neighbors, or even strangers. If this happens, you can speak to the people doing the teasing, asking them to talk to you and not your child about any feelings they have about the appropriateness of your child's nursing. You can also speak to your child directly, reassuring her that it's perfectly fine for her to continue nursing, but that some people don't understand how important this is to children. You can also give her the option of nursing in private to avoid public comment. If she wants to give up nursing, you can let her know that this is fine with you, that this is a decision she can certainly make.

Whatever your choice, when people ask you "What? Still nursing?" or, on the other hand, exclaim "You stopped already?" you might point out that the average age of weaning worldwide is between two and four years. You might also share that WHO and UNICEF both recommend nursing until age two or later. Or you might answer that you think this is a decision every nursing couple needs to make for themselves and that you feel that your choice is the best one for you and your child.

If you don't want to go into all of this, you can always use humor. The box on page 372 lists some retorts that women who practice extended breastfeeding have come up with. They represent ways to end a conversation you don't want to be having.

How Should You Wean?

There may not be a right time to wean, but there is definitely a right way—gradually if possible, sympathetically, and with a loving attitude. Weaning is a natural process; the natural way to help it along is to do it little by little, over a period of some weeks or even months.

Gradual weaning is best for both of you. If you wean slowly, you should have little or no discomfort from milk pressure. If you can possibly avoid the physical and emotional discomfort that would result from weaning cold turkey, do so. If there's no alternative, see "Sudden Weaning" on page 376.

You'll want to make yourself as available as possible to your child during the weaning process. Since he's losing something he has valued greatly—the pleasure of suckling at your breast—he needs the reassurance of your love and comforting. If you can devote extra time to him now, this should be heartening. While you don't need to feel guilty or apologetic, you do want to recognize the adjustment he's making and, through your loving understanding, help him make it more smoothly.

Child-Led Weaning

If you're still enjoying breastfeeding and are in no hurry to stop, but feel that weaning would be appropriate at this time in your child's life, you can let your child lead the way. One phrase that governs the process for many mothers is "Don't offer, don't refuse."

This way, you nurse when your child asks to, but you don't suggest it at other times. While it sometimes seems hard to believe, even the most eager nurser will eventually find other activities and foods and comforts that are more interesting than nursing. No child nurses forever. With an older child, the end of nursing sometimes happens so gradually that you may not even think of it as weaning. One day, you may suddenly realize that it's been several days since you've nursed. Typically, your child may ask to nurse a few more times, but by that time you may have no milk and the charm will be gone. Still a loving couple, you're no longer a nursing couple.

Mother-Led Weaning

If you're ready to wean, but your child hasn't shown any sign of losing interest, you may want to start the ball rolling yourself.

Try to initiate weaning at a time when your child doesn't have to make other adjustments. If he's teething or has a cold, if you've just gone back to work, if there's a new babysitter, if the family has just moved, or if there's some other major disruption of routine, put off the weaning for a few weeks. It's always easier to manage only one change at a time.

✤ Pinpoint the nursing session your child shows the least interest in, probably the early evening or noontime feeding. Eliminate this one first. Using the "don't offer, don't refuse" method can often identify the child's least favorite nursing session.

Babies under a year old need the nutrition in breast milk or formula even if they're drinking some juice and eating some solid foods. If your baby is under a year, you'll need to substitute formula (rather than whole milk) for the missed feeding. Most babies enjoy sucking on a bottle, but not all find it appealing. If your baby doesn't seem interested in drinking from a bottle, try a cup.

For an older child, the substitution can be any of a number of things— a game, a cuddle, a walk to the park, a reading session with a favorite book, a cup of milk, or a healthful snack. Most important is your involvement with the activity, so that you show your child in many ways that you love him. For suggestions on weaning the older nursing child, see the following section.

✤ Wait several days (up to two weeks) and then eliminate the next-lightest feeding of the day. Keep doing this until you're down to one nursing a day, probably the first one of the morning or the last one at night. By now, you'll be producing very little milk and your child may give up this last feeding easily. Or you may decide to continue this one favorite feeding for a while longer. Many children wean easily from daytime feedings but want to continue nursing at bedtime for some time. Weaning this way should take from a couple of weeks to a couple of months or longer.

Suggestions for Weaning the Older Child

✤ Focus on eliminating the nursing sessions that are least important to your child and most inconvenient for you, and let the others continue for a while.

✤ The best way to end this stage in your child's life is to reach an agreement between the two of you—even if that agreement originates with you rather than your child. For example, make an agreement with your child about the places where you will nurse. These places may be your home, in the car, or in a friend's house, but not in a restaurant or other public place.

✤ Make nursing sessions shorter.

✤ Use distraction. Involve her in an interesting activity at a time when she might ordinarily nurse, or as you're bringing a brief nursing session to an end.

✤ Talk to your child about weaning as a definite occurrence in the future (after the next birthday, perhaps, or after Santa Claus comes). Even if there's some backsliding after these events, your child will think of nursing as ending someday. One mother told her three-year-old a story about a little rabbit whose mother said, "I love you and I love to nurse you, but my milk is going away and it's really special milk for babies."

✤ Offer your child something she likes to eat just before she would ordinarily nurse. It's better to forestall a request to nurse than to deny it.

✤ Change your routine. At a usual nursing time, go out for a walk or a ride, invite a playmate over, or bring out a new toy.

✤ Stay away from the places where you ordinarily nurse. If you're used to nursing in a special chair, hide it or move it out of your home temporarily.

✤ Don't sit down in front of your child, since many little ones associate sitting down with nursing time. Just keep on the move in the early days or weeks of weaning. Think of it as another opportunity to exercise.

✤ Don't uncover your breasts in front of your child. This will remind her of nursing when she may not have been thinking about it.

✤ Lavish physical affection on your child during activities not associated with breastfeeding, such as reading a picture book, telling stories, or singing.

✤ Emphasize how big your child is. Stress some of the benefits of getting older, like going to nursery school, having play dates, and not wearing diapers anymore. Focus on the many things she can do for herself, like dressing herself and using the potty. Talk about nursing as something that's important for little children but not for big ones.

❖ Give one week's notice and count down every night. Then give a special present on the last night.

❖ If your child is over three, you might be able to make a contract—to promise some special outing or treat one week (or whatever time period you set) after the last nursing. A child younger than this won't be able to keep her end of the bargain—and even a three-year-old might not be able to.

❖ Ask your child to postpone a nursing; this will sometimes lead to her forgetting it. A child who asks to nurse in public, for example, can often accept waiting "until we get home." If you're already home, you can say "Yes, but first I'm going to get a drink of water." Then get her involved in some activity with you, don't sit down, and maybe she'll become interested in something other than nursing. Meanwhile, you haven't said no, and you've made a start.

❖ Enlist your child's favorite people. Ask your partner, your child's grandmother, or an adored babysitter to get her up in the morning, put her to bed, or go to her in the middle of the night, if she still wants to nurse at those times. The first time I (Sally Olds) put my eighteen-month-old granddaughter to bed when her mother, who had

always nursed her to sleep, wasn't around, I helped Anna fall asleep by taking her into my arms in a rocking chair and singing every song I could possibly remember. I think she went to sleep in self-defense, so she wouldn't have to put up with my singing!

❖ Don't try to deter your child from nursing by coating your breasts with foul-tasting substances. Allow her to keep her happy memories and her trust in you.

❖ Explain that your milk is "all gone," "went bye-bye," or something similar.

❖ While you're weaning, continue to be willing to nurse your child at times when she's especially needy. If she hurts herself or is sick or unhappy, depriving her of the comfort she's used to will only create more unhappiness for both of you. Remember that nursing through an illness is a great way to get food and immunities to an ill child.

As one mother says, "A lot of times when she asks to nurse I can distract her, but when she really needs it, I nurse—and then she's in a super mood and so it's good for both of us."

Sudden Weaning

Sometimes a circumstance comes up that requires abrupt weaning—a mother's need to be hospitalized or to take a medication incompatible with breastfeeding, a family crisis that involves travel without a child, or some other emergency.

In some cases, a situation that, at first glance, seems to call for sudden weaning can be modified. You may, for example, be able to postpone a surgical procedure for a few weeks, which will give you time to cut down nursing sessions more gradually. Or you may be able to take a different medication, take your baby with you on a trip, or make some other change. It's worth exploring other options, since sudden weaning is hard on both mother and child.

If you do have to wean suddenly, you're likely to be quite uncomfortable for several days unless you're producing very little milk. You can hasten the drying-up process and minimize discomfort in a few ways. Wear a firm, but not too tight, bra. You can also relieve discomfort by expressing just enough milk to ease the pressure on your breasts. And you may also get relief from ice packs applied to the breasts several times a day. Ask your doctor to prescribe a pain reliever. The pain reliever can be relatively strong, since now that nursing has ended, you don't have to worry about the medication reaching your child.

Occasionally, a mother under stress will make a spur-of-the-moment decision ("Okay, this has gone on long enough. Today's the day!") and will go the cold turkey route. This is almost always a mistake. If you don't have to wean abruptly, reconsider your decision. Are you doing it because of other people's criticism, because you think your child will sleep better at night (he probably won't), or because you're just tired of breastfeeding? Even if after reconsideration, you decide to begin the process, do it gradually, if at all possible. Both you and he will benefit.

How Weaning Affects You

As you transition into weaning your child, you'll experience both physical and emotional changes.

Physical Changes

When you stop breastfeeding, your body will undergo a number of physiological changes as your hormonal balance reverts to what it was before you became pregnant. As soon as you added foods other than breast milk to your child's diet, it became easier for you to become pregnant again. If you have not already adopted a method of birth control and if you don't want to conceive right away, you'll now need to use some means of contraception (see Chapter 13).

The most obvious change will be in your breasts. It may take several months for you to lose the bulk of your milk, even though none may be apparent within days after the last nursing session. Some women are able to express a drop or two of milk from their breasts up to several years after weaning. Remember that nipple stimulation promotes milk production, so if you're always checking for milk, you're likely to find some. Also, consistent nipple stimulation during sexual activity can result in slight milk secretion for some time.

It may also take several months for your breasts to return to their former size. They'll most likely be less firm than they were before you became pregnant. This is the result of child-bearing, not breastfeeding. They'll probably seem to be the same size they were before your pregnancy, although some women feel that their breasts become larger or smaller after nursing. This may have something to do with the amount of weight gained or lost. Some women become so accustomed to having larger breasts that after they wean, their breasts seem smaller to them.

You'll gradually produce less and less milk until there's virtually none at all. If at any point during weaning your breasts become overfull, you can express just enough milk to ease your discomfort, or you can put your child to the breast for a minute or two (if she's willing to stop at that). Don't overdo it or you'll just encourage your breasts to continue producing copious amounts of milk. If you're uncomfortably full most of the time, slow down the pace of weaning, if possible.

Two once popular remedies are no longer recommended. One, binding your breasts, can actually make you feel worse and cause a plugged duct. And since medicine to dry up a woman's milk usually didn't work and often had unpleasant and even harmful side effects, it was taken off the market.

Emotional Responses

Your emotional reactions to weaning may be even more apparent than your physical ones. Much of your feeling about weaning will depend on your particular circumstances. If your baby is setting the pace for weaning earlier than you had expected, you may be feeling sad, surprised, and rejected. Rejoice, instead, in your child's push for independence and in his demonstration that he can take the initiative toward starting a new chapter in his life. One of the primary goals of parenthood is to help our children become self-sufficient, in small stages appropriate to their level of development. This is only the first of many steps toward self-reliance that he'll take in his lifetime.

While it can be a blow to realize that your child doesn't need you in this particular way as much as he did before, don't lose sight of the fact that he'll need you even more in other ways. Right now, for example, he may have special needs for the comfort of your arms and the reassurance of your love. Parenthood involves learning what our children need at different stages in their lives—and being willing to give it.

If you have to wean abruptly, earlier than you had expected or wanted to, you will most likely feel the grief of unrealized expectations, of having to give up a joyful activity, and of depriving your child of something that means so much to him. As you mourn what you both have lost, however, you need to tell yourself that you have done the best you could for your child, and that you will have many opportunities throughout his life to show your love for him in an infinite number of ways.

Even if you yourself initiated the weaning process and it has gone smoothly and gradually, you may be surprised to find that you feel more than a little sad as nursing draws to a close. This feeling is common and normal. No longer will you enjoy this close physical bond, this symbiosis between you and your child in which each of you needs the other in a very special way. You'll probably have the same kind of mixed emotions the first time you leave each of your children playing happily in preschool or kindergarten, the day they go off to sleepaway camp, the day you leave them in their college dorms, or the day they say "I do" and go off to start their own families. A lump in the parental throat often accompanies our feelings of accomplishment for having helped our children to meet life's challenges with confidence and enthusiasm.

Other Food and Drink

As you introduce other foods and drinks into your baby's diet, she can begin to eat like the rest of your family.

Other Milk

If you offer any milk other than breast milk in the first year of life, you should be giving your baby a specially constituted infant formula. Most infant formulas consist of modified cow's milk, but if your baby has special needs (for example, an allergy to cow's milk), she might need a soybean-based formula. If she's allergic to the soy formula, your doctor may recommend a hypoallergenic protein hydrolysate formula. If you plan to wean your baby before six to eight months of age, begin offering an occasional bottle or cup by about three months (see Chapter 6 for suggestions on bottle-feeding the breastfed baby).

You should not offer plain cow's milk before one year of age for several

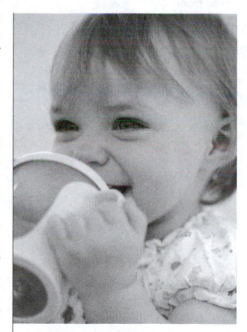

Holding a cup and drinking from it are two more signs of a developing independence.

reasons. For one thing, babies fed on whole milk before this time sometimes suffer from iron-deficiency anemia. Cow's milk contains very little iron and sometimes causes intestinal bleeding, which contributes to further iron loss. And the high intake of sodium, potassium, chloride, and protein from cow's milk can burden a baby's system.

Also, you should not offer skim or reduced-fat milk (1 or 2 percent) until your child is over two years of age. These milks don't provide the necessary fatty acids that babies need for brain growth and for the development of hormones and enzyme systems. Furthermore, since they are too high in protein concentration for the baby's digestive system to handle easily, they can overload the baby's kidney excretory capacity and cause medical problems.

Water and Juice

While breastfed babies don't need water, even in hot and dry climates (except if it fulfills the fluoride requirements for babies over six months old), some enjoy it. If you want to give your baby an occasional sip of water after breastfeeding is well established, try offering it in a cup.

Some babies like fruit juice, which can be offered after six months of age. It isn't necessary, though, and babies who drink a lot of juice tend to take less breast milk. If you do feed your baby fruit juice, be sure to dilute it with at least 50 percent water, and give only small amounts. One study of toddlers who had failed to grow normally found that they had been drinking large quantities of juice, which filled them up so much that they had too little appetite for higher-calorie, more nutritious foods. Some also had diarrhea. Children two or three years old should drink no more than 4 to 8 ounces of juice

a day, and younger babies should have less. Letting babies take a bottle of juice to bed with them or walk around sucking from it for a long period of time can lead to tooth decay.

Solid Foods

Some years ago, mothers were advised to begin feeding their babies solid foods when they were only a couple of weeks old. We now know that this is not only unnecessary but unwise, as well as a waste of time and money. Such foods may strain an infant's immature digestive system. Furthermore, they can fill up his baby's stomach so much that he doesn't nurse as vigorously, thereby not getting enough breast milk. There's also a chance that he may gain too much weight too quickly. The nutrients in solid foods often go right through the baby's system, exiting in the stool.

While breast milk is an ideal total food for the young infant, older babies need additional foods to meet their growing nutritional requirements. Sometime around four to six months of age, your baby may signal his readiness to add solid foods to his diet. A baby need not have teeth, but he must have reached the following aspects of development.

❖ He should be able to sit up with support and should have good control of his head and neck muscles. This way, he'll be able to show you when he wants food by leaning forward and opening his mouth, and to show when he doesn't by leaning back and turning away. If he can't do this, pushing food into his mouth will amount to a kind of forced feeding. Eating solid food should be something that a baby actively engages in, not just passively accepts.

❖ Be sure that he is not pushing the spoon out of his mouth with his tongue. This tongue-extrusion reflex is usually no longer operative by about five months. To test this, give your baby a quarter-teaspoon of a simple food (like mashed ripe banana or sweet potato—excellent early foods, which most babies love). If the food goes from the front of his mouth to the back of his throat and he swallows it, he's clearly ready for solids. But if he spits it out, wait a few days and try again. Watch your baby carefully to be sure he doesn't choke, but don't be alarmed if he gags a little. This is part of the learning process.

❖ Finally, your baby may be giving you very clear signals of interest in solid food by reaching for the food on your plate, making noises, or pointing.

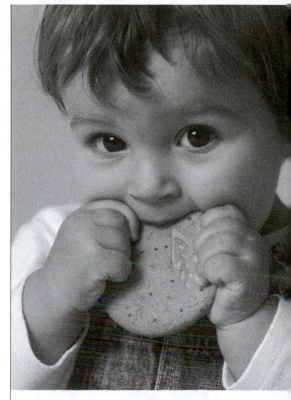

Easy-to-grasp and easy-to-eat finger foods, like this not-too-sweet biscuit, are popular early solids.

Advantages to introducing solid foods early on include both the openness to new experience that is more characteristic of younger babies and the extra time your baby will have to learn how to handle these new foods before he needs them to provide nourishment. Until recently, advice to parents with a family history of food allergy was to hold off giving their baby any foods other than breast milk for at least six to eight months. But recent research suggests that babies exposed to new foods fairly early are less likely to become allergic to them; however, the jury is still out on this one. Check with your doctor regarding the newest developments to find out whether more definite conclusions have been reached.

Remember that adding solid foods is a gradual process that occurs over a period of months as new foods are offered and your baby increases the amounts he wants to eat.

Just as you learned to read your baby's cues for hunger and readiness for nursings, you can now pay attention to the signals that mean "Hey, Mom, I want some of that!" For suggestions on feeding the first few solid "meals," see the box on page 382.

Offering Solid Foods

Following are some suggestions for introducing solid food to your baby:

❖ Use a spoon—the traditional baby spoon with a small bowl and a long handle works best.

❖ Nurse your baby before you offer her food by spoon. She'll be more open to this new experience if she isn't wildly hungry. Solid foods in the early months are more of a sensory experiment than a nutritional necessity. If you nurse her first, she'll be getting the nourishment she needs from breast milk.

❖ Pick a time when there are few distractions and both you and your baby are relaxed.

❖ If she can't sit up by herself, sit her on your lap, in a high chair that reclines slightly, or in a bouncy seat.

❖ Introduce a single-ingredient food first, and then introduce new foods one at a time, waiting three to four days between each introduction. This way, if your baby develops a rash or any other allergic symptom, you'll be able to identify a possible cause.

❖ Start spoon-feeding by putting a little food into the bowl of the spoon, turning the spoon upside down, and depositing the food onto the top of the baby's tongue. She will easily propel the food to the back of her mouth, where she'll swallow it. She'll probably like it and want more.

❖ At first, servings should be between 1 and 2 tablespoons once a day. Within a short time, your baby will be taking up to 3 tablespoons three times a day. Watch your baby very closely for signals: If she seems interested, keep feeding, but if she turns away or closes her mouth, wait for another time.

❖ One good first food is iron-fortified rice cereal mixed with expressed breast milk, water, or formula; after your baby is a year old you can use homogenized milk. Rice cereal is a good starter, since babies are least likely to be allergic to it.

❖ A good progression after iron-fortified rice cereal includes other cereals, and mashed or pureed fruits and vegetables, but there's no hard-and-fast rule about the order of foods. Among the flavors most enjoyed by babies are applesauce, ripe banana, pears, peaches, peas, carrots, avocado, sweet potato, and squash.

❖ The more different fruits and vegetables you have in your diet, the more your breastfed baby is likely to accept in hers.

❖ If you make your own baby food, put a small portion in a dish and don't save any leftovers. If you're giving commercial baby food, don't feed your baby directly from the jar. Take out the amount you plan to feed, and refrigerate the rest. If your baby doesn't eat all of the dished-out food, throw away whatever is left. The saliva in the food can foster the growth of bacteria.

❖ Do not heat food in a microwave;

it may heat unevenly and make food too hot.

❖ Consider these first few feedings of solid foods "practice feeds," just like those first few nursings so many months ago. Your baby now has to learn how to master a completely new set of muscle movements to take the food from a spoon and to swallow it. At first, she'll get more food on her face, her bib, and you than she'll get in her mouth. You'll be surprised, though, at how quickly she'll catch on and how soon she'll be ready to start eating foods she can pick up with her fingers.

❖ Don't worry if your baby doesn't take to solids right away. She's getting the nutrition she needs from breast milk. If she refuses other foods at first, let it go—and try again another day.

❖ As soon as babies can pick them up, they usually like feeding themselves soft-cooked peas, chunks of tofu, pieces of soft-cooked carrots and potatoes, and little circles of oat cereal. Just put a few pieces on the feeding tray, and wait until she eats them before giving more.

❖ Some finger foods can cause choking if they're given to a baby who cannot yet chew properly and swallow small enough amounts: raw fruit or vegetable chunks, meat or fish with bones, popcorn, seeds or nuts, marshmallows, hard candy, or other hard or crunchy foods. Because peanut butter is thick and sticky, don't give it to baby until she's over two years old. You can give your baby grapes or hot dogs only if they are cut in *very* small pieces.

❖ Don't leave your baby alone while she's eating. And don't give her solid foods while she's lying down or moving around.

❖ Do not give your baby honey until she's over a year old. Although it's safe for older children and adults, it can make infants very sick.

❖ Although a baby may initially refuse to eat a certain food, she may learn to like it if you feed it to her again, especially if you feed it along with something she already likes. It may take many tries before she's willing to eat the new food. One study found that babies who initially didn't like green beans eventually came to eat them, especially if the babies were fed peaches right after the beans. The researchers suggest focusing not only on your baby's facial expression (the squint, curled lip, or furrowed brow that means "yuck!") but also on her willingness to continue eating.

❖ Avoid, as much as possible, foods that contain added sugar, salt, and starch. You can make your own baby foods (which can be as easy as using a fork to mash a ripe banana or cooked peas). Or you can buy organic baby foods. Jarred foods may be more convenient when you're traveling, or when your table food is not appropriate for your baby.

❖ In any case, read the labels and graduate your child to table food as soon as she's ready. Commercial "stage 3," "junior," or "toddler" foods are unnecessary and costly.

Staying Close with Your Child

When your child weans and takes this first big step toward independence, you will very likely look back over his young life. You think of the months you carried him under your heart, nourishing him through your body, wondering who he was, what kind of a person he would be. You remember the exertion on both your parts as he burst into the world as an individual human being, breathing through his own lungs, making his own efforts to draw nourishment, learning how to cope with a strange world. You dwell on the time you spent together as a nursing couple, reliving the many happy moments you knew as you held your child in your arms and gave deeply of yourself.

And then you look forward. You think of the many other ways you'll give of yourself to this child: the guidance you'll provide to help him find his way in life, the love that will support him, the courage you'll give him to let go of you and be his own person, the happy hours you'll spend enjoying each other's company, playing together, having fun. You accept the fact that as a mother you'll know tears and anger, as well as laughter and delight. But just as you now remember not the minor setbacks or worries about breastfeeding but its heartfelt joys, so, too, will you balance out the stresses and demands of motherhood with the love and the warmth and the personal growth that you gain from your relationship with your children.

Breastfeeding
and the Law

L egal issues intersect with a baby's right to be breastfed in a number of areas. We'll discuss public nursing, custody conflicts, and extended breastfeeding here. Employment issues are covered in Chapter 12. Should you encounter problems in any of these areas, you may want to contact your local La Leche League leader, who should be able to offer some help in handling legal issues surrounding breastfeeding. To get the name of a local leader, first look under "La Leche League" in the white pages of your telephone directory. If you need further help, contact the main office of the league (you'll find their phone number and website in the Resource Appendix) or a lactation specialist.

Breastfeeding Laws by State

Why are laws to protect a woman's right to breastfeed necessary? Not because it is illegal anywhere to nurse in public, but because some people—fortunately, a minority—consider it indecent exposure and therefore criminal behavior. A major irony is that in many cases the harassed nursing mother's breasts are not even visible, and people who complain about her are simply uncomfortable with the very idea of breastfeeding. As attorneys Kenneth A. Friedman and the late Elizabeth N. Baldwin have written, "Most mothers who are harassed for breastfeeding are trying hard to be discreet. Although nothing shows, everyone knows what she is doing. These new mothers, breastfeeding for the first time in public, are often the ones who are picked on. [These mothers] are more likely to wean as a result of embarrassment and humiliation."

At this writing, forty-four states, the District of Columbia, and the Virgin Islands have laws whose language specifically permits women to breastfeed in any public or private location. Twenty-eight states, the District of Columbia, and the Virgin Islands exempt breastfeeding from public indecency laws. Florida law specifically states, "A mother may breastfeed her baby in any location, public or private, where the mother is otherwise authorized to be, irrespective of whether the nipple of the mother's breast is uncovered during or incidental to the breastfeeding."

Connecticut law protects breastfeeding as a mother's civil right and stipulates that no person shall restrict or limit the right of a mother to breastfeed her child.

State laws are not uniform and most are not comprehensive, and there's a need for a national policy that will synthesize them all.

In very rare circumstances, you may need an attorney to help defend your right to breastfeed. These circumstances can include challenges to your right to breastfeed in public, custody conflicts, charges of abuse, or instances in which a conflict at work may result in job loss or a need to file suit. Each case, of course, is unique and has to be dealt with on its own merits.

We need to protest every case of discrimination—after all, bottle-feeding mothers are not asked to feed their babies in private. We need to rally community support. And we need to make the point that breastfeeding is never illegal. We also need to see mothers nursing in public more often, so that young people seeing them will accept this as the natural way to feed infants, an attitude that will serve the next generation of babies. If women are not made to feel as if they have to hide when they're doing the best they can for their babies, more women will follow suit.

Remember that the law is often no more than a reflection of society-wide values and customs. As our culture becomes increasingly more nursing-friendly, many of these conflicts will cease to pose problems.

Protecting Your Nursing Baby in a Custody Case

Family breakups can occur while small children are still being nursed, and sometimes the nursing becomes an issue in custody conflicts. If you are involved in such an issue, whether with the baby's father (the term we use thoughout these appendixes) or any life partner, you need to address it firmly and reasonably, and whenever possible, by settling your disputes out of court.

Some judges pursue the laudable goal of promoting bonding between a child and a noncustodial father by mandating a certain number of hours or days of visitation with the father, away from the mother. Judges do not always take into account that a child is still nursing, and in some cases have ordered that breastfed infants spend the weekend, a week, or even longer with their fathers, ignoring the nursing relationship.

Judges who don't know much about breastfeeding often think that as long as the baby gets her mother's milk, separation from her mother doesn't matter. They think that an easy solution would be for the mother to express enough milk for the visit and send the required number of bottles with the baby. This "solution" does not take into account the loss of physical closeness and the cherished sense of comfort that both mom and baby derive from the breastfeeding experience.

In any such scenario, you need to prepare well and you need to have good, competent legal advice. Many times, it is essential to show not just the importance of breastfeeding, but the current recommendations regarding breastfeeding. You could inform the court of WHO and UNICEF recommendations that all babies be breastfed until age two or beyond, and the recommendation of the American Academy of Pediatrics that all babies be breastfed for a minimum of 12 months, and then after that for as long as it is mutually desirable.

Often it's helpful to show the judge in your case that you are your child's primary caretaker. Make sure to tell your attorney all the ways you care for and nurture your child so that he or she can help to prove this.

It's most important that you make the court understand that breastfeeding is not incompatible with your child's bond with her father. Unfortunately, many in the legal field mistakenly think that they have to give preference either to the father or to breastfeeding. It may be helpful to create a schedule that gives your baby maximum time with her father while not endangering the course of breastfeeding. When you plan this schedule, keep in mind that, sooner or later, your baby will be sleeping through the night. Suggest that when that time comes, she can join her father for an overnight stay.

It's well worth making the effort to work with your child's father. Even if he is uncooperative and unpleasant, you need to be reasonable, polite, and informative. You may want to do some or all of the following:

1. First, explain to your child's father that you'll encourage his bond with your child because you know that's best for the child (only, of course, if this is actually the case). Refrain from angry words and name-calling.

2. Decide what you want and try to come to an agreement before you file any papers with the court. If you and the father can't agree, meet with a counselor or a mediator.

3. Develop a visitation plan that provides for frequent contact between your child and her father, while still respecting your child's breastfeeding needs.

4. If you absolutely cannot work it out yourselves, providing expert evidence may be essential to prove the importance of breastfeeding specifically regarding your child. Obtain testimony from your pediatrician, a psychologist, a lactation consultant, or some other authority.

Breastfeeding an Older Child

Over the past several years, a few rare instances have arisen in which social service agencies have questioned the propriety of extended breastfeeding. A mother's decision to breastfeed her child beyond age one or two may give rise to an accusation that she is "enmeshed," or too entangled in her child's care, or is nursing for her own neurotic reasons, or is using breastfeeding to keep her child away from his father. However, no court has ever upheld a finding that extended breastfeeding constitutes abuse or neglect, or is in any way harmful to the child, regardless of the age of the nursing child.

What should you do if you are reported for abuse because of extended breastfeeding? First, remember that a social service agency must investigate every report of abuse, and this investigation does *not* constitute criminal indictment. Be polite and cooperative with the investigator. Don't volunteer information or agree to anything. Write down the accusations being made. If it seems that the matter is not going to be resolved easily, you may need to contact an attorney experienced in social service agency cases, or a criminal lawyer. To find such an attorney, see the Resource Appendix.

Educate your lawyer about the benefits and normality of extended breastfeeding. You might cite recommendations of the American Academy of Pediatrics and the World Health Organization.

Resource Appendix:

Helpful Organizations and Sources of Information

For Information and Help About Breastfeeding

La Leche League International
957 North Plum Grove Road, P.O. Box 4079
Schaumburg, IL 60173
Phone: 800-525-3243 or 847-519-7730 Fax: 847-969-0460
Email: llli@llli.org Website: www.llli.org

La Leche League International is the largest organization in the world devoted specifically to providing mother-to-mother support and education about breastfeeding. Local chapters, which hold monthly gatherings, are listed on the website. To find a chapter near you, go to www.llli.org/webindex.html or call the league. You can submit questions through the online help form on the website at www.llli.org/help_form. You can also take part in online forums. Go to http://forums.llli.org.

Through the league's Health Advisory Council, knowledgeable physicians provide guidance on medication during lactation and other medical issues. And the league's professional liaisons can offer information about legal issues and may be able to refer you to a knowledgeable attorney in your state. Go to www.llli.org/Law/LawUS.html?m=0,1,0.

International Childbirth Education Association (ICEA)
1500 Sunday Drive, Suite 102
Raleigh, NC 27607
Phone: 800-624-4934 or 919-863-9487 Fax: 919-787-4916
E-mail: info@icea.org Website: www.icea.org

ICEA promotes family-centered maternity care, offers professional certification and training programs for educators and health care providers, and publishes a quarterly journal and many smaller publications, many of which deal with breastfeeding. It also has a comprehensive mail-order catalog of audiotapes, CDs, DVDs, books, and pamphlets related to pregnancy, birth, breastfeeding, and other family issues.

World Alliance for Breastfeeding Action (WABA)
P.O. Box 1200
10850 Penang, Malaysia
Phone: 011-604-658-4816 Fax: 011-604-657-2655
E-mail: waba@waba.org.my Website: www.waba.org.my

This international umbrella organization advocates for breastfeeding and serves as a liaison among various agencies and individuals around the world. In connection with its annual World Breastfeeding Week (August 1–7), it distributes an action folder with information and ideas for actions that individuals and organizations can take in their own communities to support the year's theme.

The National Women's Health Information Center
Phone: 800-994-9662
TDD (telecommunications device for the deaf): 888-220-5446
Website: www.womenshealth.gov/breastfeeding

This U.S. government source for women's health information offers free information and encouragement on breastfeeding, either by telephone or online.

Newman Breastfeeding Clinic and Institute
Canadian College of Naturopathic Medicine
1225 Shepherd Avenue East
Toronto, Ontario M2K 1E2
Phone: 416-498-0002 Fax: 416-498-0012
E-mail: institute@nbci.ca Website: www.drjacknewman.com

Dr. Jack Newman and Edith Kernerman offer a wealth of helpful information on their website through video clips and information sheets.

To Find Professionals in a Field

OBSTETRICIAN

American College of Obstetricians and Gynecologists (ACOG)
P.O. Box 96920
Washington, DC 20090-6920
Phone: 202-638-5537
E-mail: resources@acog.org Website: www.acog.org

ACOG can refer you to an obstetrician in your area. Contact by phone, fax, e-mail, or postal mail.

PEDIATRICIAN

American Academy of Pediatrics (AAP)
141 Northwest Point Boulevard
Elk Grove Village, IL 60007-1098
Phone: 800-433-9016 or 847-434-4000 Fax: 847-434-8000
E-mail: kidsdocs@aap.org Website: www.aap.org

To find a qualified general pediatrician, pediatric subspecialist, or pediatric surgical specialist near you, go to www.healthychildren.org.
For information on health topics, go to www.aap.org/topics.html.
The AAP's 2005 policy statement on breastfeeding urges exclusive nursing for six months and continued nursing until at least one year of age. For information about current breastfeeding initiatives, e-mail: lactation@aap.org.

NURSE-MIDWIFE

American College of Nurse-Midwives
8403 Colesville Road, Suite 1550
Silver Spring, MD 20910
Phone: 240-485-1800 Fax: 240-485-1818
E-mail: info@acnm.org Website: www.midwife.org

To find a midwife in your area, go to www.midwife.org/find.cfm or call 888-643-9433.

Midwives Alliance of North America (MANA)
611 Pennsylvania Avenue, SE, Suite 1700
Washington, DC 20003-4303
Phone: 888-923-6262
E-mail: info@mana.org Website: www.mana.org

MANA is a membership organization of practicing and student midwives, supportive health care providers, and families. If you e-mail membership@mana .org, a member will provide you with the names of four members in your state or North American province. Go to mana.org/memberlist.html for more information.

FAMILY PHYSICIAN

Family physicians are medical specialists who are trained to care for everyone in your family. They can see you through your pregnancy and then care for your newborn while continuing to care for other family members. To find a family doctor, ask family and friends to recommend the doctor they use and like, or ask your local hospital for a list of family practitioners in your area. The American Academy of Family Physicians (www.familydoctor.org) is the professional organization for these doctors, but at this time it does not give medical or personal advice or answer e-mails that include individual medical questions or personal information.

NUTRITIONIST

American Dietetic Association (ADA)
120 South Riverside Plaza, Suite 2000
Chicago, IL 60606-6995
Phone: 800-877-1600 or 312-899-0040
E-mail: findnrd@eatright.org Website: www.eatright.org

Members of the ADA are nutritionists who have met stringent requirements entitling them to put the letters RD (for Registered Dietitian) after their names. The organization can help you find a nutritionist in your area. Go to www.eatright .org and click on "Find a Registered Dietician." The ADA also provides a wealth of information on food and nutrition on its website.

CHILDBIRTH EDUCATOR

Lamaze International
2025 M Street, NW, Suite 800
Washington, DC 20036-3309
Phone: 800-368-4404 or 202-367-1128 Fax: 202-367-2128
E-mail: info@lamaze.org Website: www.lamaze.org

One of the oldest childbirth education organizations, Lamaze International encourages birthing experiences in which the mother is awake and aware, supported by her family and friends, and is not separated from her baby. The organization trains and certifies childbirth educators and breastfeeding support specialists and provides information for expectant and new parents. To find a Lamaze class in your area, go to www.lamaze.org/default.aspx?tabid=62.

LACTATION CONSULTANT

International Board of Lactation Consultant Examiners (IBLCE)
6402 Arlington Boulevard, Suite 350
Falls Church, VA 22042
Phone: 703-560-7330 Fax: 703-560-7332
E-mail: iblce@iblce.org Website: www.iblce.org

IBLCE is the professional accrediting association for lactation consultants, recognized by the International Lactation Consultant Association (ILCA). IBLCE sets standards by developing yearly certifying examinations, which are given in several languages. Lactation consultants who have met IBLCE's requirements may add the letters IBCLC after their names.

International Lactation Consultant Association (ILCA)
2501 Aerial Center Parkway, Suite 103
Morrisville, NC 27560
Phone: 888-452-2478 or 919-861-5577 Fax: 919-459-2075
E-mail: info@ilca.org Website: www.ilca.org

ILCA conducts ongoing education programs and publishes a peer-reviewed journal, among its other activities. It has affiliate groups in many countries and localities and can refer you to a lactation consultant in your area who has been certified by the International Board of Lactation Consultant Examiners via a directory that is updated every two weeks. Go to www.ilca.org/i4a/pages/index .cfm?pageid=3337.

DOULA

Doulas of North America (DONA) International
100 East Washington Street
Springfield, IL 62701
Phone: 888-788-3662 Fax: 217-528-6545
E-mail: info@dona.org Website: www.dona.org

DONA's website allows you to search for pregnancy, birth, and postpartum doulas in your area.

INFANT MASSAGE

Infant Massage USA
7481 Huntsman Boulevard, Suite 635
Springfield, VA 22153
Phone: 800-497-5996 or 703-455-3455
E-mail: general.info@infantmassageusa.org Website: www.infantmassageusa.org

This is the United States chapter of the International Association of Infant Massage, based in Sweden (www.iaim.net). The organization trains instructors of infant massage and can put you in touch with a certified teacher near you.

For Mothers of Multiples

National Organization of Mothers of Twins Clubs, Inc.
2000 Mallory Lane, Suite 130-600
Franklin, TN 37067-8231
Phone: 248-231-4480
E-mail: info@nomotc.org Website: www.nomotc.org

This network of more than 450 local clubs representing multiple-birth families publishes a quarterly magazine and other literature, participates in research projects, fosters networking, and puts families in touch with local chapters.

For Mothers of Babies with Special Needs

Cleft Palate Foundation (CPF)
1504 East Franklin Street, Suite 102
Chapel Hill, NC 27514-2820
Phone: 919-933-9044 24-hour toll-free helpline: 800-242-5338 Fax: 919-933-9604
E-mail: info@cleftline.org Website: www.cleftline.org

To enhance the quality of life for people affected by cleft lip and palate and other facial birth defects, CPF provides free information to individuals and health-care professionals, and awards scholarships and research grants.

National Down Syndrome Society (NDSS)
666 Broadway, 8th floor
New York, NY 10012
Phone: 800-221-4602 Fax: 212-979-2873
E-mail: info@ndss.org Website: www.ndss.org

NDSS provides education and services for people with Down syndrome and their families, including helpful suggestions for breastfeeding babies with the syndrome.

Human Milk Banks

Human Milk Banking Association of North America
1500 Sunday Drive, Suite 102
Raleigh, NC 27607
Phone: 919-861-4530
E-mail: info@hmbana.org Website: www.hmbana.org

At this writing, only ten human milk banks exist in North America: nine in the United States and one in Canada. Four additional banks are under development: three in the United States and one in Canada. These banks carefully screen volunteer donors; collect, screen, and process milk; and dispense it to critically ill infants and children. Recipients pay a processing fee on a per-ounce basis, but no one is denied access for inability to pay. Uses of donor milk have included prematurity, failure to thrive, immuno-deficiencies, chronic renal failure, infant botulism, and management of chronic diarrhea. To donate or obtain breast milk, contact the closest milk bank. A list and a map showing locations are on the website.

The Internet

The Web is a valuable source of information about breastfeeding and child care as well as a route to networking with professionals and with other parents. One important caution: You need to consider the trustworthiness of the websites you consult and to evaluate carefully any information you receive online. See page 401.

Help in the Workplace

MCH Services, Inc.
P.O. Box 6241
Beverly Hills, CA 90212
Phone: 800-822-6688 Fax: 310-552-2100
Rona Cohen, RN, MN, IBCLC, President
E-mail: mchservices@mchservicesinc.com Website: www.mchservicesinc.com

MCH Services provides comprehensive corporate lactation programs to employers and their workers. Services include offering access to prenatal information, to breastfeeding products, and to a network of lactation consultants, as well as professional support and encouragement.

National Business Group on Health (NBGH)
50 F Street, NW, Suite 600
Washington, DC 20001
Phone: 202-628-9320 Fax: 202-628-9244
E-mail: info@businessgrouphealth.org Website: www.businessgrouphealth.org

This national nonprofit organization analyzes health policy and related worksite issues from the perspective of large employers. It promotes employer-sponsored services and benefits that support the health and well-being of workers as an investment in the company's productivity. Go to www.businessgrouphealth.org/benefitstopics/breastfeeding.cfm for a free tool kit for employers and employees, including case histories of successful workplace programs.

National Healthy Mothers, Healthy Babies Coalition
2000 North Beauregard Street, 6th Floor
Alexandria, VA 22311
Phone: 703-837-4792 Fax: 703-684-5968
E-mail: info@hmhb.org Website: www.hmhb.org

This consortium of public and private organizations, employers, policy makers, and consumers works to promote and improve community-based services for healthy mothers, babies, and families. It publishes weekly newsletters, "Fast

Facts" pamphlets on family health issues, maintains programs, and holds local and national meetings.

The National Women's Health Information Center

The Health, Resources, and Services Administration (HRSA) of the U.S. Department of Health and Human Services offers the free kit The Business Case for Breastfeeding: Steps for Creating a Breastfeeding Friendly Worksite. It includes: The Business Case for Breastfeeding brochure; Easy Steps for Supporting Employees, an educational booklet; Tool Kit: Resources for Building a Lactation Support Program; Employee's Guide to Breastfeeding and Working; and materials for lactation specialists and health professionals. Go to www .womenshealth.gov/breastfeeding/programs/business-case/index.cfm.

Sources for Breast Pumps

Besides the following manufacturers, lactation consultants, retail stores, and online retailers sell pumps, often at discount prices.

Ameda
475 Half Day Road, Lincolnshire, IL 60069
Phone: 866-992-6332
Website: www.ameda.com

Phone or go to the website for information on buying or renting Ameda's breast pumps and other products, milk storage guidelines, breastfeeding suggestions, and to speak to a lactation consultant.

Avent Philips Corporation
Phone: 800-542-8368
Website: www.avent.com

For electronic and manual breast pumps.

Hygeia II Medical Group, Inc.
1370 Division Street, Suite C, Vista, CA 92081
Phone: 888-786-7466 or 760-597-8811 Fax: 760-597-8848
E-mail: Sales@hygeiababy.com Website: www.hygeiababy.com

A variety of pumps, including a hospital-grade rental pump and a piston-driven personal-use (not hospital-grade) electric pump that has been FDA-cleared for use by more than one mother (each of whom needs to have her own accessory kit, the only part of the pump that touches her body or breast milk). All Hygeia pumps have a button that can record and play back the baby's cry or cooing to help stimulate milk flow.

Medela, Inc. Breastfeeding USA
1101 Corporate Drive
McHenry, IL 60050
Phone: 800-435-8316 or 800-835-5968 Fax: 835-363-1246
E-mail: customer.service@medela.com Website: www.medelabreastfeedingus.com

For information on buying and renting breast pumps and other products and access to a lactation consultant, go to www.medelabreastfeedingus.com/bnn. For information about insurance issues related to breastfeeding, go to www .breastfeedinginsurance.com

Bailey Medical Engineering
2216 Sunset Drive
Los Osos, CA 93402
Phone: 800-413-3216 or 805-528-5781 Fax: 805-528-1461
E-mail: folks@baileymed.com Website: www.baileymed.com

To find the Nurture III double electric breast pump.

Supplementation

INFORMATION ABOUT
DEE KASSING'S SYSTEM OF BOTTLE-FEEDING

Access her article "Bottle-Feeding as a Tool to Reinforce Breastfeeding" in the *Journal of Human Lactation* (Volume 18, No. 1, published February 2002). You can find it at www.bfar.org/bottlefeeding.pdf.

SOURCES FOR NURSING SUPPLEMENTERS

See Chapter 15 for descriptions of nursing supplementers. Both companies listed below sell direct, can refer you to local outlets, and offer consultation on the use of their products.

Lact-Aid International
P.O. Box 1066, Athens, TN 37371-1066
Phone: 866-866-1239 (toll-free in the U.S.) or 423-744-9090
E-mail: feedback@lact-aid.com Website: www.lact-aid.com

The Lact-Aid NursingTrainer System was introduced in 1971. The company's website maintains a growing online library of free articles, FAQs, and a bibliography on breastfeeding and related topics for parents and health practitioners. Free user help is also available via phone.

Medela, Inc. (See facing page.)

Medela makes several different nursing supplementers: the Supplemental Nursing System (SNS), the Starter SNS (meant for short-term disposable use), and the SpecialNeeds Feeder for babies whose facial or oral problems hamper their ability to maintain adequate suction for feeding. Because it's smaller, the Mini-SpecialNeeds nipple is especially helpful for small babies. The company also makes a specially designed flexible silicone cup designed for cup-feeding infants.

Helpful Books

SPECIAL CONCERNS

Flais, Shelly Vaziri, MD, FAAP. *Raising Twins: From Pregnancy to Preschool.* Elk Grove Village, IL: American Academy of Pediatrics, 2009. Practical suggestions for developing schedules, strategies, and socialization, among other twin-raising issues, along with personal experiences of the author, a pediatrician and a mother of twins.

Gruman-Trinkner, Carrie T. *Your Cleft-Affected Child: The Complete Book of Information, Resources, and Hope.* Alameda, CA: Hunter House, 2001. Written by the mother of a child born with a cleft lip and palate, the book contains a glossary of terminology, a bibliography, and a list of helpful resources.

Hormann, Elizabeth. *Breastfeeding an Adopted Baby and Relactation.* Schaumburg, IL: La Leche League International, 2007. Help in making the decision to pursue this path and suggestions on techniques, with the principal emphasis on the mother–baby relationship, by a lactation consultant who nursed her own adopted child.

Skallerup, Susan J. *Babies with Down Syndrome: A New Parents' Guide,* 3rd edition. Bethesda, MD: Woodbine House, 2008. With up-to-date factual information and personal stories from contributors, including a young man with Down syndrome, the book contains a glossary, a reading list, and a resource guide.

West, Diana. *Defining Your Own Success: Breastfeeding After Breast Reduction Surgery.* Schaumburg, IL: La Leche League International, 2001. Contains a compilation of ways to increase milk supply, which can also help mothers who have not had breast surgery.

Comprehensive Professional References

Hale, Thomas W., and Peter E. Hartmann. *Hale and Hartmann's Textbook of Human Lactation.* Amarillo, TX: Hale Publishing, 2007.

Lawrence, Ruth A., and Robert M. Lawrence. *Breastfeeding: A Guide for the Medical Profession,* 6th edition. St. Louis: C. V. Mosby, 2005.

Mohrbacher, Nancy, and Julie Stock. *The Breastfeeding Answer Book,* 3rd revised edition. Schaumburg, IL: La Leche League International, 2003.

Website Appendix

The following websites are a very small sampling of the many online resources that can help nursing moms. They're all accurate at the time of this writing—but things move fast on the Internet. To find a website about any topic, type your topic into a search engine, and you'll come up with enough sites to keep you at your computer for the rest of your life.

The Internet is a valuable source of information about breastfeeding and child care and a route to networking with professionals and with other parents. In addition to the websites of the organizations listed in the Resource Appendix and those listed here, you can find a wealth of information by typing *breastfeeding, lactation,* or other specified topics into your search box.

One important caution: You need to consider the trustworthiness of the websites you consult and to evaluate carefully any information you receive online.

General Information

www.babyfriendlyusa.org/eng/01.html Information about baby-friendly hospitals in the United States and around the world.

www.babygooroo.com News, information, products, and helpful suggestions.

www.breastfeeding.com Articles, Q & A with advice from experts and moms, photos and stories about breastfeeding celebrity moms, a directory of lactation consultants, and an online store. Click on "Things to Do While Breastfeeding" for activities to do with one hand while nursing or pumping.

www.drjacknewman.com Downloadable handouts on specific topics from an eminent authority.

www.internationalbreastfeedingjournal.com Articles about current research.

www.uppitysciencechick.com Up-to-date scientific information about depression in new mothers, among other topics.

www.usbreastfeeding.org United States Breastfeeding Committee, a partnership of medical and lay organizations.

U. S. Government Sites

www.cdc.gov/breastfeeding Provides news, statistics, links to helpful organizations, phone numbers to call for help with problems, and a link for printing a crib chart for your baby in the hospital, where you can record your and your baby's medical information.

www.cfsan.fda.gov/~dms/wh-toc.html Information on women's health, including food safety.

www.fda.gov/medwatch/index.html U.S. Food and Drug Administration, with information on drugs, breast pumps, and other medical products regulated by the FDA.

www.mchb.hrsa.gov/pregnancyandbeyond Free booklets with suggestions for working moms and employers.

www.ncbi.nlm.nih.gov/sites/entrez Search for biomedical articles dating back to the 1950s. Search for topic, author, or journal.

Working Moms

http://wfnetwork.bc.edu The Sloan Work and Family Research Network provides information about research, government involvement, and other aspects of work and family. Type "breastfeeding" into the search box.

Special Interests and Situations

www.apta.org The American Physical Therapy Association offers free downloadable brochures, including "Posture: Tips for Mom" (type "posture" into the search box).

http://arhp.org Reproductive health professionals offer free brochures and information about birth control.

www.biologicalnurturing.com/index.html Positions and techniques that trigger babies' basic reflexes.

www.bymomsformoms.blogspot.com Maintained by the company that makes Lansinoh HPA Lanolin nipple ointment, forums for moms to ask questions and share experiences.

www.chej.org Grassroots organization of people working to protect communities from environmental contaminants.

www.center4research.org Promotes the health and safety of women, children, and families, by using objective, research-based information to encourage new, more effective programs and policies.

www.cribsforkids.org A safe-sleep education program for low-income families that may provide a crib and educational materials.

www.edf.org The Environmental Defense Fund works to solve a variety of environmental problems. Discussions of safety about eating fish.

www.hsph.harvard.edu/nutritionsource/what-should-you-eat/pyramid Healthy Eating Pyramid from Harvard University School of Public Health.

www.kangaroomothercare.com Research, how-to suggestions, and products to further the practice of kangaroo care.

www.lifecare.com/services/worklife/mothersatwork.html LifeCare and its corporate lactation program.

www.llli.org/llleaderweb/LV/LVMayJun89p35.html and
www.breastfeeding.asn.au/bfinfo/large.html Suggestions for women with large breasts.

http://neonatal.ttuhsc.edu/lact/lactationregistrypage.html Pregnant or nursing women with particular health conditions or taking specific drugs can volunteer to take part in research projects.

www.shakenbaby.org Help in preventing shaken baby syndrome, which results from a caregiver's shaking a baby and can cause serious brain damage or even death. For emergency telephone support, call 877-636-3727 (or in Texas: 817-882-8686).

www.tsa.gov/travelers/airtravel/children/formula.shtm U.S. air travel regulations.

PRODUCT PURCHASING

www.armsreach.com The Arms Reach Co-Sleeper is an adjustable baby bassinet that can be set up so that one open side faces the parental bed, so that a mom can reach baby without getting out of bed.

www.blossumz.com Therapeutic breast gel packs to use for engorgement, mastitis, clogged ducts, or sudden weaning.

www.breastfeedingbooks.com/?s=dvd/ DVD: "Breastfeeding: You Can Do It!"

www.lansinoh.com Maintained by the company that makes Lansinoh HPA Lanolin nipple ointment, the site has information on Soothies gel pads, which are designed to soothe and protect the nipple for a temporary period.

www.milkscreen-moms.com A test for alcohol in breast milk.

www.simplylily.com/product1.html Medical-grade silicone breast pads that reduce leaking, stick to your breasts so you don't need a bra, and can be worn overnight or even swimming.

Postpartum Depression

www.ppdsupportpage.com

www.postpartumdads.org

A Comparison of Cow's Milk and Human Milk

Most infant formulas are made from a base of cow's milk that has been modified to suit the digestive systems of babies under one year of age. Although a baby will not drink straight cow's milk, the comparisons in this table indicate what some of the differences are between cow's milk formulas and human milk.

	COW'S MILK	HUMAN MILK
COLOR	Creamy, white, possibly because of high levels of casein.	Bluish cast reflects lower fat content. Toward the end of a feeding, when fat content is higher, it looks creamier.
BIOACTIVITY	Affects living tissue in cows and calves.	Affects living tissue in human mothers and babies.
VITAMINS	More vitamins D and K. Virtually no vitamin C.	More A and E, which may protect against anemia. Mother who eats well produces enough vitamin C for her baby. Exclusively breastfed babies need vitamin D drops to prevent softening of the bones. This is especially urgent for all babies, who should not be exposed to the sun, and for babies whose nursing mothers are strict vegans. Vitamin K should be administered to newborns to aid in blood clotting.
IRON	Very little.	About the same amount of iron as in cow's milk. However, the iron in human milk is better absorbed by the breastfed baby: 50% of the iron in human milk, compared to only 10% in cow's milk, and only 4% in iron-fortified formula. Breast milk usually meets a baby's iron requirements for at least the first six months of life. Hemoglobin should be checked at six months.
OTHER MINERALS	Four times the amount of *calcium,* seven times the *phosphorus,* and twice the *sulfur* as human milk. The formula-fed baby excretes a large portion of these minerals as excess because they cannot be used.	*Zinc* is more available in breast milk, preventing a zinc-deficiency disorder rarely seen in breastfed babies. Two to three times the amount of *selenium* as in formulas. This mineral helps form a protective enzyme and is critical to developing and protecting a growing child's lungs.
PROTEIN	More than twice as much as in human milk, and in a form utilized less efficiently by the baby. About half the protein in cow's milk is passed in the stool.	Virtually all the protein in breast milk is used by the baby. Also, human milk has different kinds of proteins: Whey proteins (such as alpha-lactalbumin, lactoferrin, and secretory IgA) are abundant. Also present are *Lactobacillus bifidus* and an antistaphylococcal factor. The whey protein portion of human milk contains most of its protective substances. Other small proteins present in human milk and absent from formula are growth factors that promote a baby's growth and development. Two sugar-based proteins in human milk that coat fat particles help to prevent infection; these proteins are not in cow's milk.

	COW'S MILK	HUMAN MILK
SUGAR	Half that in human milk.	*Lactose,* the predominant sugar in human milk, (1) provides an important source of energy; (2) is essential for brain cell functions and enhances the development of the central nervous system; (3) is responsible for the beneficial acidity of the breastfed baby's intestinal tract (which, along with the presence of *L. bifidus,* makes it harder for harmful bacteria to flourish); and (4) being less sweet than other sugars, may help in appetite control and the development of taste. Furthermore, the complex sugars in human milk seem to protect breastfed babies from a number of disease-causing bacteria and fungi.
FATS	Usually *polyunsaturated vegetable fats* are put into formulas to replace saturated fats in cow's milk. Although DHA and ARA, fatty acids essential for brain and eye development, are now added to some formulas, there is no convincing evidence that they are beneficial in this form.	High in *essential saturated fats* (which are largely converted to cholesterol in the body). Breastfed babies have higher cholesterol levels during the first year of life, which may be the way nature programs them to help them handle cholesterol later in life. Human milk provides the long-chain *fatty acids* DHA (docosahexaenoic acid) and ARA (arachidonic acid), which are not only essential for brain and eye development but which are thought to raise IQ scores in childhood. Babies digest human milk fat more efficiently than cow's milk fat because of the presence of the enzyme lipase.
ENZYMES	Appropriate for calves.	Contains *lipase,* an enzyme that helps babies digest the fat of human milk more efficiently.
GROWTH MODULATORS	Appropriate for calves.	Constituents in human milk that help various cells develop and differentiate, these factors may have other roles, too. *Taurine,* an amino acid, aids in digestion and is also thought to be important in brain and nervous system development.
HORMONES	Appropriate for calves.	Human milk contains *oxytocin* (may help foster a loving mother-baby bond), *melatonin* (helps regulate the baby's biological clock, letting the baby know when to eat), *gonadotropin-releasing* hormone (influences sexual development), *thyroid* hormones (may prevent certain disorders), *prostaglandins* (help to regulate body functions), *endorphins* (painkillers and contributors to feelings of well-being), and other hormones.

Index

A

AAP. *see* American
   Academy of Pediatrics
acetaminophen
   (Tylenol), 222, 224
aching, 130
acid reflux, 121
ACME. *see* American
   College of Nurse-
   Midwives Accreditation
   Commission for
   Midwifery Education
ACOG. *see* American
   College of
   Obstetricians and
   Gynecologists
acquired immune
   deficiency syndrome
   (AIDS), 349
active nursing, signs of,
   113, 114, 119, 146–47
acute otitis media, 147

see also ear infections
ADA. *see* American
   Dietetic Association
adopted baby, nursing,
   359
Advil. *see* ibuprofen
afterpains, 114
   see also uterine
   contractions
AIDS. *see* acquired
   immune deficiency
   syndrome
alcohol intake, 39
   bed-sharing and, 161
   during pregnancy, 232
Aleve. *see* naproxen
allergic reactions
   breastfeeding and
   protection against, 12,
   181
   to cow's milk, 12
   to dairy, 181, 182–83
   diet, mother's and, 12,
   181
   food, 181
   milk protein, 183

peanut butter and, 178,
   181
alternative remedies, 199
alveoli, 47, 51
Ambien. *see* zolpidem
Ameda, 397
American Academy of
   Pediatrics (AAP), 391
   *Breastfeeding Handbook
   for Physicians*, 219
breastfeeding
   supported by, 27
first nursing
   recommendations
   from, 93
nursing
   recommendations by,
   31–32
recommendations for
   successful
   breastfeeding from,
   91, 92
statement on
   breastfeeding by, 7
American Board of
   Medical Specialties, 69

American College of
Nurse-Midwives
Accreditation
Commission for
Midwifery Education
(ACME), 66
see also midwives
American College of
Nurse-Midwives, 392
see also midwives
American College of
Obstetricians and
Gynecologists (ACOG),
391
see also obstetrician-
gynecologist
American Dietetic
Association (ADA), 392
American Public Health
Association, 27
amoxicillin, 224
amphetamines, 233
anemia, 379
anesthesia
dental, 224
dose, 221
general, 220
regional, 220
antibiotics, 224, 228,
320, 323
antidepressants,
200–202, 225, 226–27
antiepileptic drugs, 224
antihistamines, 224
antihypertensives, 224
appearance, baby's, 126
appearance, mother's,
209–11, 304
nursing-friendly
clothing and, 210–11
your hair and, 209–10
your nails and, 210
your skin and, 210
appetite spurts, 142,
324–25
ARA, 9
arching back, 169, 327

areola, 50–51
artificial sweeteners, 188
asthma, breastfeeding
and, 12
asymmetric latch, 112
atenolol, 225
attractiveness, mother's
feelings about, 304
Avent Phillips
Corporation, 397
azithromycin, 224

B

"baby and me" classes, 77
"baby blues," 196–200
causes, 196–97
duration, 201
incidence, 201
measures to help with,
198–99
postpartum depression
v., 201
symptoms, 201
time of onset, 201
treatment, 201
baby massage, 152, 306,
394
baby nurse, 68
Baby-Friendly Hospital
Initiative, 74–75, 95
babywearing, 149–50
advantages, 149
crying and, 153
by fathers, 306
safety, 150
see also kangaroo care
backache, 190, 209
Bailey Medical
Engineering, 398
barbiturates, 233–34
bathing baby, 153
bed wetting, 13
bed-sharing

benefits of, 157–58
safe, 160–61
SIDS and, 158
behavior, baby's, 126
benefits of breastfeeding
for baby, 3–15
bond formed as, 3
for mother, 16–23
Bergman, Nils, MD,
14–15, 344
Berlin, Cheston M., Jr.,
MD, 144
bifidobacteria, 224
bilirubin, 59–60, 94, 127
bilirubin encephalopathy,
127–28
bioactive breast milk, 58
birth control, 229,
286–91
coitus interruptus, 290
conditionally
recommended,
289–91
diaphragm, 288
emergency
contraception pill, 291
female condom, 288
IUD, 289
LAM, 286–88
male condom, 288
minipill, 289
natural family planning,
290
NuvaRing, 290
pill with estrogen and
progestin, 291
progestin-only implant,
290
progestin-only pills, 289
skin patch, 291
spermicide, 289
sponge, 288
sterilization, 289
weaning and, 377
birth control pill with
estrogen and progestin,
291

birth disorders, testing
for, 102
birth plan, 77
birthing centers, 77,
92–93
birthing experience,
92–93
bisphenol A (BPA), 5,
136, 245
biting, 168, 370
bleeding nipples, 204–5,
315
blood pressure, 19–20
bonding, 3, 15
husband/partner-baby,
139
with newborn, 90
oxytocin and, 55
bone density, 7, 193
bone loss, 190
bottle(s)
baby's refusal of, 264
BPA in, 5, 136, 245
nipples, 134, 136,
264
sterilizing, 248, 249
washing, 248
bottle-feeding, 133–37
bottles for, 136
breastfeeding combined
with, 31
breastfeeding-
compatible, 133–36
by father, 308
introducing, 262–63
nipple confusion and,
95–96
nipples for, 134, 136
positions for, 134–35
practicing, 144–45
premature infant, 337
bowel movements, 122
bilirubin excretion and,
127
breastfed baby's, 20, 165
color, 122, 124
consistency, 124

frequency, 165
log, 124, 142
milk intake and,
124–26
smell, 124
BPA. see bisphenol A
bra, supportive, 53
see also nursing bra
brain development,
12–13
breaking the suction,
115, 316
breast(s)
after childbirth, 48
anatomy of, 49–53
cancer of, 7, 18,
350–51
care, 204–09
cells, 58
development, 45–49
glandular insufficiency,
47
hard, swollen, 312–14
lactating, 52
during pregnancy,
47–48
preparation of, 80–83
sagging, 30, 53
sexual activity and,
280–81
sexualization of, 25
shape, 49
size, 30, 34, 49–50
small, 34
supporting structure, 53
surgery, 21, 41–42
tissue, 49–50
trauma, 21
weaning and, 377–78
breast augmentation,
352–53
breast cancer, 350–51
breastfed babies and
risk of, 7
breastfeeding and
protection from, 18
breast changes, 17

after childbirth, 48–49
during menstrual cycle,
46–47
during pregnancy, 30,
47–48
during puberty, 46
breast compression, 325
breast infection. see
mastitis
breast lumps
clogged ducts and, 322
infection and, 208
painful, 130
plugged duct and, 208
breast milk, 58–62
availability of, 14
in baby's eyes, 9
baby's growth stages
and changes in, 9
bioactive, 58
bluish tint, 35, 61
cholesterol in, 10
on circumcised penis, 9
complex sugars in, 11
composition of, change
in, 8, 60, 61
cow's milk compared
with, 60–61, 404–07
delivery of, 51–52
digestibility of, 8
drinking cow's milk and
making, 38
drying up, 49, 377
elements in, 4
essential fatty acids in, 4,
12
exercise and taste of,
192–93
fat composition, 4–5,
8–9
immunity for baby and,
4
infections treated with,
148
mother's custom-
designed, 8
in newborn, 45

nutrient value of,
  beyond one year, 61
premature infants and
  composition of, 8, 62,
  338–39
production of, 51–52
protective substances
  in, 9–11
protein content, 4, 61
richness, 35
smells, 5–6
storing collected,
  248–51
"structure" of, 61
tastes, 5–6
tint, 60
uniqueness of, 61–62
uses, 148
breast milk jaundice,
  128–29
breast pads, 204, 207,
  208, 272
breast pumps
  battery-operated, 237
  choosing, 237–43
  cleaning, 266
  closed systems, 239
  comfort, 238
  comparisons, 237
  convenience, 239
  cost, 241
  economy electric, 241
  effectiveness, 238
  electric, 237, 239–41
  FDA regulations, 237
  fit, 238
  foot-operated, 237, 241
  hands-free pumping
    bra, 241–42
  high-quality electric,
    237, 240–41
  hospital-grade double
    electric, 236, 240
  inverted nipples and, 83
  manual (handheld),
    237, 241
  open systems, 239

renting, 240
safety, 238
sources for, 397–98
types, 236–37, 239
used, 239
breast reduction, 353
breast shells, 81–82,
  208, 243, 314, 318
breast shields, 314, 318
breast surgery, 351–53
breastfed babies
  bowel movements, 20,
    165
  breast cancer and, 7
  diarrhea and, 6, 8, 11
  digestive problems in, 8
  discrimination against,
    261
  ear infections in, 11
  formula-fed babies and,
    differences between,
    10
  formula-fed baby health
    and, 7–8
  growth of, 10
  heart disease and, 7, 10
  infectious diseases in, 7
  obesity and, 4, 7
  SIDS in, 7
  smell, 20
  survival rates, 6
breastfeeding
  AAP recommendations
    for successful, 91, 92
  AAP statement on, 7
  another woman's baby,
    358–59
  away from home,
    203–16
  beginning, 90–91,
    103–37
  benefits of, in first six
    months of life, 6
  bottle-feeding
    combined with, 31
  comforting baby and,
    15

convenience, 17
cost-saving with, 19, 20
cultural influence on,
  23, 24–25
cultural shift away
  from, 24
deciding against, 22–23
deciding on, 1–28
disease protection,
  9–12
as earth-friendly, 20–22
embarrassment and,
  32–33
emotional gratification
  from, 14–15
emotional preparation
  for, 56
emotional upset and,
  35–36
extended, 371–73, 388
factors influencing
  decision for, 1–2
father's negative
  feelings about, 25
formula-feeding and
  switching to, 2
health in adulthood
  and, 6–8
health in childhood
  and, 6–8
at home, 140–48,
  203–16
hospital staff and
  support of, 26–27
immediate, 91
as impossibility, 21, 33
inadvisability of, 21
infant nutrition and,
  3–6
learning, 42
length of time, 4, 31–32
mental preparation for,
  56
for mother's health,
  17–20
opposition to, 37
pain and, 34–35

postpartum, 18, 91,
93–96
postpartum depression
and, 19, 200
preparing for, 63–88
in public, 26, 32–33,
212–16
questions about,
29–43
reasons against, 2–3
reasons for, 2–3
reasons women give for
not wanting to, 22–23
rediscovery of, 2
resources, 390–91
sensuous nature of,
284–86
as sexual passage,
275–96
society and, 25–27
solid foods and
continuing, 4
30-day guarantee, 2
weight gain and, 30–31
*Breastfeeding an Adopted
Baby and Relactation*
(Hormann), 359
breastfeeding
consultants, 67
see also lactation
consultants
*Breastfeeding Handbook
for Physicians* (AAP),
219
Breastfeeding
Pharmacology website,
219
breathing disorders, 6–7
"brick dust" stain,
125–26
broccoli, 38
bromocriptine (Parlodel),
225
burping, 120–22, 152
methods, 121–22
spit up and, 122
Butler, Robert, MD, 189

C

cabbage, 38, 183
cabbage leaves,
engorgement and, 313
caffeine, 184, 230–31
"caked" breasts, 321–22
see also clogged ducts
calcium, 38, 176
caloric intake, mother's,
38, 173, 174, 179
see also diet, mother's
cancer
breast, 18, 350–51
ovarian, 18
see also breast cancer
car safety, 212
car seat safety, 212
carbamazepine, 224
caregivers, interviewing
potential, 260
cauliflower, 38
Celexa, 227
celiac disease, 12
cephalosporins, 224
Certified Lactation
Consultant (CLC), 67
see also lactation
consultants
certified nurse-midwife
(CNM), 66
see also midwives
cesarean birth, 96–97
cesarean section, 39, 79
chemotherapeutic
agents, 225
chicken pox, 347
child care, finding,
260–61
childbirth, pain relief
during, 220–21
childbirth educators,
resources for finding
professional, 393
chills, 130

cholesterol
in breast milk, 10
in colostrum, 59
cimetidine (Tagamet),
224
CLC. *see* Certified
Lactation Consultant
cleft lip/palate, 362
Cleft Palate Foundation
(CPF), 395
clogged ducts, 130,
321–22
alternating positions
and, 105
continuing to nurse,
321
lumps and, 322
tight clothing and, 211
cloth diapers, 124
clothing, nursing-
friendly, 210–11
working mother and,
272
clutch hold, 107–8
CMV. *see*
cytomegalovirus
CNM. *see* certified
nurse-midwife
cocaine, 233
codeine, 225
coitus interruptus, 290
cold, in baby, 346–47
nose breathing and,
114, 333
nursing strike and, 333
cold remedies, over-the-
counter, 227
colic, 151–57
causes, 155–56
dairy in mother's diet
and, 183
dealing with, 156–57
definition of, 154–55
growing out of, 154
mother's diet and,
155–56
rule of three, 154

treatment, 155
colic hold, 156
collecting milk, 243–47
    storage, 248–51
    see also expressing milk;
        hand-expression;
        pumping milk
coloring your hair, 209
colostrum, 31, 58–60
    antibodies, 60
    cholesterol in, 59
    components, 59
    fat content, 59
    function of, 59
    IgA, 59
    laxative function of,
        59–60
    milk supply and,
        establishing, 94
    pregnancy and, 47,
        58–60
    production of, 48
communication, 293–94
    husband/partner and,
        305
condoms, 288
constipation, 8, 165–66
contraception, 20, 229,
    288–91
    recommended, 288–89
    types, 286–87
    use of, 40–41
    see also birth control
Cooper's droopers, 53
co-sleeping
    benefits of, 157–58
    sex and, 295
    SIDS and, 158
cough and cold OTC
    remedies, 227
cow's milk
    adverse effects of, 181
    allergy, 12
    breast milk compared
        with, 60–61, 405–7
    formula and, 8
    mineral levels in, 60–61

in mother's diet, 12, 38
    offering your baby,
        379–80
    protein levels in, 60–61
CPF. *see* Cleft Palate
    Foundation
cracked nipples, 204–5,
    315
    infection and, 315
    moist wound healing
        for, 315–16
cradle hold, 106–07
crib safety, 159
cross-cradle hold, 106
cross-over hold, 106
crying, 150–51
    babywearing and, 153
    comforting for, 152–54
    different types of, 140
    pacifiers and, 154
    responding to, 150–51
    serious problems and,
        151
C-section. *see* cesarean
    birth
cue(s), baby's hunger,
    119, 140–41
    breastfeeding on, 91
    rooming-in and, 97
    solid foods and, 381
cultural norms, 23
cup feeding, introducing,
    262–63
custody cases, 387–88
cytomegalovirus (CMV),
    348

D

dairy
    allergy to, 181–83
    colic and, 182
    in mother's diet,
        155–56

see also cow's milk
day-care centers, 261
defrosting milk, 252
dehydration, signs of,
    130–31
dental anesthetics, 224
dental cavities
    juice and, 380
    prolonged breastfeeding
        and, 39–40
    sleeping on breast and,
        163
Depo-Provera, 290
depression, 195
    baby blues and, 196
    measures to help with,
        198–99
    nipple pain and, 315
    see also postpartum
        depression
DHA
    in breast milk, 6, 9
    mother's intake of,
        178
diabetes, 350
    type 2, 19
diaper rash, 6
diapers, 165–66
    cloth, 124
    disposable, 125
diaphragm, 288
diarrhea, 165, 346
    breastfeeding and
        protection against, 6,
        8, 11
diet, mother's, 20, 30–31,
    173–74
    allergic reactions of
        baby to, 12
    baby's reaction to, 38
    calcium in, 176
    caloric intake and, 38,
        173, 174
    colic and, 155–56
    components warranting
        special attention,
        176–78

cost and, 185–86
cow's milk in, 12, 38
dairy in, 155–56
DHA in, 178
folic acid in, 178
foods to avoid, 181–84
guidelines for health,
 174–76
iron in, 177
liquids, 180
milk production and,
 143
milk-coloring foods
 and, 184
protein in, 177–78
supplementation, 180,
 218, 367
vegetarian, 179–80
vitamin D in, 176–77
your health and, 173
Diflucan. *see* fluconazole
disease protection,
 breastfeeding and,
 9–12
disposable diapers, 125
doctor's appointment,
 baby's first, 122–23
"doll's eyes" technique,
 116
domperidone, 227
DONA International. *see*
 Doulas of North
 America International
donor milk, 357–58
doula(s), 67–68
 cost of, 68
 hospital births and, 77
 postpartum, 68, 84
 questions to ask, 72
 resources for finding
 professional, 394
Doulas of North America
 (DONA) International,
 67, 394
Down syndrome, 363,
 395
draught, 53

see also let-down reflex
drinks, introducing,
 379–82
 cow's milk, 379–80
 juice, 380
 water, 380
drugs
 during childbirth,
 220–21
 hard, 230–34
 nursing and, resources
 for information on,
 219
 pregnancy and, 218
 recreational, 218,
 230–34
 see also medicines/
 medications
Drugs and Lactation
 Database (LactMed),
 219
drying up your milk, 49,
 377

E

ear infections, 11, 147
eczema, 12
Eiger, Marvin S., MD,
 124
emergency contraception
 pill, 291
emotions
 breastfeeding and,
 14–15, 35–36
 let-down reflex
 inhibited by, 35, 56
employer benefits of
 breastfeeding, 258
"emptying" the breast,
 120
endocrine glands, 45
endorphins, release of,
 190

engorgement, 48,
 312–14
 latching on and,
 113–14
 relieving, 313–14
 sudden weaning and,
 314
environmental
 chemicals, 43, 184–85
epidurals, 220
episiotomy, 278
Ergomar. *see* ergotamine
Ergostat. *see* ergotamine
ergotamine (Ergomar,
 Ergostat, Gynergen),
 225
erythromycin, 224
essential fatty acids, 4,
 12
 see also DHA
estrogen, 46
 birth control pill with,
 291
eszopiclone (Lunesta),
 227
exchange transfusion,
 132
exclusive pumping, 133
exercise, 181–82
 beginning to, 189–92
 breast milk taste and,
 192–93
 guide for nursing
 mother, 192–95
 postpartum, 191
 schedule, 190–92
 strenuous, 192–93
 types of, 193–94
 variation, 192
 warm-up, 194
 weight loss and, 187
exocrine glands, 45
expressed milk
 defrosting, 252
 feeding, 251–52
 flying with, 215
 handling, 247–48

medicines and
 discarding, 222
for premature infants,
 340–41
quantity of, 267–68
separation of, 251
smell of, 251
storing, 248–51
transporting, 251
expressing milk, 91,
 235–52
 alcohol consumption
 and, 233
 engorgement and, 313
 learning, 264–65
 milk production and,
 246–47
 ovulation and, 57
 at work, 267
extended breastfeeding,
 371–73
 dental cavities and,
 39–40
 legality of, 388
 recommendations for,
 373
eye drops, newborn, 101

F

Family and Medical
 Leave Act, 256
family members, support
 from, 68–69
family physicians, 65
 questions to ask, 71
 resources for finding
 professional, 392
fast-gaining infant,
 330–31
 solid foods and, 380
fasting, 180
fat composition
 breast milk, 4–5, 8–9

colostrum, 59
fathers, 297–307
 babywearing, 306
 becoming, 298
 being a complete,
 307–08
 boot camp for, 302
 bottle-feeding, 308
 "breastfeeding," and
 nurturing your baby,
 306
 breastfeeding benefits
 for, 298
 importance of, in
 family, 300–01
 kangaroo care and,
 344–45
 learning how to cope,
 303–04
 mothering for, 292
 night duty, 307
 older children and, 308
 skin-to-skin contact
 and, 306
 special meetings for,
 301
 support for, 309
 see also husband/
 partner
fatigue, 165
 exercise and, 191
 sex and, 276
feeding(s)
 let-downs during,
 number of, 54
 log, 142
 offering both breasts
 per, 115–17
 offering one breast per,
 115, 117
 relaxation and, 145,
 333
 routines, 139
 working mother and,
 265–69
feeding, duration of,
 119–20, 146–48

"emptying" breast and,
 120
 hind milk and, 120
 let-down reflex and,
 120
 short, 119–20
feeding frequency,
 117–19
 benefits of, 118
 jaundice and, 118
 milk production and,
 143
 premature infants and,
 343
 relactation/induced
 lactation and, 360
 slow-gaining infant and,
 325
 sore nipples and, 118
feeding on cue, 91
feeding schedules, 141
 for working mothers,
 271–73
female sexuality, 282–84
 five phases of, 282–83
 hormones and, 283–84
 outside pressures/
 emotions influencing,
 283
fever
 baby's, 131
 mother's, 130
first nursing, 18, 91,
 93–96
fish, contaminants in,
 182
Flagyl. see metronidazole
fluconazole (Diflucan),
 224, 320
fluoride, 367
flying with baby, 214–15
 airline's breastfeeding
 policy and, 214
 breastfeeding and,
 214–15
 bringing expressed
 breast milk and, 215

folic acid (folate), 178
Folley, S. J., 55
fontanel, sunken, 126, 131
Food and Drug Administration (FDA), 237
Food Guide Pyramid, 174
food labels, 187, 188
football hold. *see* clutch hold
fore milk, 4–5, 52
  too much, 149
formula
  cow's milk as base for, 8, 379
  hospitals and, 95
  hypoallergenic protein hydrolysate, 379
  jaundice and, 131–32
  nutrition, 61–62
  soybean-based, 379
  supplementation with, 127, 129, 131, 144
formula-fed babies
  breastfed babies and, differences between, 10
  breastfed baby health and, 7–8
  digestion of formula in, 5
  growth of, 10
  insulin concentrations in, 5
  leptin production in, 5
  obesity and, 4
formula-feeding
  breastfeeding and switching from, 2
  cost of, 5
  disadvantages of, 5
  expiration dates and, 5
  hospitals and, 92
  overfeeding and, 5
  popularity of, 2

storing prepared bottles of formula and, 5
working mothers and, 268
frequency of feedings, 98
fussiness, 151
  daily, 155

G

galactagogues, 143–44
galactocele (milk-retention cyst), 324, 351
galactosemia, 363
gastroesophageal reflux (GER), 121
  colic and, 155
  crying and, 151
gastroesophageal reflux disease/disorder (GERD), 155
gastrointestinal disorders, 6
gastrointestinal tract, baby's, 155
gavage, 337
general anesthesia, 220
gentamicin, 224
GER. *see* gastroesophageal reflux
GERD. *see* gastroesophageal reflux disease/disorder
glandular insufficiency, 47
glandular tissue, 51
going out with baby, 212
grandmothers, helping new mother and, 83, 85
growth spurts, 142, 324–25
growth stages in babies, 9
Gynergen. *see* ergotamine
György, Paul, MD, 12

H

hair loss, 210
hand-expression, 236, 242–43
  see also expressing milk
hand-to-eye coordination, 11
hard drugs, 231
harmful substances
  environmental, 183
  in food, 182–83
Hartmann, Peter E., 49
health care provider(s)
  changing, 72
  choosing your, 64
  consultations, 70
  disagreeing with your, 311–12
  fees, 72
  group practice, 71
  hospital affiliations, 70
  questions to ask, 70–71
  trusting your, 69–73
  types of, 64–74
  see also specific types of health care providers
health insurance
  breastfeeding benefits, 73–74
  lactation consultants covered under, 74
  midwives covered under, 66
Healthy Eating Pyramid, 174–75
hearing test, 102
heart disease
  in babies, 363–64
  breastfed babies and risk of, 7, 10
  breastfeeding and protection against, 19
help
  for new mother, 83–88

asking for, 198
finding, 84–86
seeking, 130–31
hemorrhage, 278
hepatitis B, 349
hepatitis C, 349
herbal remedies, 199,
 229–30
 nursing and, 218
 postpartum, 222
herbal tea, 184, 230
heroin, 234
herpes, 348–49
herpes simplex virus
 (HSV), 348
high-risk pregnancies, 77
hind milk, 4–5, 52
 feeding duration and,
 120
 offering one breast
 during feeding and,
 117
 too little, 149
HIV. see human
 immunodeficiency virus
HMF. see human milk
 fortifier
HMOs, 74
Hoffman technique, 81
home birth, 77–79
 back-up plan, 79
homeopathics, 199,
 229–30
Hormann, Elizabeth, 359
hormones
 balance, 48
 female sexuality and,
 283–84
 placenta and
 production of, 47
 secretion, 16–17, 45
hospital(s)
 advantages, 76–77
 "baby and me" classes,
 77
 Baby-Friendly Hospital
 Initiative, 74–75

birth plan and, 77
birthing rooms, 75
breastfeeding in, 76,
 92–93
breastfeeding
 premature infant in,
 341–43
breastfeeding
 resistance, 99–101
breastfeeding support
 in, 74–75
 disadvantages, 99
 doulas and, 77
 environment, 99–101
 formula practices at, 95
 giving birth in, 74–77
 interruptions, 99
 lactation professionals
 in, 98
 rooming-in, 75
 visitors, 101
hospital staff
 breastfeeding
 supported by, 26–27,
 98–99
 communicating with,
 100
hospitalization
 of baby, 347
 of mother, 348
HSV. see herpes simplex
 virus
human
 immunodeficiency virus
 (HIV), 349
Human Milk Banking
 Association of North
 America, 395
human milk fortifier
 (HMF), 338
human placental
 lactogen, 47
Human Sexual Response
 (Masters, Johnson),
 285
hunger, signs of, 119
hunger strikes, 264

husband/partner,
 297–307
 baby bonding with, 139
 breastfeeding support
 and, 36, 300, 301–03
 communication,
 293–94, 305
 helping new mother,
 83, 85–86, 305–07
 involvement of, 139
 is still your lover,
 292–96
 jealousy of new baby,
 293, 299
 mother as lover and,
 304–05
 prenatal classes, 301
 sexual interest, 304
 working mothers and
 help from, 254
hydrogel pads, 318
Hygela II Medical
 Group, Inc., 397
hypoallergenic protein
 hydrolysate formula, 379
hypoglycemia, 363
hypothalamus, 55–56

I

IBLCE. see International
 Board of Lactation
 Consultant Examiners
ibuprofen (Advil,
 Motrin), 224
ICEA. see International
 Childbirth Education
 Association
IgA. see immunoglobulin
 A
ILCA. see International
 Lactation Consultant
 Association
illness, in baby, 346–47

illness, in mother, 347–51
  recommendations
    against breastfeeding
    and, 347–48
immunity, breast milk
  and, 4
immunoglobulin A (IgA)
  breast milk
    transmission of,
    9–10
  in colostrum, 59
Imodium. see loperamide
Implanon, 290
induced lactation, 359
  succeeding at, 360–61
Infant Massage USA,
  394
infections
  breast, 322–23
  breast lumps and, 208
  breast milk and
    treating, 148
  cracked nipples and,
    315
  ear, 11, 147
  respiratory, 6
  sexual intercourse and
    risk of, 278
  vaginal yeast, 228
infectious diseases, in
  breastfed baby, 7
inflammatory breast
  cancer, 351
information sources,
  389–400
insulin, 224
  in formula-fed babies, 5
International Board of
  Lactation Consultant
  Examiners (IBLCE),
  67, 393
International Childbirth
  Education Association
  (ICEA), 390
International Lactation
  Consultant Association
  (ILCA), 393

Internet as resource, 396
  website appendix,
    401–04
intrauterine device
  (IUD)
  copper, 289
  with levonorgestrel, 289
inverted nipples, 35, 50,
  81–83
  breast pumps and, 83
  Hoffman technique for,
    81
  test for, 81–82
iron, 368
  in cow's milk, 379–80
  mother's intake of, 177
  vitamin C and
    absorption of, 177
IUD. see intrauterine
  device

J

jaundice, 59–60, 94
  breast milk, 128–29
  evaluation for presence
    of, 123
  feeding frequency and,
    118
  in infants, 127–32
  pathologic, 130
  physiologic, 128
  signs, 128
  starvation, of newborn,
    129
  treatment, 131–32
  types of infant, 128–30
jaw development, 13
Johnson, Virginia E., 284
  Human Sexual
    Response, 285
juice, 380

K

kangaroo care, 15, 152
  fathers and, 344–45
  for premature infants,
    15, 337, 344–45
Karp, Harvey, MD, 154
Kegel, Arnold, 279
Kegel exercises, 279, 280
kernicterus, 127–28
Kinsey, Alfred C., 285

L

La Leche League
  International, 28, 390
  breastfeeding
    consultants, 67
  drugs and breastfeeding
    information, 219
Lact-Aid International,
  398–99
Lact-Aid Nursing Trainer
  System, 328–29
lactation, 52
  eating during, 185–86
  induced, 359–61
  menstruation and,
    57–58
  miracle of, 44–62
  ovulation and, 57–58
  pregnancy and, 57–58
lactation consultants
  (LCs), 27, 66–67
  health insurance
    coverage of, 74
  resources for finding
    professional, 393
lactation professionals
  employer-provided, 259
  hospital, 98
lactation programs,

employer-supported, 257–59
Lactational Amenorrhea Method (LAM), 20, 40, 57, 229, 286–88
effectiveness, 287
lactic acid, 192–93
LactMed. *see* Drugs and Lactation Database
Lactobacillus acidophilus, 224
lactose, 4
LAM. *see* Lactational Amenorrhea Method
Lamaze International, 393
lamotrigine, 224
lanolin, 204, 316
Lansinoh HPA Lanolin, 204, 316
latching on, 110–14
engorgement and, 113–14
first nursing and, 94
holding your breast for, 110–11
pain and, 34
latch-on
assessing baby's, 98
asymmetric, 112
breathing and, 114
correct/incorrect, 112
sore nipples and, 112–13, 316
late-preterm infants, 345–46
laws, breastfeeding, 385–88
custody cases and, 387–88
extended breastfeeding and, 388
public nursing, 214
by state, 386–87
workplace and, 269
LCs. *see* lactation consultants

leaking milk, 206–8
working mothers and, 274
leptin, 5
let-down reflex, 53–56
emotions inhibiting, 35, 56
feeding length and, 120
feeling your, 114
forceful, 148
medicines, influence on, 223
problems, 55
pumping milk and triggering, 266
signs of active, 56, 114
timing, 53
working, 54
levothyroxine (Synthroid), 224
Lexapro, 227
licensed practical nurse (LPN), 68
licorice, 230
LilyPadz, 208, 318
liquids, mother's consumption of, 180–81
lithium, 225
loperamide (Imodium), 224
low-risk pregnancies, 65
LPN. *see* licensed practical nurse
Lunesta. *see* eszopiclone
lysozyme, 10

M

macrophages, 11
MANA. *see* Midwives Alliance of North America
marijuana, 233

Marks, David, MD, 344–45
Marks, Laura, MD, 139
massage
baby, 152, 306, 394
engorgement and, 313
Masters, William H., 284
Human Sexual Response, 285
mastitis, 110, 130, 322–23
antibiotics for, 323
continuing to nurse with, 323
symptoms, 322
treatment, 323
maternity centers, 77
maternity leave, 79, 256
lactation programs and, employer-supported, 258
planning ahead and, 260–65
mature milk, 48, 60–61
see also breast milk
MCH Services, Inc., 396
McKenna, James J., 161
Mead, Margaret, 295
meconium, 122
colostrum's laxative function and, 59–60
expulsion of, 94
see also bowel movements
Medela, Inc.
Breastfeeding U.S., 398, 399
medicines/medications
bed-sharing and, 161
breastfeeding and, 221–28
of concern, 226–27
dosage, 228
half-life, 223, 228
nursing and, 218
postpartum, 222–23

postpartum depression, 200–202
pumping and discarding milk while taking, 222
questions to ask before taking, 223, 228
safe, 224
temporary cessation of breastfeeding, 226
unsafe, 225
unusual symptoms in baby and, 228
weaning and, 22
see also over-the-counter remedies
menstruation
breast changes and, 46–47
breastfeeding during, 39
lactation and, 57–58
suspension of, 17, 18
MER. *see* milk-ejection reflex
methadone, 234
methamphetamine, 234
metronidazole (Flagyl), 224
middle ear infections, 11, 147
see also ear infections
midwives, 65–66
medical back-up, 65
questions to ask, 70–72
resources for finding professional, 392
training/accreditation, 65
Midwives Alliance of North America (MANA), 392
milk. *see* breast milk; cow's milk
milk banks, 357–58, 395
milk ducts, 51
milk delivery and, 52

size, 51–52
see also clogged ducts; plugged duct
milk intake, 124–27
adequate, 141–43
appearance and, baby's, 126
behavior and, baby's, 126
bowel movements and adequate, 124–26
nursing experience and, 126–27
urine and adequate, 124–26
weight, baby's and, 126
milk production
building up, 142–45
fluid intake and, 181
hormonal contraceptives and, 229
nicotine and, 231
pumping/expressing and, 246–47
milk protein allergy, 183
milk supply, 17, 33–34
abundant, 148–49
diminished, 325
establishing, 94, 115
increased demand and, 325–26
increasing, 268, 324–25
offering both breasts during feeding and, 115
prolactin levels and, 119
tandem nursing and, 357
milk-ejection reflex (MER), 53, 114
see also let-down reflex
milk-retention cyst, 324
Milkscreen, 232
mineral supplementation, 367
minipill, 289
Montgomery's glands, 51

mother-baby contact, postpartum, 97–98
mothering the mother, 83–88
mother's health
baby's health and, 92
breastfeeding and, 17–20
Motrin. *see* ibuprofen
mucin, 9
multiples, 354–56
breastfeeding, 42–43
resources for mothers of, 394
My Pyramid, 174

N

naproxen (Aleve), 224
National Business Group on Health (NBGH), 396
National Down Syndrome Society (NDSS), 395
see also Down syndrome
National Healthy Mothers, Healthy Babies Coalition, 396–97
National Organization of Mothers of Twins Clubs, Inc., 394
National Women's Health Information Center, The, 391, 397
natural family planning, 290
natural remedies, 229–30
NBGH. *see* National Business Group on Health

NDSS. *see* National
Down Syndrome
Society
near-term infants,
345–46
neonatal intensive care
unit (NICU), 336
neonatologist, 66
newborn
birth disorders test for,
102
bonding with, 90
bottles given to, 95–96
breast milk in, 45
breastfeeding, 91
doctor's follow-up, 91,
98–99
eye drops, 101
first doctor's
appointment, 102
health measures,
101–02
hearing test, 102
nipple confusion and,
95–96
nursing strike of,
331–32
pacifiers and, 95–96
starvation jaundice of,
129
tests, 102
vitamin K shot, 101
water bottles given to,
95
weight loss,
postpartum, 99, 103
Newman, Jack, MD, 325
Newman Breastfeeding
Clinic and Institute,
391
Newton, Niles, PhD, 282
nicotine, 231–32
NICU. *see* neonatal
intensive care unit
night and day confusion,
baby's, 145–46
night feedings, 161–65

encouraging baby to
give up, 162–63
joys of, 164–65
"nip and nap," 146
nipple(s), 50
bleeding, 204–05, 315
bottle, 5, 134, 136,
148, 249, 264
chewing on, 316
cracked, 204–05,
315–16
inverted, 35, 50
painful, 130, 204–5,
314–15
"pseudo-inverted," 50
rash around, 319
shapes, 50
size, 238
sore, 107, 110, 112–13,
118, 204, 314–19
nipple confusion, 95–96,
136
pacifiers and, 147
slow-gaining infant and,
326
nipple creams, 316
nipple shields, 82, 346
nitrous oxide, 224
nose breathing, 114,
333
novacaine, 224
nursing bra, 30, 204–6,
272
finding right, 206–7
the nursing family, life as
part of, 171
nursing strike, 331–34,
370
of baby, 332–34
menstruation and, 39
of newborn, 331–32
nursing supplementers,
328–29
relactation/induced
lactation and, 361
nursing-related
problems, 310–34

baby who gains too fast,
330–31
baby who gains too
slowly, 325–30
clogged ducts, 321–22
dealing with, 198
disagreeing with your
doctor, 311–12
engorgement, 312–14
galactocele, 324
mastitis, 322–23
sore nipples, 314–19
sudden increase in
baby's demand,
324–25
temporary rejection of
breast, 331–34
thrush, 319–21
nutrition, infant, 3–6
nutritional supplements,
218
nutritionists, resources
for finding professional,
392
nuts, allergy, 181
NuvaRing, 290
nystatin, 224
for thrush, 320

O

obesity, 4, 7
obstetrician-gynecologist
(ob/gyn), 64–65
questions to ask, 70–71
resources for finding
professional, 391
older children, 37, 86–88
fathers and, 308
Olds, Sally, 16, 295
omega-3 fatty acids, 6, 9
see also DHA
organizations, helpful,
389–400

orientation period for nursing, 139
Orinase. *see* tolbutamide
Ortho Evra, 291
osteoporosis, 18–19
OTC remedies. *see* over-the-counter remedies
other milk, introducing, 379–80
ovarian cancer, 18
overfeeding, 5
overstimulation of baby, 151
oversupply of milk, 148
 leaking milk and, 207
 see also milk supply
over-the-counter (OTC) remedies
 cough and cold, 227
 nursing and, 218
 postpartum, 222
overweight mother, 188
 breastfeeding positioning and, 105
ovulation, 20, 40, 57
 expressing milk and, 57
 lactation and, 57–58
 pumping milk and, 57, 341
oxytocin
 bonding and, 55
 production, 54
 release of, 55
 secretion, 16–17

P

pacifiers, 95–96, 147
 crying and use of, 154
 night feeding and, 163
 nipple confusion and, 147

SIDS prevention and, 147
Paget's disease, 351
pain medication
 cesarean birth and, 97
 engorgement and, 314
painful nipples, 130, 204–05, 314–15
Parlodel. *see* bromocriptine
paroxetine (Paxil), 225, 227
partner. s*ee* fathers; husband/partner
Paxil. *see* paroxetine
PCA. *see* personal care aide
PCP. *see* phencyclidine
peanut allergy, 178, 181
pediatrician, 66
 first visit to, 122–23
 questions to ask, 71
 resources for finding professional, 391
pelvic floor (Kegel) exercises, 279, 280
penicillin, 224
perinatologist, 65
personal care aide (PCA), 68
personality, baby's, 166–70
 the alarm clock, 167
 the biter, 169
 colic and, 155
 the dawdler, 167
 development of, 15
 the dozer, 167–69
 the good eater, 167
 the lopsided nurser, 169
 the nonconformist, 167
 the overeager beaver, 169
 the playgirl/playboy, 170

the spitter, 169
 the unhappy archer, 169–70
 the waiter, 167
phencyclidine (PCP), 234
phenobarbital, 224
phenylketonuria (PKU), 102, 363
phenytoin, 224
phototherapy, 129, 132
physiologic jaundice, 128
PIF. *see* prolactin-release inhibiting factor
pillows, breastfeeding-specific, 105–06
pituitary gland, 55–56
PKU. *see* phenylketonuria
placenta
 delivery of, 95
 hormone production by, 47
plugged duct, 110, 321–22
 breast lump and, 208
 see also clogged ducts
positions, breastfeeding, 104–17
 alternating, 104–5
 cesarean birth and, 97
 good, 107
 lying down, 108–10
 obese mother and, 105
 oversupply and, 149
 pillows for, 105–06
 for premature infants, 341–42
 sitting up, 105–08
 sore nipples and, 107, 315, 317
 see also bottle-feeding; *specific positions*
postpartum
 breastfeeding, 18, 91, 93–96

breastfeeding
immediately, 58–59,
94–95
doulas, 68, 84
medicine, 222–23
mother-baby contact,
97–98
period, 93
skin-to-skin, 94
postpartum blues, 201
see also "baby blues"
postpartum depression,
196, 200–202
"baby blues" v., 201
breastfeeding and
protection against, 19,
200
causes, 196–97
duration, 201
getting help for, 200
incidence, 201
measures to help with,
198–99
medication for, 200
nondrug treatments for,
202
risk factors, 200
stress and, 197
symptoms, 201
time of onset, 201
treatment, 201
postpartum exam, 278
pregnancy
alcohol intake during,
232
areola darkening
during, 51
breast changes during,
30, 47–48
breastfeeding and
prevention of, 40
breastfeeding during, 41
cocaine use during, 233
colostrum and, 47,
58–60
drugs and, 218
high-risk, 77

lactation and, 57–58
low-risk, 65
nursing through,
356–57
prolactin and, 47–48
smoking during, 232
weaning during, 356
weight gain during, 189
working mothers and
planning during,
255–57
premature infants
bottle-feeding of, 337
breast milk composition
for, 8, 62, 338–39
breastfeeding, 41,
336–46
breastfeeding, in
hospital, 341–43
breastfeeding mother,
support for, 340
expressed milk for,
340–41
feeding by gavage for,
337
feeding sequences for,
343–44
kangaroo care for, 15,
337, 344–45
nursing positions for,
341–42
taking your baby home,
343–44
prenatal classes, 79–80,
301
preterm infant. see
premature infants
probiotics, 224, 228
antibiotics and, 320
progesterone, 46
progestin, birth control
pill with, 291
progestin-only
contraceptive,
injectable, 290
progestin-only implant,
290

progestin-only pills, 229,
289
projectile vomiting,
120–21
prolactin
milk production and, 55
milk supply and, 119
offering both breasts
during feeding and,
115
ovaries and, 57
pregnancy and levels of,
47–48
production, 54
psychological effects,
48
release of, 36
prolactin-release
inhibiting factor (PIF),
47
protein
in breast milk, 4, 61,
406
in cow's milk, 60–61,
406
milk, allergy, 183
mother's intake of,
177–78
sources, 177–78
vegetarian diet and, 179
Prozac, 227
pseudoephedrine, 225
"pseudo-inverted"
nipples, 50
see also inverted nipples
ptosis, 53
public nursing, 26,
32–33, 212–16
acceptance of, 212
legality of, 214,
386–87
locations for, 216
privacy and, 216
pumped milk
handling, 247–48
medicines and
discarding, 222

storing, 248–51
thermos or cooler for
storing, 266
pumping bras, 241–42
pumping milk, 91,
235–52
alcohol consumption
and, 233
employer-provided
places for, 270
equipment for, 266–67
exclusively, 133
learning, 264–65
let-down reflex and,
triggering, 266
milk production and,
246–47
nursing while, 244–46
ovulation and, 57, 341
sore nipples and, 318
temporary cessation of
breastfeeding and,
226
see also expressing milk

R

RA. see rheumatoid
arthritis
radioactive compounds,
226
recreational drugs, 218,
230–34
reflux, 121
see also
gastroesophageal
reflux
refusal to nurse, from
one breast, 115
regional (local)
anesthesia, 220
registered nurse (RN), 68
rejection of breast,
temporary, 331–34

see also nursing strike
rejection of milk, 184
relactation, 359
succeeding at, 360–61
relaxation
feedings and, 145,
333
milk production and,
143
resources, 389–400
respiratory infections, 6
Retin-A. see tretinoin
rheumatoid arthritis
(RA), 19
rickets, 177
RN. see registered nurse
romance, 294–95
rooming-in, 75, 91, 97
rooting reflex, 116, 140
Rossi, Alice, 284

S

sage, 230
scent signal, nursing, 51
scheduled deliveries, 79
seafood, 181
seashells, 319
secondhand smoke,
231–32
selective serotonin
reuptake inhibitors
(SSRIs), 227
separation of mother and
baby, 346
sexual activity
appearance of mother
and, 296
breastfeeding and,
275–96
breasts and, 280–81
co-sleeping and, 295
husband/father and,
304

lubrication, 279–80
noncoital activities and,
283
orgasm, 282
pain and, 278–80
resuming, 277–81
spurting milk during,
280–81
your interest in, 276–77
sexual arousal, 284–86
Sexual Behavior in the
Human Female
(Kinsey), 285
sexual recovery, 190
sexuality
breastfeeding and, 40
maternal role and, 284
sexualization of breasts,
25
SIDS. see sudden and
unexpected death of an
infant
single mothers, 37–38
sippy cup, 262
sitting up positions,
105–08
clutch (football) hold,
107–08
cradle hold, 106–07
cross-cradle, cross-over,
transitional hold, 106
skin patch, 291
skin-to-skin contact
father and, 306
kangaroo mother care
and, 15
pluses of, 15
postpartum, 94
for premature infants,
344–45
see also kangaroo care
sleeping arrangements,
157–61
bed sharing, 157
co-sleeping, 157
safety, 159–60
separate rooms, 157

sleeping on the breast, 115–17
  dental cavities and, 163
sleeping pills, 227
slide-over technique, 169
slow-gaining infant, 325–30
slow-gaining older baby, 326–27
smell, baby's, 153
smoking, 231–32
  breast sagging and, 53
  passive, 231–32
  during pregnancy, 232
SNS. see Supplemental Nursing System
soft spot. see fontanel
solid foods
  baby's interest in, 381
  breastfeeding and introducing, 4
  introducing, 379–83
  starting, 92
  suggestions for offering, 382–83
Sonata. see zaleplon
sore nipples, 107, 110, 314–19
  depression and, 315
  feeding frequency and, 118
  lanolin for, 204
  latch-on and, 112–13, 316
  pain reliever for, 319
  positioning and, 315, 317
  treating, 316–19
soybean-based formula, 379
special needs babies, 362–64
  resources, 395
special situations, 335–64
  babies with special needs, 362–64
  baby gets sick, 346–47

breast surgery, 351–53
breastfeeding another woman's baby, 358–59
  helpful books on, 399–400
  late-preterm infants, 345–46
  milk banks, 357–58
  mother gets sick, 347–51
  near-term infants, 345–46
  nursing adopted baby, 359
  nursing through pregnancy, 356–57
  piercing, 353–54
  relactation, 359
  separation of mother and baby, 346
  tandem nursing, 356–57
  tattooing, 353–54
  websites for, 403–04
Special Supplemental Nutrition Program for Women, Infants, and Children (WIC), 4, 19
spermicide, 289
spitting up, 120
  burping and, 122
  cutting down on, 170
spoiling your baby, 150
sponge, birth control, 289
SSRIs. see selective serotonin reuptake inhibitors
starvation jaundice of the newborn, 129
sterilization, birth control, 289
sterilizing bottles and nipples, 5, 148, 249
Stewart, David, PhD, 308
stomach upset, 155
storing milk, 235–52

cleaning and sterilizing containers, 249
  containers for, 248–49
  in freezer, 250
  helpful suggestions for, 249–50
  in refrigerator, 250
  at room temperature, 250
  thermos or cooler for, 266
stress
  breastfeeding and reducing, 197
  children's ability to deal with, 15
  depression and, 197
stretch marks, 210
suck confusion, 136
suckling, baby's
  signs of active, 113
  slow-gaining infant and, 328–30
sudden infant death syndrome (SIDS)
  in breastfed baby, 7
  pacifiers and preventing, 147
  shared sleeping and, 158
sudden and unexpected death of an infant. see sudden infant death syndrome
Supplemental Nursing System (SNS), 328–29
supplementation
  with formula, 127, 129, 131, 144
  resources, 398–99
supply and demand, 140, 324–25
support
  for new mother, 83–88
  finding, 84–86
  husband/partner and, 36, 300–303

working mother, 254–55
support networks
  breastfeeding, 85–86, 199
  for breastfeeding mothers of premature infants, 340
  for single mother, 38
swaddling, 152
  sleeping and, 159
Synthroid. *see* levothyroxine

T

Tagamet. *see* cimetidine
taking baby off the breast, 114–15, 316
  breaking suction and, 115, 316
tandem nursing, 87, 356–57
TB. *see* tuberculosis
teeth, baby, 35
teething
  nursing strike and, 333
  slow-gaining baby and, 326
temperature
  baby's, 152
  room, sleeping and, 160
tetracycline, 224
  long-term use, 225
thirdhand smoke, 232
30-day breastfeeding guarantee, 2
thrush, 228, 319–21
  antibiotics and, 224
tight frenulum, 332
time for yourself, 198
tobacco, 231–32
tolbutamide (Orinase), 224

tongue thrust, 13
tongue-extrusion reflex, 381
too much milk, 148, 207
tooth development, 13
touch, importance of, 14–15
"touched-out" feeling, 277
transitional hold, 106
transitional milk, 48, 60, 140
  see also breast milk
traveling
  air, 214–15
  with baby, 17
  car safety, 212
  working mothers and, 273
tretinoin (Retin-A), 224
tricyclics, 225, 227
tuberculosis (TB), 347
tumors, breast, 208
twins, 354–56
  breastfeeding, 42–43
  simultaneous nursing of, 355–56
  see also multiples
Tylenol. *see* acetaminophen
type 2 diabetes, 19

U

ultrasound, 322
UNICEF. *see* United Nations Children's Fund
United Nations Children's Fund (UNICEF)
  Baby-Friendly Hospital Initiative, 74–75

breastfeeding supported by, 27
  extended breastfeeding recommendations, 373
urination/urine
  log, 142
  milk intake and, 124–26
uterine contractions, 16–17, 35, 94–95
  let-down reflex and, 114

V

vaginal yeast infection, 228
valproate, 224
vegan diet, 179
vegetarian diet, 179–80
visiting nurses, 68
vitamins, 366–68
vitamin C, iron absorption and, 177
vitamin D, 366
  for baby, 177
  mother's intake of, 176–77
vitamin K, 101
vomiting, 120–21

W

WABA. *see* World Alliance for Breastfeeding Action
waking your baby, 116, 145–46
  slow-gaining infant and, 326
water

bottles of, given to
newborn, 95
offering your baby, 380
WBW. *see* World
Breastfeeding Week
weaning, 32, 368–71
affects on you, 377–79
birth control and, 377
breasts and, 377–78
child-led, 370, 373–74
early, 222
emotional responses to,
378–79
how should you wean,
373–74
making the decision,
370–71
medicines and, 222
mother-led, 374
nursing strike and, 333
of older child, 375–77
phases, 368
physical changes in you
and, 377–78
during pregnancy, 356
sudden, 376–77
sudden, engorgement
and, 314
when should you start,
369–70
websites, 401–04
weight, baby's
fast-gaining infant,
330–31
loss, 99, 103, 123
milk intake and, 126
not gaining enough, 146
nursing adequacy and,
123–24
postpartum, 123–24
regaining birth, 123
slowly gaining, 325–30

solid foods and, 380
weight gain, mother's
breastfeeding and,
30–31
during pregnancy, 189
weight loss, mother's,
16–17, 30–31, 186–89
portion sizes, 187
rate of, 187
weight-bearing activities,
190, 193
well-baby visits, 102
wet nurses, 358
WHO. *see* World Health
Organization
whole grains, 174
WIC. *see* Special
Supplemental Nutrition
Program for Women,
Infants, and Children
women's roles, 24–25
Woolwich shield, 314
working mothers, 31, 32,
253–74
baby's feedings and,
265–69
breastfeeding wardrobe
for, 272
coworkers and, 273–74
employer-supported
breastfeeding for,
256–57
expressing milk, 267–68
formula-feeding and,
268
help for, 396–97
lactation programs,
employer-supported,
257–59
leaking and, 274
making transition to,
261–62

milk supply and, 244
negotiating with
employer and,
268–69
nursing schedule for,
271–73
places for pumping
milk, 270
planning ahead,
255–57
support for, 254–55
travel and, 273
websites for, 403
work schedule, 269–71
World Alliance for
Breastfeeding Action
(WABA), 390
World Breastfeeding
Week (WBW), 269
World Health
Organization (WHO)
Baby-Friendly Hospital
Initiative, 74–75
breastfeeding
encouraged by, 25
breastfeeding
supported by, 27
extended breastfeeding
recommendations,
373
nursing
recommendations by,
32

Z

zaleplon (Sonata), 227
Zoloft, 227
zolpidem (Ambien), 227

About the Authors

Sally Wendkos Olds has written extensively about relationships, health, and personal growth. She has won national awards for her writing, including the Career Achievement Award of the American Society of Journalists and Authors, of which she is a member and a past president. Ms. Olds's college textbooks on child and adult development, coauthored with psychologist Diane E. Papalia, PhD, have been read by more than two million students and are the leading texts in their fields. She is also the author of *Super Granny: Great Stuff to Do with Your Grandkids, The Working Parents' Survival Guide,* and *The Eternal Garden: Seasons of Our Sexuality,* and the coauthor of *Helping Your Child Find Values to Live By* and *Raising a Hyperactive Child.*

A graduate of the University of Pennsylvania, Ms. Olds is a member of La Leche League International, International Childbirth Education Association, the Authors Guild, and other professional and civic organizations. She nursed her three daughters and is the proud grandmother of five breastfed children. Visit her at her website: www.SallyWendkosOlds.com.

Laura M. Marks, MD, a pediatrician at Willows Pediatric Group in Westport, Connecticut, breastfed her own three children and is expert at guiding other women through the process. A graduate of the University of Pennsylvania and Yale University School of Medicine, she is a member of the Alpha Omega Alpha medical honor society. She interned at Harvard University Medical School and Massachusetts General Hospital, and completed her residency at Children's Hospital at Yale New Haven Medical Center.

With her husband, David Marks, MD, Dr. Marks coauthored *The Headache Prevention Cookbook: Eating Right to Prevent Migraines and Other Headaches.* She is the medical advisor to the Weston (Connecticut) School District and is on the Pediatric Executive Committee of Norwalk Hospital. Dr. Marks is a member of the American Academy of Pediatrics's Section on Breastfeeding Medicine, the Academy of Breastfeeding Medicine, and La Leche League International.

Marvin S. Eiger, MD, coauthor of the first three editions of this book, is a graduate of Harvard University and New York University School of Medicine and practiced pediatrics in New York City for thirty years. Dr. Eiger established the Comprehensive Lactation Program at New York's Beth Israel Hospital, serving as its medical director until he retired from practice. He is the father of two children and grandfather of three.